Chemical and Biological
Warfare Agents

A Review of the Scientific Literature As It Pertains to Gulf War Illnesses

VOLUME 5

CHEMICAL AND BIOLOGICAL WARFARE AGENTS

William S. Augerson

Prepared for the Office of the Secretary of Defense

National Defense Research Institute

RAND

This literature review, one of eight commissioned by the Special Assistant to the Deputy Secretary of Defense for Gulf War illnesses, summarizes the existing unclassified scientific literature on the health effects of selected chemical and biological warfare agents that may have affected service members who served in Operations Desert Shield and Desert Storm. The eight RAND reviews are intended to complement efforts by the Department of Defense and other federal agencies as they attempt to understand the full range of health implications of service in that conflict. The reviews largely reflect data from 1997 and earlier but contain some from 1998 and later.

While many veterans have reported an array of physical and mental health complaints since the war, the extent to which veterans are experiencing either unusual rates of identifiable illnesses with known etiologies or any other illnesses from as yet unidentified origins is not yet clear.

The other seven RAND literature reviews deal with oil fire pollution, depleted uranium, pesticides, pyridostigmine bromide, immunizations, infectious diseases (which includes review of two biological warfare agents, anthrax and botulinum toxin), and stress, all potential factors in some of the illnesses Gulf War veterans have reported.

These reviews are intended principally to summarize the scientific literature on the known health effects of given exposures to these risk factors. Where available evidence permits, the reviews also summarize what is known about the range of actual exposures in the Gulf and assess the plausibility of the risk factor as a cause of illnesses. These broader statements should be regarded as suggestive rather than definitive because much more research both on health effects and exposures remains to be completed before more definitive statements are made. Recommendations on necessary additional research are also made when appropriate.

These reviews are limited to literature published or accepted for publication in peer-reviewed journals, books, government publications, and conference proceedings. Unpublished information, such as reports or Internet notes, was occasionally used, but only to develop hypotheses or, in the case of press reports, for historical background. The reports are written for a professional and technical audience using unclassified sources.

This monograph was submitted for peer review in summer 1998. Some selected articles that appeared in the literature after that date are also referenced in the monograph, principally to accommodate reviewer recommendations.

This work is sponsored by the Office of the Special Assistant and was carried out jointly by RAND Health's Center for Military Health Policy Research and the Forces and Resources Policy Center of the National Defense Research Institute. The latter is a federally funded research and development center sponsored by the Office of the Secretary of Defense, the Joint Staff, the unified commands, and the defense agencies.

CONTENTS

FIGURES

TABLES

After the Persian Gulf War (1990–1991), many veterans reported such signs and symptoms as rashes, fatigue, muscle and joint pain, headaches, loss of memory, depression, abdominal pain and diarrhea, coughing, sneezing, choking sensations, chest pain, sleep disturbance, and hair loss.[1] Surveys indicate that roughly 4 percent developed their symptoms before the war, 25 percent during the war, and 25 percent in the year following the war. Nearly 50 percent developed their symptoms in the second and third years after the war—and beyond (Kroenke, 1998). This report reviews the scientific literature related to the health effects of one of the possible causes of these illnesses, chemical and biological warfare agents.[2] These are grouped as follows, with a chapter devoted to each group:

- skin damaging agents (mustards, lewisite, phosgene oxime)
- toxins (ricin, trichothecenes, aflatoxins)
- nerve agents (tabun, sarin, soman, cyclosarin, and VX).[3]

POSSIBLE EXPOSURE

Before the Gulf War, Iraq had made extensive use of chemical warfare against Iran and its own people (United Nations [UN], 1984; Cordesman and Wagner, 1990). It is also known that Iraq conducted a program of research and devel-

---

[1]Although the press has used the term "Gulf War Syndrome" to describe these illnesses, no single definition has been developed, and no new disease entity has been established (Gibbons 1998; Marshall, 1997; NIH 1994). This review uses the term Gulf War illnesses to refer to the health problems reported by Gulf War veterans.

[2]This report concentrates on chemical warfare agents and one class of biological warfare agents, called toxins. Toxins are produced by living organisms (microbes, fungi, plants, and animals), but it is actually the chemical they produce that is used, which makes these toxins different from other biological agents, such as anthrax, that kill as a result of their biological properties. Other biological warfare agents, anthrax and botulism, are reviewed in a separate RAND report on infectious diseases (Hilborne and Golomb, 2000).

[3]Little information was found on the chemical thiosarin.

opment of chemical and biological weapons. This capability was a major concern for coalition forces, which made great efforts to minimize the risk of exposure to chemical and biological warfare weapons by providing protective equipment, detectors, medications, and immunizations and by addressing the issue in troop training (Clancy and Franks, 1997).

During the air war (which began in mid-January 1991) and the short ground war (which ended in early March 1991), there were no obvious chemical or biological attacks on coalition forces. However, there were a number of alarms and ambiguous events involving chemical agents, and it is know that U.S. troops did blow up a large ammunition depot at Khamisiyah that contained chemical weapons. Many reports of detector alarms—which seem primarily to have stemmed from known interfering substances, such as smoke and engine exhausts—undoubtedly contributed to the perception of some veterans that they were exposed to chemical agents.

Coalition air attacks did strike some Iraqi chemical and biological facilities. However, studies modeling the release of nerve agents and mustards from such attacks indicate that significant transport of agent to the vicinity of U.S. forces was unlikely (Central Intelligence Agency [CIA], 1996). Some concern remains that low levels of exposure might have occurred from such attacks (U.S. General Accounting Office, 1997; Riegle and D'Amato, 1994).

We know of at least one chemical weapon exposure that involved U.S. forces, which took place shortly after the defeat of Iraqi forces. In the process of destroying an Iraqi weapon depot at Khamisiyah, U.S. forces blew up a bunker and stocks of rockets that contained the nerve agents sarin and cyclosarin without knowing that the rockets contained chemical warheads. No casualties occurred, and it was only much later determined that nerve agents were destroyed and probably released during the demolition. This event has been studied and modeled extensively. A number of models were developed to estimate exposures, which yielded estimates indicating that a large number of U.S. troops (perhaps as many as 100,000) were potentially exposed to very low levels of nerve agents—levels unlikely to cause any acute clinical symptoms.

A second incident has also been investigated extensively (OSAGWI, 1997d[4]). In that incident, a single U.S. soldier developed typical mustard agent–like blisters on his arm several hours after being in an Iraqi bunker while he was assisting in the destruction of Iraqi vehicles and military equipment. Whether the cause of the blisters was mustard agent or some other source is currently unresolved and continues to be investigated.

---

[4]OSAGWI has made a large number of Gulf War–related documents available on line in addition to its own products For simplicity, all are listed under OSAGWI in the Bibliography.

As part of conditions imposed at the termination of hostilities, Iraqis were required to declare their holdings of chemicals and biological weapons and to permit UN inspectors to access facilities and oversee destruction of all chemical and biological weapons. As a result of UN Special Commission efforts, much more is known about Iraqi capabilities at the time of the war (Zilinskas, 1997). Still, the picture is far from complete, and the Iraqis have been far from candid.

APPROACH

This report describes the medical effects of the chemical and biological agents it was believed Iraq could have possessed. These agents are intended to kill or disable humans. Although we describe the effects of militarily effective higher-dose exposures, the primary focus of the paper is on the effects of lower-dose exposures, especially long-term or delayed effects. The information is intended to assist in the analysis of possible exposures, but this review does not attempt to determine if such exposures occurred or to determine their relationship to Gulf War illnesses. Such determinations are the responsibility of OSAGWI and others.

The literature did not yield either examples of clinical problems arising two or more years after agent exposure or mechanisms for such health developments. There were reviews of some longer-term medical problems that can arise from lower levels of exposure and of mechanisms that could persist for some time after exposure ceases.

PROBLEMS OF RECOGNITION

The ability of U.S. forces to recognize exposures, especially at low levels, depended on chemical detection and clinical recognition of the signs and symptoms of agent exposure. The review found that there might be situations in which health effects from exposures might not be recognized clinically.

U.S. detectors were unable to recognize toxins or biological agents. "Dusty" mustard (or "dusty" nerve agent) also would probably not have been recognized by CAM or M8A1 detectors because they act on an ion mobility principle (OSAGWI, 1990). Nerve agents would probably have been detected by monitors at concentrations below those that affect the eyes. This is certainly the case for tabun and sarin, but it is less certain for VX and other potent agents (Defense Science Board, 1994; NRC, 1997). These detection systems produced a large number of apparently false alarms (from smoke exhausts and other interfering chemicals), which perhaps caused some veterans to believe they had been exposed to agents.

Although exact agent identification would have been more difficult, clinical recognition of militarily efficient attacks would have been straightforward. The recognition of lower-level exposures is more complex and uncertain for the following reasons:

- The signs and symptoms of lower-level exposures are not specific and can resemble other common health problems. Historically, victims may have misinterpreted many low-level exposures as common headaches, respiratory or gastrointestinal illness, asthma, or conjunctivitis (Gaon and Werne, 1955). As will be discussed with separate agents, there may be subtle points to help differentiate agent exposures from common problems. Table S.1 indicates the overlapping effects of the agents under review.

- Significant biological effects can occur from acute or cumulative exposures that do not produce obvious signs and symptoms (Gaon and Werne, 1955; Holmes, 1959; Bowers, Goodman, and Sim, 1964; Wolthuis, Groen, et al., 1995; Burchfiel, 1976; Stephens, Spurgeon, and Berry, 1996; Mayer, 1953a; Steyn, 1995). (Similar effects have been reported from structurally similar organophosphate pesticides.)

- Several of the agents do not have immediate effects following exposure. For example, effects from mustard exposure may not occur for several hours to several days (Wachtel, 1941; Vedder, 1925); ricin effects may not be apparent for hours to a day (Franz and Jaax, 1997); and even massive exposures to aflatoxin produce symptoms only after an 8- to 16-hour delay (Chao et al., 1991).

- Responses to agent exposure can vary substantially because of such factors as race, temperature, diet, gender, and time of day (Vedder, 1925). For example, circadian variations can produce changes such that exposure at one time of day may result in distinct illness, while an identical exposure 12 hours later there may be little sign from the same exposure (Elsmore, 1981).

- In the case of nerve agents, it is possible that prior administration of pyridostigmine bromide may decrease and shorten the clinical response (Gall, 1981; Husain, Kumar, Vijayaraghavan, et al., 1993; Vijayaraghavan et al., 1992). This has not been extensively studied at low dosages.

- There is also a condition of tolerance in which exposure to anticholinesterase chemicals results in decreased response to subsequent exposure to chemicals of the same class—so that exposures do not produce typical signs and symptoms. Single and repeated subclinical exposures produce tolerance (Costa, Schwab, and Murphy, 1982).

SKIN DAMAGING AGENTS

Lewisite, phosgene oxime, and mustard agents are all skin-damaging agents. Although they have some distinct chemical properties, they all affect the skin, eyes, and respiratory tract and, once absorbed, have systemic toxicity.

Table S.1

Signs and Symptoms of Agent Exposure

	Skin[a]	Eye[b]	Respiratory[c]	Gastrointestinal[d]	Musculoskeletal[e]	Systemic[f]	Mental[g]
Lewisite	X	X	X	X		X	
Phosgene-oxime	X	X	X				
Mustards	X	X	X	X		X	X
Ricin		X	X	X	X	X	
Trichothecenes	X	X	X	X		X	X
Aflatoxins		?	X	X	X	?	?
Nerve agents	X[h]	X	X	X	X	X	X

[a]Rash irritation, erythema, blisters, and itching.

[b]Irritation, tearing, redness, and blurred vision.

[c]Rhinorrhea, sore red throat, cough, tight chest, and wheezing.

[d]Nausea, vomiting, cramping, and diarrhea.

[e]Muscle cramps, aching joints, and muscles.

[f]Malaise, lethargy, and low fevers.

[g]Difficulty thinking or remembering, and sleep disorders.

[h]Local sweating, itching, and erythema.

Lewisite

Lewisite was developed during World War I and has not received much recent study. In high concentrations, this arsenic-containing agent produces irritation and blistering of the skin and injury to the eyes and lungs promptly after exposure. At lower levels, the effects resemble exposure to tear gas, with irritation of skin, eyes, and respiratory tract, which could be misinterpreted as being due to other irritants or infection. Chronically exposed munitions workers have developed chronic bronchitis, but arsenic-based neuropathy was not reported. Chronic exposure to lewisite may predispose to Bowen's squamous cell intraepithelial cancer of the skin. There is no indication that brief exposures to low levels of lewisite are associated with long-term problems. Lewisite degrades rapidly in the environment, making hazard from long-range transport unlikely. Some Fox vehicles reported detecting lewisite during the Gulf War, but these findings were not confirmed. Interference from petroleum products and oil fires explains the false readings (OSAGWI, 1997c).

Phosgene Oxime (Agent CX)

Phosgene oxime, which was developed before World War II, has not been studied extensively. Iraq may have used it against Iran (OSAGWI, undated a). This chemical is highly reactive and unstable, making it an unlikely hazard if transported long distances through the atmosphere. It is unusual in that it can harm materials as well as people. Phosgene oxime is very painful and irritating, especially to the skin and eyes, so exposure is likely to be noticed. Higher levels of exposure cause severe skin burns that heal slowly and may result in fatal pulmonary edema. No information on the effects of long-term or low-level exposure to phosgene oxime was found in the unclassified literature. In an incident after the Gulf War, a coalition officer sustained a severe, painful chemical burn that was suspected of being due to exposure to phosgene oxime, but was later determined to be from some kind of nitric acid (OSAGWI, 1998a).

Mustards (Agents H, HD, T, HT, Q, and HN)

The mustard agents (first used during World War I) have similar chemical structures and are effective military agents. Their mechanism of action is not fully understood, but it is known that they interact with DNA to cause cell death in ways that resemble radiation injury. This review concentrates on sulfur mustard (H), which Iraq used widely against Iran (UN, 1984). Mustard agents are quite persistent and stable in the environment. Because of the delayed onset of effects (as much as a day), exposure is not immediately obvious. Iraq was thought to have used a "dusty" form of mustard (mustard absorbed on fine silica particles) in its war with Iran. This form is said to produce more-rapid skin effects and more-lethal pulmonary injury and may be more difficult to detect (OSAGWI, 1996).

Mustards are primarily incapacitating agents, producing skin blisters and eye injuries that are disabling for a time, although recovery usually occurs. More-severe pulmonary, skin, and systemic poisoning can be fatal. Mustards injured thousands of soldiers during World War I. While some of the injured had respiratory complaints, the other complaints associated with Gulf War illnesses were not noted. With the repeated exposures munitions workers encounter, serious delayed effects can occur. Long-term mustard workers are in poorer health than their peers, reporting depression, nervousness, autonomic disorders, bronchitis, and frequent infections. They have a higher prevalence of skin and lung cancer (Yamakido et al., 1996; Pechura and Rall, 1993; Dacre and Goldman, 1996; Lohs, 1975).[5]

Low-level exposure to mustards can produce skin erythema resembling sunburn, with eye irritation, runny nose, sore throat, cough, and lethargy, which could be misdiagnosed or overlooked. However, loss of taste and smell is commonly associated with respiratory symptoms, which is not typical of colds or irritants. Scrotal inflammation strongly suggests mustard exposure.

There are a number of Iranian reports on the results of civilian exposures to mustards. These include changes in male-to-female birth ratios (Pour-Jafari, 1994) and increases in cleft lip and other congenital malformations (Taher, 1992). However, other environmental and nutritional factors could not be excluded. Mustards suppress the immune system but are immunogenic in their own right, including hypersensitivity reactions to later exposures (Grunnet, 1976).

Although early clinicians thought that mustards injured the nervous system, the neurological effects of mustard exposures have not been well studied (Vedder, 1925, Dacre and Goldman, 1996). It is known that mustards inhibit cholinesterase, and early mustard casualties were depressed and lethargic. Recently, there have been reports of a high prevalence of post-traumatic stress disorder (PTSD) in veterans who were subjects of World War II experimental mustard exposures (Schnurr, Friedman, and Green, 1996). The matter is still under study, and the mechanism of the disorder is not understood.

There is evidence that combined exposures to mustards and nerve agents have greater toxicity than expected from either alone (Krustanov, 1962). There are no data on combined effects of mustards and pyridostigmine bromide.

---

[5]Mustards are mutagens and carcinogens, but the risk from brief low-level exposures is small (Pechura and Rall, 1993; Dacre, 1996).

There are now sensitive measurement techniques to detect mustard adducts with hemoglobin and with DNA in tissues (Ludlum and Austin-Ritchie, 1994; Ehrenberg and Osterman-Golkar, 1980). It may be possible to detect such effects in the blood and tissues obtained during and after the Gulf War and now housed at the Armed Forces Institutes of Pathology (AFIP).

BIOLOGICAL TOXINS

Biological toxins are poisons produced by living organisms. The most potent poison known is botulinum toxin, a toxin reviewed in the RAND infectious disease report (Hilborne et al., 2000). The toxins reviewed in this report are ricin (which is extracted from the castor bean) and the trichothecene toxins and aflatoxins (which are produced by fungi). All of these toxins are capable of producing fatal illnesses that are virtually untreatable. None of these agents could be detected by the systems available to U.S. forces during the Gulf War.[6] Therefore, clinical recognition was the means of toxin detection. We are unaware of reports of illness attributed to toxins.

More is known about ricin and the trichothecene toxins as military agents than about aflatoxin, which was considered a public health problem until it was revealed after the war that Iraq had placed aflatoxin in missiles and rockets (Zilinskas, 1997).

Ricin (Agent W)

Ricin is a protein that can be extracted from the castor bean. Its toxicity has been known and used since ancient times. Although it was not used in World War II, it was developed to weapon status by the United Kingdom and the United States during that war (OSRD, 1946). Ricin is a powerful weapon—the same dose of a crude ricin aerosol extract or the nerve agent sarin both kill 50 percent of the exposed population.

Ricin is not stable in the environment (degrading in a few days), so it is unlikely that ricin would be a threat after long-distance travel through the atmosphere. Effective military attack with ricin would produce, after a delay of hours, eye inflammation, severe pulmonary edema, and death from respiratory failure, as is seen in nonhuman primates exposed to ricin aerosols (Wilhelmsen, 1996). When injected, ricin produces a fever, high white blood cell count, seizures, and multiple organ failures. It does not apparently damage or penetrate the skin.

---

[6]Specialized units were deployed to collect, sample, and evaluate biological agents possibly used during the war, but in some cases, material was referred to U.S. laboratories for analysis.

The clinical effects of low-level inhalation exposure were observed in research and production workers in World War II (OSRD, 1946). Symptoms of coughing, dyspnea, inflammation and burning of the trachea, aching joints, and nausea began four to eight hours after exposure. Several hours later, profuse sweating usually preceded the abatement of symptoms. Muscle cramps and weakness are common after ricin exposure. No long-term follow-up information was found.

Ricin is highly immunogenic. Laboratory workers responded to second exposures with apparent hypersensitivity reactions—sneezing, coughing, and other asthmatic symptoms. If U.S. forces were exposed to ricin, it should be possible to find ricin antibodies in the exposed persons. Iraq admitted testing it in artillery shells but claimed not to have deployed it as a weapon (Zilinskas, 1997).

Trichothecene Mycotoxins

This family of toxins was used as military agents in Southeast Asia, where they were referred to as "yellow rain," and later in Afghanistan, where they were used by Soviet forces. Iraq admitted to the UN that it had produced some trichothecene toxins and tested them on animals but contended that they had not proceeded to weapon development (Zilinskas, 1997). There were reports that Iraq had used these toxins against Iran (such as Heyndrickx, 1984, pp. 132–146), but other laboratories could not detect trichothecene mycotoxins in Iranian casualties. The toxins are very stable in the environment and resist decontamination, so continued toxicity after long-distance atmospheric transport is possible. There are many tricothecene mycotoxins, and it is not known which ones Iraq produced.

Trichothecene toxins (T-2 being the most important and most studied) can be lethal when inhaled or ingested and are damaging to the skin and eyes at very low concentrations (nanograms to micrograms). Vomiting and nervous system effects after low-level exposures are common.

After substantial acute exposures (cancer therapy; yellow rain), sequelae have included rashes, joint pain, fatigue (Schultz, 1982), fever, chills, hypotension, confusion, somnolence, memory loss, hallucinations (Belt et al., 1979), dyspnea, diarrhea, and recurrent infections (Yap et al., 1979; Murphy et al., 1978; Crossland and Townsend, 1984). Laboratory findings show low white-cell counts, low platelet levels, and decreased coagulation factors.

Chronic low-level exposure of a family in a house contaminated with tricothecene mycotoxins (probably verrucarin, roridan, and satratoxin) produced frequent respiratory illness, flu-like symptoms, sore throat, diarrhea, headache, fatigue, and alopecia (hair loss). The family had marked changes in hematological values. These problems defied diagnosis for a long time (Croft, Jarvis, and Yatawara, 1986; Jarvis, 1985).

Memory loss has been seen in survivors of yellow rain, in cancer chemotherapy patients, and in tests on experimental animals. Such cases were usually accompanied by hematological changes, which have not been an apparent feature in Gulf War veterans suffering from Gulf War illnesses.

If trichothecenes were prevalent in the Gulf theater environment, one would expect a high prevalence of eye irritations and skin inflammations, since these agents act on the skin and eyes so powerfully at low concentrations (nanogram to microgram amounts).

It is theoretically possible to detect trichothecene metabolites in tissues collected during and after the Gulf War. These tissues are available to the AFIP. Since trichothecene exposure can occur naturally, suitable controls and a sophisticated experimental design would be required. Such studies would be technically difficult. The views of the AFIP on this matter should be determined.

Aflatoxins

Because aflatoxins can contaminate food and grain, causing illness in domestic animals and perhaps liver cancer in humans, they have long been of concern as a public health threat. Before the Gulf War, aflatoxins (of which the type designated AFB_1 is the most toxic) had not been used in war and had received only passing mention in discussions of biological warfare (U.S. Army, 1990). Thus, the report that Iraq had produced substantial amounts of these toxins to fill Scud missiles and 122 mm rockets was surprising. The intended effect is unknown, and some analysts were uncertain about why these toxins were selected as a weapon (Zilinskas, 1997).

These toxins are very stable, are resistant to decontamination, and would retain their toxicity after long-distance atmospheric transport (although they would be diluted in concentration). They do not represent a hazard to the skin, which appears to be an effective barrier against them. Since metabolic activation is required for their toxicity to manifest itself, their effects are delayed for several hours after exposure.

Experience with heavily contaminated food indicates that human acute lethal doses are in the range of 2 mg/kg (Harrison and Garner, 1991). The toxin is well absorbed from the lungs, and it would be feasible to create an aerosol to deliver 140 mg, a fatal dose for a 150-pound man. Orally intoxicated humans acutely show vomiting, seizures, fever, respiratory distress, liver failure, and coma (Chao et al., 1991; Bourgeois, Olson, et al., 1971). There are no follow-up data from the known acute oral poisonings.

We do not have a clinical picture of low-level respiratory exposure to aflatoxins. One could expect nausea, vomiting, cough, and respiratory symptoms. Animal studies indicate that inhaled aflatoxins at low levels are immunosuppressive (Jakab et al., 1994). However, grain workers exposed to such toxins are not reported to have high prevalence of pulmonary infections (Autrup, Schmidt, and Autrup, 1993). Indeed, grain workers who encounter these toxins also have other complex exposures and primarily report nonspecific respiratory symptoms.

Some animal data hint at respiratory toxicity from low doses. Although no primate aerosol studies were found, other animal studies have shown pulmonary damage from nanogram and microgram amounts (Northup et al., 1995; Jakab et al., 1994).

Chronic oral intake of low concentrations of aflatoxins is associated with increased risk of liver cancer, impaired child health and development, and frequent infections (Groopman, Scholl, and Wang, 1996). Neurological problems have not been described. The increased cancer risk from short-term exposure is small.

Persons exposed to aflatoxins develop antibodies to the toxin. It is possible to identify aflatoxins and their adducts in formalin-fixed tissue of poisoned victims (Harrison and Garner, 1991). Whether it would be possible to detect the toxin in tissues available to the AFIP is a matter for discussion with that organization. The expense and complexity of such studies do not commend them as a screening method, but such studies might be valuable if there are indications of possible exposure. Care in the design of such studies is essential, since western European populations have been shown to have low levels of these antibodies (Autrup and Seremet, 1990).

NERVE AGENTS

The nerve agents are part of a group of organophosphorus compounds, which are potent inhibitors of the enzyme acetylcholinesterase. This enzyme regulates neural function by inactivating the neurotransmitter acetylcholine. This group of chemicals also includes organophosphate pesticides, which are chemically similar to the nerve agents but less toxic.[7]

This study reviewed the nerve agents tabun (GA), sarin (GB), soman (GD), cyclosarin (GF), and VX.[8] The agents reviewed differ in various respects. Tabun is

---

[7]Another class of chemicals can also inhibit acetylcholinesterase: the carbamates, of which pyridostigmine bromide is a member.

[8]We attempted to review thiosarin, an analog of sarin that replaces the oxygen attached to the phosphorus molecule with sulfur, but could find little information on this chemical.

the least toxic. Sarin is highly volatile, which makes it less of a skin-exposure hazard. Soman is of intermediate volatility and is resistant to treatment. VX is potent but not volatile. Cyclosarin is more persistent than sarin. Still, there are sufficient similarities in the biochemistry of these agents to treat them as a group in this review. Although the class of agent would be evident, it is unlikely that a clinician seeing a mild or severe casualty from a nerve agent would be able to discern which agent produced the illness.

The Germans discovered nerve agents shortly before World War II. This class of chemicals remains the most toxic ever known. Two agents (tabun and sarin) reached weapon status, but were not used, during World War II. In the years after World War II, hundreds of military agents and thousands of pesticides in this class were tested. There is considerable information about the effects of these agents on humans from accidents during research, development, and production; from warfare; and from studies on volunteers. Sarin is the best documented and cyclosarin the least well documented. There is an enormous literature about the effects of nerve agents on animals and *in vitro*.

Militarily efficient attacks with vapor or aerosols have very rapid effects, including collapse, respiratory distress and failure, seizures, and paralysis. Less severely exposed persons experience confusion, dim vision, respiratory difficulty, marked salivation, vomiting, diarrhea, weakness, tremors, and incoordination. Milder exposures produce acute symptoms including dim vision (impaired night vision is a distinctive result), difficulty and pain with focusing, headache, red eyes, runny nose, tight chest, and cough, followed by nausea, cramps, diarrhea, and muscle weakness. Confusion, irritability, depression, difficulty thinking, poor coordination, and sleep disturbances are also common. Although not extensively studied, people who have been exposed to nerve agents are known to be accident prone, although most seem to recover from this in a few days or about two to three weeks (Gaon and Werne, 1955; Holmes, 1959).

During research and production of these nerve agents, it was noted that some persons who did not report illness were found to have very low levels of acetylcholinesterase, indicating unrecognized exposure. Such persons have not been the subjects of long-term follow-up studies. A study of agricultural workers exposed to organophosphorus pesticides detected impaired mental performance in workers who reported no symptoms and whose exposure to these pesticides was documented (Stephens, Spurgeon, and Berry, 1996).

Iraq used tabun against Iranian forces in the Iran-Iraq war (UN, 1984) and may have used other nerve agents (sarin, cyclosarin) later in that war (OSAGWI, undated e). It was known that Iraq conducted research on and had chemical agents, but there remains no absolute certainty about the numbers or types of Iraqi chemical and biological weapons that were in existence at the time of the

Gulf War. (It was several years after the war that the UN documented Iraqi possession of VX, tabun, sarin, and cyclosarin). Before the war, it was suspected that Iraq had stocks of soman, but this has not been proven. Exposure to this agent is hard to treat, and this was the threat that inspired the use of pyridostigmine bromide. There may have been some low-level exposures of U.S. forces to sarin and cyclosarin after the war as a result of the demolitions at Khamisiyah. The CIA estimated that any exposure was an amount unlikely to produce any acute clinical effect (CIA, 1997; OSAGWI, 1997a).

Longer-Term Effects

Both human and animal research data indicate that low-level exposures to nerve agents have long-term effects. The prevailing view of experts in the 1950s and 1960s was that complete recovery always occurred following nerve agent exposure (other than in severe cases in which anoxic brain damage occurs) (Grob, 1956). This view is supported by the fact that no long-term health problems due to agent exposure were seen in volunteers exposed to the agents (NRC, 1985). The prevalent view may have decreased the recognition of longer-term effects, although these were occasionally reported (Gaon and Werne, 1955; Craig and Freeman, 1953). Furthermore, the Japanese experience with moderate and mild exposures indicates that subtle neurological dysfunction can be detected at six months and a year for some individuals (Yokoyama et al., 1998; Nakajima, Ohta, et al., 1998).

Nonhuman primates showed electroencephalogram (EEG) changes lasting over a year following a short series of doses of sarin, which did not make them sick (Burchfiel and Duffy, 1982). Longer-term studies of production workers exposed to sarin indicated that muscle aches and pains, drowsiness, and fatigue were significant problems. Continued study of others a year after their last exposure showed disturbed memory, difficulty in maintaining alertness and attention, and "soft" neurological findings suggesting coordination defects. Computer-interpreted EEGs were abnormal (Metcalf and Holmes, 1969; Duffy and Burchfiel, 1980).

Delayed Neuropathy

Some organophosphorus compounds produce a delayed injury to the nervous system that becomes obvious weeks to months after exposure. This produces paralysis from a peripheral neuropathy, although occasionally effects may resemble other neurological disorders (Hayes, 1982; Johnson, 1975; Abou-Donia, 1981). There is no treatment. Inhibition of an enzyme, neuropathy target esterase (NTE), is required to produce the neuropathy.[9] There had been concern that nerve agents might produce this disorder. However, it was only possible to produce delayed neuropathy in animals when they were dosed with levels of sarin and soman many times the LD_{50} dose (it was necessary to treat the animals to keep them alive) (Gordon, Inns, et al., 1983). More recently, Husain, Vijayaraghavan, et al. (1993) have shown that mice exposed to ten daily doses of sarin that did not make them sick from anticholinesterase effects had typical delayed neuropathy lesions.

Although the main weight of the evidence suggests that nerve agents have little ability to produce delayed neuropathy, the complexity of this phenomenon and the complexity of the interactions with other chemicals make it impossible to reject it on clinical grounds alone and suggest more research is needed in this area.[10]

Tolerance and Other Adjustments to Exposure

Exposures to a variety of chemicals that inactivate acetylcholinesterase (even when not clinically apparent) can induce a condition of tolerance, in which signs and symptoms of further acute exposure are greatly diminished or lacking. This condition is associated with a decrease in the abundance and sensitivity of acetylcholine receptors (Costa, Schwab, and Murphy, 1982). This condition may also be a pathological process with impairments in memory and learning (Taylor, El-Fakahony, and Richelson, 1979; Buccafusco et al., 1997). Although humans have shown tolerance to pesticides and nerve agents, we have no information about the recovery from this condition. Repeated exposures to anticholinesterases (such as pesticides or pyridostigmine bromide) could induce a condition of tolerance that would make clinical recognition of low-level nerve agent exposure more difficult and that would further increase the level of tolerance. Tolerant animals and people are very sensitive to the effects of anticholinergic drugs such as atropine, antihistamines and other like drugs (Chippendale et al., 1972).

Anticholinesterase chemicals may produce longer-term changes in brain chemistry by affecting the expression of immediate early genes (such as c-fos) and the proteins they encode. Alternation of the expression of immediate early genes can affect how many other genes respond to environmental stimuli. Kaufer et al. (1998) observed that, in animals, robust cholinergic stimulators

---

[9]The function of NTE is unknown; it is found in the spinal cord, brain, sciatic nerve, platelets, and lymphocytes.

[10]As of late 1999, no findings of typical axonal neuropathy have been reported in Gulf veteran studies.

(including stress, pyridostigmine bromide, pesticides, and nerve agents) can all induce increased expression of c-fos in the brain. Kaufer et al. contend that alternation of c-fos expression may induce "convergent" mechanisms that contribute to longer-term brain effects and specifically mention Gulf War illnesses. Developments in this field deserve close attention, although the duration and consequence of such changes in gene expression and their clinical significance have not yet been determined.

Possible Long-Term Consequences from Unrecognized Exposure

Earlier reviews generally discounted a role for nerve agent exposures in contributing to undiagnosed illness in Gulf War veterans because no recognized exposures had produced signs and symptoms. This review identified biological mechanisms that can sequester or actively degrade nerve agents, so there is some (unknown) level of agent exposure that would have no effect because of detoxification. The levels of exposure calculated from the Khamisiyah event are so low that enduring responses would not be expected, and indeed, the exposure may have been at the no-effect level (CIA, 1997).

Still, low-level exposures to nerve agents are difficult to recognize. Animal research and human experience with nerve agents and organophosphorus pesticides show altered neurological function from doses that do not produce overt signs or symptoms (Gaon and Werne, 1955; Brody and Gammill, 1954; Craig and Freeman, 1953; Bowers et al., 1964; Korsak and Sato, 1977; Sirkka, Nieminen, and Ylitalo, 1990; Wolthuis, Groen, et al., 1990; Stephens, Spurgeon, and Berry, 1996; Burchfiel, 1976). Indeed, mild to moderate nerve agent exposures seem capable of producing biological changes and health effects lasting over a year. No reports were found in the literature of disorders attributed to nerve agents that began two or more years after exposure.

Some long-term follow-up studies of nerve agent exposures report signs and symptoms similar to those reported by those suffering from Gulf War illnesses (Metcalf and Holmes, 1969). Japanese reports a year after exposure do not indicate similar problems, although there are subtle neurological findings and persisting eye pain and irritation (asthenopia) (Yokoyama et al., 1998a, b; Nakajima, Ohta, et al., 1998).

There is little evidence to asses the long-term consequences of exposure to levels of nerve agent that are too low to produce any acute effects. This possibility remains an area needing further research

It may be possible to determine directly if soldiers were exposed to nerve agents during the Gulf War. Measurement of nerve agent metabolites in formalin-fixed tissues has been reported in Japan (Matsuda et al., 1998). Whether these techniques are sensitive enough to detect metabolites from low-level exposures in tissues available to AFIP is uncertain.

STRESS

Responses to stress are the subject of another RAND review (Marshall, Davis, and Sherbourne, 1999). However, because the threat of chemical and biological agents arouses concern in most people, this review of such agents also touches on this topic.

The operational activity to prepare for chemical and biological attacks during the Gulf War occupied considerable training and other activities involving most personnel (Clancy and Franks, 1997). Many persons find wearing the necessary protective equipment to be physically demanding (Teitlebaum and Goldman, 1972; Joy and Goldman, 1964) and psychologically stressful (Brooks et al., 1983, Carter and Cammermeyer, 1985). During the war, agent alarms and other precautions raised the possibility of chemical and biological weapons attack and caused personnel to wear full protection for sustained periods. These events were certainly the source of stress for some individuals.

It is not easy to separate late clinical effects of agent exposure from late stress effects of PTSD. There are indications that veterans who participated in World War II mustard experiments have a high prevalence of PTSD (Horvath, 1997; Schnurr, Friedman, and Green, 1996). The Hmong survivors of trichothecene attacks (yellow rain) in Southeast Asia showed prolonged problems of apathy, anxiety, and disordered memory (they had also been severely traumatized by attacks and harrowing refugee experiences) (Crossland and Townsend, 1984). PTSD has been seen in survivors of the Japanese sarin attacks and has complicated analyses of other subtle late effects of nerve agent exposure (Yokoyama, Araki, et al., 1998a, 1998b).

Animal data indicate that the use of steroids can potentially alter responses to nerve agents and vice versa (Clement, 1985; Stabile, 1967). There is evidence, which has been challenged by some recent studies, that stress in animals can increase the permeability of the blood-brain barrier (Sharma, 1991), permitting entrance to the brain of chemicals normally excluded. Although the full clinical significance has yet to be determined, the observation in animals that stress and several anticholinesterases (including pyridostigmine bromide, nerve agents and pesticides) have a common reaction mechanism (promoting the expression of the immediate early gene c-fos in the brain) is noteworthy (Kaufer et al., 1998).

CONCLUSIONS AND FURTHER RESEARCH

This review describes the properties and health effects of chemical and biological agents that might have been available to Iraq at the time of the Gulf War. The review is intended to provide information on the health effects of these chemical warfare agents and toxins, and to help determine on clinical grounds if personnel were exposed to these agents during and shortly after the Gulf War. The review found gaps in the literature, including inadequate or no useful information on thiosarin, long-term follow-up on exposure to phosgene oxime and the toxins, and follow-up data on persons who had become tolerant of nerve agents. Additionally recommended research areas are provided at the end of this section.

A number of conclusions can be drawn from the study:

1. Militarily effective exposure to any of the agents reviewed would have produced severe health effects that would have required clinical treatment or resulted in death. Although some differential diagnosis between agents might have been difficult, no such symptoms consistent with large-dose exposure were reported during the Gulf War, with the exception of the possible exposure of one individual to mustard gas residual in an Iraqi bunker.

2. Low-level exposure to many of these chemical weapon agents could have produced mild clinical signs that could have been overlooked or misinterpreted as arising from other common sources, such as irritation from dust and sand, upper respiratory infections, gastroenteritis, asthma, and the flu. The possibility of low-level exposure to a number of agents more or less at the same time makes diagnosis very difficult. There can be problems of recognition, of modifications of response, or of distinct effects from unrecognized exposures. Therefore, on clinical grounds alone, it is not possible to rule out low-dose exposures to one or several classes of agents or the possibility of some resultant contribution to some of the symptoms Gulf War veterans have experienced. Still, it is difficult to believe that exposures affecting large numbers of persons would escape clinical recognition.

3. No references in the literature report clinical symptoms developing years after exposure, as was the case in about 50 percent of the health problems Gulf War veterans have reported.

4. There is very little literature on the long-term effects of exposure to doses below those that would cause any acute clinical symptoms. The possibility that such exposure could possibly produce chronic health effects cannot be ruled out based on the current state of the literature and needs to be investigated, both for one-time exposure and for longer-term, very-low-dose exposures over an extended period.

The report also reviewed some literature on the possible interaction effects of chemical warfare agents and other factors. Kaufer et al. (1998) discuss several factors that may contribute to symptoms seen in Gulf War veterans—including stress, pyridostigmine bromide, and anticholinesterase nerve agents—are capable of activating regulatory genes (such as c-fos) in the brains of animals. Because of the potential long-term effects of these genes, this observation may be important. However, the long-term effects in animals and the clinical significance of these studies for humans remain to be determined. Epidemiological studies of illnesses in veterans of the Gulf War might consider the possibility of aggregate effects arising from the varied factors noted above. Since mustards and trichothecene toxins (as well as nerve agents) also inhibit acetylcholinesterase, it may be useful to examine their effects on regulatory gene expression as well.

Finally, there are significant gaps in our knowledge that warrant additional research. The most obvious area in need of a great deal of additional research is the health effects from exposure to low levels of chemical warfare agents and toxins. Little is known about the long-term effects of either a single exposure or longer-term exposures to low doses of chemical warfare agents and toxins that result in either mild symptoms or no acute symptoms at the time of exposure.[11]

Further research in many other areas would also be very useful; these areas include the following:

- A better understanding is needed of the effects of mustard agents on the functioning of the central nervous system, including the brain effects of low doses of mustard agents in combination with nerve agents and pretreatments.

- Long-term follow-up studies of the Japanese exposed to sarin—particularly at low levels—in the subway attack would be useful.

- A better understanding is needed of the acute respiratory toxicity of aflatoxin in nonhuman primates, as well as a better understanding of aflatoxin's role in seizures and neurotoxicity. Follow-up information from survivors of the Malaysian poisoning event would be valuable.

- Research is needed to determine the long-term effects of converging cholinergic activation of c-fos. Likewise, the understanding of the consequences of receptor downregulations from cholinergic stimuli must be improved.

---

[11]It should be noted that the Department of Defense and the Veterans' Administration also recognize this need and have initiated a good deal of such research.

- The work of Kaufer et al. (1998) on the duration of the response in the convergent response mechanism of nerve agent action should be followed up, and the relative effects of low levels of known nerve agents in this model should be documented.

- The observations of Buccafusco et al. (1997) on the downregulation of nicotinic receptors in the brain from low-dose diisopropyl fluorophosphate (DFP), with subsequent impaired learning in animals, needs to be extended. Confirming the effect with low-dose nerve agents and documenting the duration of the effect appears to be important. Primate studies with more-complex performance studies could follow.

- Those involved in epidemiology studies of accidents during and immediately after the Gulf War should be made aware of the observation that sarin workers who recovered from mild exposures were noted to have many industrial and vehicular accidents.

- The capabilities of the AFIP may help rule in or out certain exposures. Autopsy and surgical material from the Gulf War and from veterans later might be reviewed, looking for tissue evidence of various agent exposures (which, since they were not an obvious cause of death, might have been overlooked in initial studies). There are indications that biochemical evidence of exposure to various agents can be detected in blood serum and even in formalin-fixed tissues. It is far from certain that existing methods are sensitive enough to identify low-level effects (e.g., DNA adducts in formalin-fixed tissues from autopsies). Whether to conduct such studies is not simple, since the expense does not commend such studies as a screening method. Perhaps such studies should be reserved for cases in which suspicion is high. There may be reasons beyond Gulf War illnesses to develop such a capability.

This report reviews the biological effects of chemical warfare agents and biological toxins that are of interest because of their possible presence in the Persian Gulf theater of war and because of later concern about their role in illnesses in Gulf War veterans. This material was primarily written in 1997; selected information from 1998, 1999, and 2000 was added later as a result of the review process. I have included the most important of these references, but have not included others because they were not germane or did not change the conclusions.

The reader should note that there is considerable mention of organophosphate and carbamate pesticides here, as there is in the pyridostigmine bromide report (Golomb, 1999a). These chemicals are discussed because they have common mechanisms of action with many military agents and to enhance understanding of the potential effects of both; these chemicals also require consideration when looking at agent interactions. Some subjects, such as delayed neurotoxicity, require analysis of pesticide experience, where they were first discovered. The report on pesticides in this series (Cecchine et al., 2000) is a definitive statement on the matter as it pertains to Gulf War use and effects. Likewise, there is some coverage of stress here, although the stress report in this series (Marshall, Davis, and Sherbourne, 1999) contains the definitive coverage of the matter.

I wish to thank Harold J. Fallon, MD, University of Alabama School of Medicine, and Robert G. Feldman, MD, Boston University School of Medicine, for their thoughtful reviews of earlier versions of this work. The report also benefited from the comments of Victor Utgoff of the Institute for Defense Analyses.

The report has benefited greatly from their comments; however, of course, any deficiencies are the fault of the author.

I wish to thank the following individuals for their help:

Ross Anthony
Pam Bromley
James Chiesa
Thomas Dashiell
Daniel Entholt
David Franz
Phyllis Gilmore
Beatrice Golomb
Brennie Hackley, Jr.
Lee Hilborne
Michael Hix
Harry Holloway
Victor Kalasinsky
Caren Kamberg
James Little
David Moore
Elaine Newton
Richard Rettig
Robert Roswell
Jeffrey Smart
Robert Ursano
Dale Vesser

The librarians and staff of the U.S. Army Medical Research Institute of Chemical Defense were also very helpful.

Accommodation	Adjustment or adaptation, especially that of the eye for various distances resulting in pupil constriction or dilation
ACh	Acetylcholine—a neurotransmitter secreted at synapses of cholinergic nerves
AChE	Acetylcholinesterase—an enzyme that hydrolyzes acetylcholine into choline and acetic acid
ACTH	Adrenocorticotropic hormone
Aerosol	A suspension or dispersion of small solid or liquid particles in air or gas
AFB_1	Aflatoxin B_1
AFG_1	Aflatoxin G_1
AFIP	Armed Forces Institute of Pathology
Agent L	Lewisite: dichloro(2-chlorovinyl) arsine
Agent Q	Sesquimustard, 1,2-bis-(2-chloroethylthio) ethane—a potent vesicant
Agent T	bis-(2-chloroethylthio ethyl) ether—an agent stockpiled during World War II as a mustard agent additive:
Alopecia	Absence of hair from skin areas where it normally is present
Analog	A chemical compound structurally similar to another chemical compound and having the same effect on body processes
Anticholinergic	A substance that inhibits the ability of nerve fibers to liberate ACh at a synapse when a nerve impulse passes
Anticholinesterase	A substance that inhibits the action of the enzyme cholinesterase
Aphonia	Inability to produce speech sounds

Apoptosis   Programmed cell death, signaled by the nuclei in nor-
                   mally functioning human and animal cells when age or
                   state of cell health and condition dictates; an active
                   process requiring metabolic activity by the dying cell

ATP   Adenosine 5´ triphosphate—a nucleotide cofactor im-
                   portant in many biological reactions where energy is
                   transferred

Blepharospasm   Twitching of an eyelid

Bronchiectasis   Persistent and progressive dilation of bronchi or bron-
                   chioles as a consequence of inflammatory disease, ob-
                   struction or congenital abnormality; symptoms in-
                   clude fetid breath and paroxysmal coughing, with the
                   expectoration of mucopurulent matter

CAM   Chemical Agent Monitor (a UK detection device)

Casualty   An individual incapable of performing normal tasks; in-
                   cludes both those who are temporarily incapacitated
                   and those who are killed

Catabolism   Any destructive metabolic process by which organisms
                   convert substances into excreted compounds

CCEP   Comprehensive Clinical Evaluation Program

Centrilobular co- A pathological change in the liver
  agulative necrosis

Cerebral edema   The presence of abnormally large amounts of fluid in
                   brain

ChE   Cholinesterase

Chemical warfare   A solid, liquid, or gas that, through its chemical proper-
  agent   ties, produces lethal or damaging effects on man, ani-
                   mals, plants, or materials

Chemotactic   A response of motile cells or organisms in which the di-
                   rection of movement is affected by the gradient of a
                   diffusible substance; differs from chemokinesis in that
                   the gradient alters probability of motion in one direc-
                   tion only, rather than rate or frequency

Chiral   A molecule that, in a given configuration, cannot be su-
                   perimposed on its mirror image; thus, a given chemical
                   formula can have many different chiral forms, which
                   may react differently in some biological processes

Chlorine gas   A lung irritant extensively used during World War I,
                   generally in admixture with phosgene

Cholinergic   Effects produced on the parasympathetic nervous system similar to those ACh produces

CIA   Central Intelligence Agency

Contamination   The presence of a foreign or unwanted substance on terrain, personnel, or equipment

CT   Product of concentration (mg/m^3) multiplied by time of exposure (min) (see Appendix A)

CX   Phosgene oxime; dichloroform oxime

Cyclosarin   Cyclohexyl methylphosphonofluoridate—a nerve agent also known as GF

DAS   Diacetoxyscipenol

Decontamination   The process of removing and destroying a contaminant

DEET   Diethyl-m-toluamide, an insecticide

Dendritic keratitis Inflammation of the cornea (and conjunctiva) due to herpes virus type I; a characteristic finding on physical examination of the eye (cornea) is a dendritic (crystalline or tree-like) pattern

DFP   Diisopropyl fluorophosphate—a weak organophosphate nerve agent, also known as agent PF3

DMSO   Dimethylsulfoxide

DNA   Deoxyribonucleic acid

DSB   Defense Science Board

DTIC   Defense Technical Information Center

EEG   Electroencephalogram—detects abnormalities in the electrical waves emanating from different areas of the brain

Electroretinogram   A graphic record of electrical activity of the retina, used especially in the diagnosis of retinal conditions

ELISA   Enzyme-linked immunoadsorbent assay

Enkephalin   Either of two molecules found in the brain of some mammals that have pain-killing properties and seem to be composed of two small peptides, but these may be the breakdown products of larger molecules

Extrapyramidal syndromes	The extrapyramidal system of the nervous system is centered on the basal ganglia and influences motor control through pyramidal pathways, generally by means of input to the thalamus. When the extrapyramidal system is disturbed, motor control is affected, and patients suffer extrapyramidal syndromes. These are a combination of neurologic effects that include tremors, chorea, athetosis, and dystonia. This is a common side effect of neuroleptic agents (phenothiazines). Other medications known to cause these reactions include haloperidol; molindone; perphenazine and amitriptyline; loxapine; pimozide; and, rarely, benzodiazepines.
GA	Tabun, O-ethyl N,N-dimethylphosphoroamidocyanidate—a nerve agent
GAO	General Accounting Office
GB	Sarin, O-isopropyl methylphosphonofluoridate—a nerve agent
GD	Soman, O-pinacolyl methylphosphonofluoridate—a nerve agent
GF	Cyclosarin, Cyclohexyl methylphosphonofluoridate—a nerve agent
Granulation	The formation in wounds of small, rounded masses of tissue composed largely of capillaries and fibroblasts, often with inflammatory cells
H	Levinstein mustard, 2,2-dicholorodiethylsulfide
HD	Distilled mustard
Hematemesis	The vomiting of blood
Hemoptysis	The expectoration of blood or of bloodstained sputum
Hemorrhagic diathesis	A constitution or condition of the blood that makes the tissues react in special ways to certain extrinsic stimuli and thus tends to make the person more than usually susceptible to certain diseases
HL	A mixture of mustard and lewisite
HMT	Hexamethylene tetramine
HT	A mixture of distilled mustard and Agent T
HT-2	Hydrolyzed T-2

Hydrolysis	The addition of the hydrogen and hydroxyl ions of water to a molecule, with its consequent splitting into two or more simpler molecules
Hypopion	An eye condition in which there is pus in the anterior chamber of the eye, usually resulting from a corneal laceration or abrasion
Hypovolemia	A condition of abnormally low intravascular volume with a decreased volume of circulating plasma in the body, which can be due to blood loss or dehydration
ICD	International Classification of Diseases code
IEG	Immediate early gene
IMPA	isopropyl methylphosphonic acid
Incapacitating agent	An agent that produces temporary physical or mental effects that will render individuals incapable of concerted effort in the performance of their assigned duties
IOM	Institute of Medicine
Keratitis	Inflammation of the cornea—a noninflamatory dystrophy of the cornea
Keratopathy	Disorder of the cornea
L	Lewisite; chlorovinyldichloroarsine—a skin blistering agent
LC_{50}	The concentration required to kill 50 percent of test individuals
LCL_0	Lowest reported lethal concentration
LCT_{50}	Product of the concentration times time that causes lethality in 50 percent of the exposed population.
LD_{50}	The dose required to kill 50 percent of test individuals
LDL_0	Lowest reported lethal dose
Macrovesicular steatosis	Fat deposits in tissue
Mediastinal lymphadenitis	Inflammation of lymph nodes in the space in the thoracic cavity behind the sternum and in between the two pleural sacs
Methenamine	An antibacterial agent, most commonly used in the treatment of urinary tract infections, whose antibacterial action derives from the slow release of formaldehyde by hydrolysis at acidic pH

Mimetic	The symptomatic imitation of one organic disease by another
Miosis	Constriction of the pupils of the eye
MMWR	Morbidity and Mortality Weekly Report
Motor end plate	The structure in which motor nerve fibers terminate with branching processes in a striated muscle fiber
Motor neuron	Nerve cell concerned with carrying impulse away from the central nervous system to an effector organ, such as a muscle or gland
MPA	Methylphosphonic acid
Mustard	bis-(2-chloroethyl)sulfide; also known as agent H or distilled mustard (HD)—a skin blister agent
MW	Molecular weight
Myelosuppression	The suppression of bone marrow activity, resulting in reduction in the number of platelets, red cells and white cells found in the circulation
N	Normal (equivalents per liter, as applied to concentration); nitrogen (as in N-methylpyridine)
Na_2CO_3	Sodium carbonate
NaCl	Sodium chloride
NAD	Nicotinamide adenine dinucleotide—a cofactor involved in various metabolic pathways as a hydrogen acceptor, forming NADH2
NADPH	Nicotinamide adenine dinucleotide phosphate reductase—a cofactor similar to NAD
NaOH	Sodium hydroxide
NAS	National Academy of Science
NATO	North Atlantic Treaty Organization
Nettle gas	An agent that causes stinging similar to that of nettles
Neuronolysis	Breakdown of nerve cells
Neurotransmitter	A chemical, such as ACh, that is secreted at a nerve ending and allows the transmission of a nervous impulse across a synapse
NH_2-	Ammonium ion
NIH	National Institutes of Health
Nonpersistent Agent	A CW agent that retains its toxicity for several hours or less under normal weather and terrain conditions

NRC	National Research Council, part of the National Academy of Science
NTE	Neuropathy target esterase
Nystagmus	An involuntary, rapid, rhythmic movement of the eyeball, which may be horizontal, vertical, rotatory or mixed
OH-	Hydroxide ion
OPIDN	Organophosphate-induced delayed neuropathy
Orthostatic hypotension	Low blood pressure when rising from a chair or bed; a drop in blood pressure precipitated by changes in body position
OSAGWI	Office of the Special Assistant for Gulf War Illnesses
OSRD	Office of Scientific Research and Development
Oxidation	Any process involving the addition of oxygen, loss of hydrogen, or loss of electrons from a compound
Oxime	A cholinesterase reactivator used in the treatment of organophosphate poisoning
P2S	Pyridine-2-aldoxime methyl methanesulfonate—a cholinesterase reactivator.
P^{32}	Chemical symbol for the radioactive isotope of phosphorus of atomic mass 32
PAC	Presidential advisory committee
PAM	Pyridine-2-aldoxime methochloride, Pralidoxime chloride, 2-PAM chloride, Protopam—a cholinesterase reactivator
Parasympathetic nervous system	A network of nerves that controls such involuntary, unconscious, automatic bodily reactions as dilation of certain blood vessels, slowdown in heartbeat, narrowing of pupils, salivation, and increased nasal secretion; the sympathetic nervous system generally has opposite effects
PB	Pyridostigmine bromide—a pretreatment compound for nerve agent, antidote-enhancing compound
PCO_2	Symbol for carbon dioxide partial pressure (tension)
PEG	Polyethylene glycol
Percutaneous	Penetration of the skin
Persistent agent	A CW agent that retains its toxicity for one to several days under normal weather and terrain conditions

Phosgene	Also known as agent CG— a choking agent
Pretreatment	An intervention that, if given before exposure, makes subsequent therapy far more effective and that modifies the manifestations of exposure favorably; includes most interventions currently used prospectively against military chemicals
Prophylaxis	An intervention that, if given before exposure, prevents the development of casualties or adverse effects; for example, immunization against yellow fever, which completely protects persons exposed to infected mosquitoes
PTSD	Post-traumatic stress disorder
Q	Sesquimustard; 1,2-bis (2-chloroethylthio) ethane
R	Alkyl, univalent hydrocarbon radical (or hydrogen)
Radiomimetic	Having effects similar to those of radiation
RBC	Red blood cells
Reduction	Decreasing the oxygen content or increasing the proportion of hydrogen in a chemical compound or adding an electron to an atom or ion
RNA	Ribonucleic acid
S4 gallop	Fourth heart sound, generally a sign of a failing ventricle
Sarin	Isopropyl methylphosphonofluoridate, also known as Trilon 46 and GB—a nerve agent
SCE	Sister chromatid exchange
Scleral	Having to do with the sclera or white of the eye
SGOT	Serum glutamic oxalacetic transaminase
SGPT	Serum glutamic pyruvic transaminase
SH	Sulfhydryl group
Sign	What the physician finds on examination; compare *symptom*
SIPRI	Stockholm International Peace Research Institute
Soman	1,2,2-Trimethylpropyl methylphosphonofluoridate; a nerve agent also known as GD
Stomatitis	Inflammation of the oral mucosa due to local or systemic factors that may involve the buccal and labial mucosa, palate, tongue, floor of the mouth, and gingivae

Sympathetic nervous system	A network of nerves that trigger constricting blood vessels, making hair stand on end, raising "gooseflesh" on the skin, widening the pupils, contracting most sphincters, and speeding up the heartbeat; these stimulants add up to the "startle reaction" by which the body mobilizes for "flight or flight" in the face of sudden danger or surprise
Symptom	What the patient complains of; the body's signal that something is wrong; compare *sign*
Synapse	The region of junction between processes of two adjacent neurons forming the place where a nerve impulse is transmitted from one neuron to another
Syndrome	A set of symptoms or signs that together characterize or identify a specific disease or disorder
Synechia	A disease of the eye, in which the iris adheres to the cornea or to the capsule of the crystalline lens
T-2	One member of the trichothecene mycotoxin family; 4⁻, 15-diacetoxy-8a-3 methylbutyryloxy-12, 13-epoxytrichothec-9-en-3a-ol
Tabun	Ethyl N, N-dimethylphosphoramidocyanidate; a nerve agent also known as Trilon 83, Le 100, gelan, MCE, and GA
TDLo	Lowest reported toxic dose
TG	Thiodiglycol
TGMTase	Thioethermethyl transferase, an enzyme
Thickening agent	A substance added to CW agents to increase their viscosity
Thrombocyto penia	A decrease in the number of platelets in the blood, resulting in the potential for increased bleeding and decreased ability for clotting
TMB-4	Trimethylene-di-(pyridine-4-aldoxim-) dibromide
TOCP	Tri-o-cresyl phosphate, tri-o-tolyl phosphate
Toxic encephalopathy	A toxic degenerative disease of the brain
Toxin	A poisonous substance generally of microbial, vegetable or animal origin
UK	United Kingdom
UN	United Nations

UNSCOM	United Nations Special Commission
Uriticant	A substance that causes itching
USAF	United States Air Force
USAMRIID	U.S. Army Medical Institute of Infectious Disease
V-agents	A family of nerve agents consisting of alkyl esters of S-dialkylamino ethylmethylphosphonothiolic acids
V-agents	A family of nerve agents consisting of alkyl esters of S-dialkylamino ethylmethylphosphonothiolic acids
VA	Veterans Administration
VE	O-ethyl S-(2-diethylaminoethyl) ethylphosphonothiolate, o-ethyl-s-(2-isopropylaminoethyl) methylphosphonothiolate
Vegetative asthenic	European designation of illness with symptoms of weakness, fatigue, and cardiovascular changes
Vesicant	Causing blisters
VX	ethyl-s-diisopropylaminoethyl methylthiophosphonate—a nerve agent
WHO	World Health Organization
Yperite	Mustard agent (also called Agent H, mustard gas)

Chapter One

INTRODUCTION

In the summer of 1990, after the Iraqi invasion of Kuwait, the United States and its coalition allies rapidly deployed large military forces to Saudi Arabia and adjacent countries, initially to prevent invasion of Saudi Arabia (Operation Desert Shield). Later that year, in November, additional large forces were deployed. In January and February 1991, the coalition conducted combined air, ground, and naval operations to eject Iraqi forces from Kuwait in Operation Desert Storm (Watson et al., 1991). The military offensive operations were rapid and successful.

Nearly 700,000 U.S. personnel served in the theater of operations. The U.S. forces had substantially fewer casualties and less illness than had been expected, despite a challenging environment (Quin, 1982) and an opponent with large, modern, and well-equipped forces experienced in combat in the region (Cordesman and Wagner, 1990; Helmkamp, 1994). Iraq's demonstrated ability to use chemical warfare and indications of its interest in biological warfare were major concerns for senior U.S. commanders (Clancy and Franks, 1997). These concerns influenced planning operations and led to very substantial defensive efforts, with extensive training, deployment of detectors, use of protective equipment, and the urgent deployment of pretreatments and immunizations.

After the termination of hostilities, coalition forces were rapidly reduced as efforts were being made to destroy Iraqi military materiel in occupied areas before withdrawal. Later, as part of international agreements, United Nations (UN) teams had access to Iraq to observe or conduct the destruction of weapons of mass destruction and the facilities associated with them, including Scud missiles and chemical facilities.

After the withdrawal of U.S. forces, it gradually became apparent that a considerable number of U.S. personnel who had served in the theater were ill with varied symptoms that in some cases did not readily fit common disease patterns. Later, some coalition countries reported similar symptoms in their personnel. In general, such reports were rare, and some countries reported none.

A later compilation from a registry of U.S. Gulf service personnel showed the following common problems, in descending order of frequency (Defense Science Board [DSB], 1994):

- skin rashes, fatigue
- muscle and joint pain
- headache
- loss of memory
- shortness of breath
- diarrhea
- cough
- choking sensation, sneezing, chest pain.

Reviews, including that of the DSB (1994), did not find chemical and biological agent exposures to be a plausible explanations for the many cases of illnesses in Gulf War veterans being reported. The information available at the time indicated that exposure to agents was not possible because of the great distances between U.S. forces and targets in Iraq where agents might have been released. Likewise, no clinical reports suggested exposures, and it was considered unlikely that long-term effects would arise from exposures that did not produce symptoms. More suspicion was directed toward stress as a basis for the illnesses.

The later disclosure that postwar demolition operations had caused some release of nerve agents proximate to U.S. forces at Khamisiyah lead to some modification of views. The Institute of Medicine (IOM) felt that further animal research and human epidemiology studies were indicated to evaluate long-term neurotoxic effects of low-level exposures (IOM, 1997), and the Presidential Advisory Committee (PAC) on Gulf War Illnesses also considered that agent exposure could not be totally excluded as playing some role, although the calculated exposures were low.

Two main registries currently deal with illnesses in Gulf War veterans:

- the Comprehensive Clinical Evaluation Program (CCEP), involving active and reserve component military personnel, administered by the Department of Defense (DoD)
- a registry of former service members, operated by the Department of Veterans Affairs (Joseph, 1997; Hallman et al., 1998).

The concerns about health problems of those who served in the Gulf region have produced a number of reviews, study efforts, and comprehensive examination efforts (IOM, 1996; National Institutes of Health [NIH], 1994; DSB, 1994).

In 1994, there was a further IOM review of the CCEP, and the Veterans Administration (VA), the U.S. Department of Health and Human Services (DHHS), and the DoD jointly established the Gulf Veterans Coordinating Board. In 1995, the President established an advisory committee on Gulf veterans' illnesses. Many possible causes of veterans' problems have been considered, and a number of research programs were inspired by the problem (PAC, 1996a, 1996b, 1997).

The long list of potential exposures that have been of concern includes fuels, smoking, chemical and biological agents, solvents and petrochemicals, tent heater fumes, non-U.S. and contaminated food and water, oil-field fires, chemical-resistant paints, pesticides, immunizations, infectious diseases, microwaves, antimalarial drugs, depleted uranium, and stress (DSB, 1994; PAC, 1996a; Kroenke et al., 1998).[1]

To date, it has not been possible to develop a coherent case definition of a "Gulf War syndrome" (NIH, 1994; Joseph, 1997; Gibbons et al., 1998; Kroenke et al., 1998; Marshall and Gass, 1998). The term "illnesses in Gulf War veterans" has been used to describe the varied signs, symptoms, and findings in ill Gulf-service personnel.

The CCEP recorded data on 18,495 registered individuals, taken from structured histories, including self-reported exposures. A recent review used the CCEP data to provide a temporal picture of the onset of common symptoms (Kroenke et al., 1998). Table 1.1 shows the overall symptom frequency for the registry.

Figure 1.1 shows the timing of the onset of the symptoms. Fewer than 5 percent of veterans reported symptoms occurring before the war, 25 to 30 percent during the war, 25 percent in the year following the war and nearly 50 percent beginning 2 or more years after the war.

Kroenke et al. (1998) analyzed the exposures to various factors that registrants in the CCEP had self-reported. Although the reports have not yet been validated, 1,145 soldiers (6 percent) thought they were exposed to nerve agents, and 422 soldiers (2 percent) reported exposures to mustards. The authors found no association between individual symptoms and self-reported exposures.

Several more focused studies concentrated on units or regions (Haley and Kurt, 1997; Haley, Kurt, and Horn, 1997; Haley, Horn, et al., 1997; Stretch et al., 1995; Penman et al., 1996; Marshall and Gass, 1998; Cowan et al., 1998; Morris, 1998).

---

[1]In addition to this report, the following of these are the subjects of RAND reviews: infectious diseases (Hilborne and Golomb, 2000), pyridostigmine bromide (Golomb, 1999), immunizations (Golomb, 2000), stress (Marshall, Davis, and Sherbourne, 1999), oil well fires (Spektor, 1998), depleted uranium (Harley et al., 1999), and pesticides (Cecchine et al., 2000).

Table 1.1

Symptom Frequency for 18,495 Gulf War Veterans Evaluated in the Comprehensive Clinical Evaluation Program

Symptom	Any Complaint (%)	Chief Complaint (%)
Joint pain	50.0	12.1
Fatigue	46.9	10.6
Headache	39.7	7.9
Memory/fatigue problems	34.0	4.1
Sleep disturbance	33.0	2.7
Rash	30.2	6.3
Concentration difficulty	26.4	0.5
Depressed mood	22.3	1.0
Muscle pain	21.2	1.1
Dyspnea	18.4	2.7
Diarrhea	18.2	1.8
Abdominal pain	16.3	1.6
Hair loss	11.8	0.5
Bleeding gums	8.2	0.1
Weight loss	6.4	0.1

SOURCE: Kroenke, Koslowe, and Roy (1998); as compiled in 1994. Reprinted with permission.

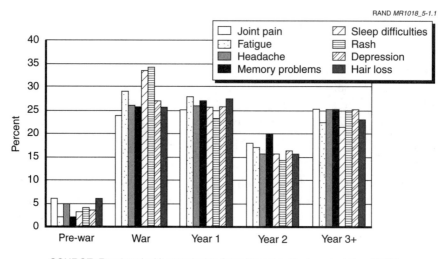

SOURCE: Reprinted with permission from Kroenke, Koslow, and Roy (1998).

Figure 1.1—Onset of Symptoms

Mortality and hospital studies have not shown differences in hospitalization rates or mortality between military personnel who deployed to the Gulf and a matched control military population that did not, but this has not eased concern about the problem (Gray et al., 1996; Kang and Bullman, 1996). Mortality from motor vehicle accidents was higher in Gulf returnees than in nondeployed control groups.

Some caution is advisable in drawing conclusions from these studies and the CCEP. Haley (1998a, 1998b) has hypothesized there may be some possible selection bias due to the "healthy warrior" effect: Illness might simply have been more prevalent in the control population, since sick persons were not deployed. He further hypothesized that hospitalization rates might not be reliable in that sick veterans might have disproportionately separated early from the service and might have received care from nonfederal health facilities, which were not included in the hospital case review. The hospital experience of veterans in nonfederal hospitals is now under study in California (Smith et al., 1998). Other researchers have questioned Haley's theories (Gray, Knoke, et al., 1998; Kang and Bullman, 1998; Cowan, Gray, and DeFraites, 1998).

An important concern has been raised that U.S. personnel may have been exposed to military chemical warfare agents and toxins, and that such exposures play a role in the ongoing problems of some who served in the region. Previous reviews have considered this possibility but did not find significant exposures plausible, given assurances that no Iraqi attacks had occurred and that the Iraqi chemical targets struck during the air war were too remote to affect U.S. personnel. This conclusion was somewhat controversial, with congressional hearings producing reports of unusual events, positive detector alarms, and other anecdotes as contrary data (Riegle and D'Amato, 1994; Senate, 1994; House, 1997).[2]

The later discovery that U.S. forces, in the course of demolition work at the Iraqi depot of Khamisiyah, had unknowingly exploded bunkers and rockets containing nerve agents has required recognition that exposures were possible. Several efforts to model this event have identified a larger exposed personnel population than earlier such attempts suggested. The levels of agent were rather low for this population. Apart from the possibility of unauthorized or unintended small-scale Iraqi employment of agents, congressional hearings and the General Accounting Office (GAO) have raised the possibility that air war attacks on Iraqi facilities where chemical or biological agents were present might have

---

[2]The Office of the Special Assistant to the Deputy Secretary of Defense for Gulf War Illnesses (OSAGWI) has been investigating thoroughly the events covered in testimony and others brought to attention using a case study approach. The office has posted completed studies on its Web site (http://www.gulflink.osd.mil/).

resulted in agent transport into areas where U.S. and coalition forces could have been exposed (Riegle and D'Amato, 1994; GAO, 1997; Senate, 1994; House, 1997).

Two small-scale events during and after the war have not been readily explained. Czech chemical defense troops supporting the Saudi army made low-level detections of nerve agent, subsequently identified as sarin, on January 19, 1991. No casualties resulted, but the origin of the small amount of sarin is unexplained (OSAGWI, 1998b[3]). After the war, a U.S. soldier engaged in destroying Iraqi equipment entered a bunker and then left. Hours later, he developed a typical mild mustard-type injury on his arm. Interpretation of detector readings from that event has been inconclusive and complicated by oil contamination on garments (OSAGWI, 1997d).

Before the war, it was known that Iraq had a substantial chemical and biological warfare program and had employed chemical agents against Kurdish dissidents and extensively against Iran during their long war (Cordesman and Wagner, 1990; Stockholm International Peace Research Institute [SIPRI], 1971; UN, 1984). Since the Gulf War, UN demilitarization efforts have yielded a clearer picture of Iraqi capabilities (Marshall, 1997; Zilinskas, 1997; United Nations Special Commission [UNSCOM], 1991, 1992, 1995).

The Special Assistant for Gulf War Illnesses asked RAND to review the scientific literature on the health effects of eight possible causes of illness among veterans of the Gulf War. This review of selected chemical and toxin agents is a part of the effort. The intention is to provide factual information about agents and issues of concern.

APPROACH

RAND was initially asked to review chemical and biological warfare agents that Iraq was thought to possess:

- sarin (GB)
- cyclosarin (GF)
- thiosarin
- mustard (presumably H or distilled mustard [HD])
- phosgene oxime (CX).

---

[3]OSAGWI has made a large number of Gulf War–related documents available on line in addition to its own products For simplicity, all are listed under OSAGWI in the Bibliography.

After studying reports of the Iran-Iraq War and unclassified post–Gulf War information, RAND added additional agents (with the concurrence of OSAGWI) but gave priority to the initial list. The author had no advice or assistance from U.S. intelligence organizations in the selection of agents for study. It was also noted there was no immediately available information on thiosarin, although there were a few references to thiosoman (SIPRI, 1973). Also noted was that there was little information on human exposures to phosgene oxime, and less on long-term or low-dose effects. The additional agents were

- tabun (GA), an agent Iraq used against Iran (UN, 1984)

- soman (GD), a very toxic nerve agent suspected to be in Iraqi stocks

- VX, an extremely toxic nerve agent attributed to Iraq (OSAGWI, 1990)

- lewisite (L), a blister agent that a Fox vehicle reportedly detected during the Gulf War (Riegle and D'Amato, 1994), which Iraq had previously been suspected of using (OSAGWI, 1997c)

- toxins, specifically trichothecene mycotoxins, which were suspected to have been used in the Iran-Iraq War (Heyndrickx, 1984; Marshall, 1997; Zilinskas, 1997)

- ricin (W), a plant toxin that Iraq acknowledged having in stock (UNSCOM, 1991, 1992, 1995; Zilinskas, 1997)

- aflatoxin, a fungal mycotoxin that Iraq admitted having in Scud warheads and bombs (UNSCOM, 1991, 1992, 1995; Marshall, 1997; Zilinskas, 1997; Sidell, Takafuji, and Franz, 1997).[4]

As the review process continued, much new information became available as a result of research inspired by Gulf War illnesses. Some references could not be retrieved. Some older U.S. government documents are no longer available from the Defense Technical Information Center (DTIC). Moreover, it has not, to date, been possible to obtain some older foreign references (Speigleberg, 1963). In addition to the many panel and study group reports (IOM, 1996; DSB, 1994; NIH, 1994; PAC, 1996b; Riegel and D'Amato, 1994), clinical and operational reports of medical experiences during the Gulf War were considered.[5] The U.S. Army Medical Research Institute of Chemical Defense staff and library were

---

[4]Botulinum toxin, which is remarkably toxic, with little chance of unrecognized exposures, is being considered in a companion piece (Hilborne and Golomb, 2000).

[5]Most of these were found in the journal *Military Medicine*, which gave a background picture of illnesses both in U.S. forces and Iraqi prisoners; see Joseph (1997), Garland (1993), Koshes and Rothberg (1995), Cook (1994), Newmark and Clayton (1995), Hines (1993), McDiarmid et al. (1995), Hyams et al. (1996), Paparello et al. (1993), Wintermeyer et al. (1994, 1996), West (1993), Longmire (1991), Keenan (1991), Pierce (1997), Wittich (1996), Wasserman et al. (1997).

very helpful in making available references that were otherwise difficult to obtain.

Discussions with staff members of the Armed Forces Institute of Pathology and the U.S. Army Medical Research Institute of Infectious Diseases (USAMRIID) provided helpful background information, as did informal discussions with Department of Veterans Affairs clinicians concerned with agents and illnesses in Gulf War veterans.[6]

The descending priority of retrieval and review was as follows:

1. **Documented human experience** (especially lower-dose, chronic, and longer-term effects). There is documented information about human exposure to most agents. The following situations can yield such information:

   - *Military and civilian casualties* can occur during operational use of agents.

   - *Accidental and occupational exposures* can give a great deal of information about clinical responses, and in some cases have had sustained follow-up. The quantitative amount and duration of exposure are, however, unknown, although rough estimates are sometimes possible. Epidemiological information, when available, is reported.

   - *Intentional exposure as part of research* has yielded a considerable amount of information from older studies, especially with nerve agents and mustards, and in some cases there have been long-term follow-up studies. (The situation is similar with respect to human experience with organophosphate pesticides.)

2. **Relevant nonhuman primate data.** Nonhuman primates are widely considered the best models for predicting human responses to chemicals and toxins. They are often used to validate studies using nonprimate animal models. As will be discussed later, there are substantial problems in extrapolating quantitative data from rodents, dogs, cats, and hens to humans. Indeed, even within a class, responses can be surprising. For example, Husain et al. (Husain, Kumar, et al., 1993; Husain, Vijayaraghavan, et al., 1993) found that chronic sarin exposure did not produce delayed neuropathy in rats but did so in mice. Even nonhuman primates are incomplete models for humans, e.g., they do not develop blisters from mustard agents.

3. **Other animal research**, especially low-dose chronic regimes.

---

[6]The comprehensive *Textbook of Military Medicine* (Sidell, Takafuji, and Franz, 1997) only became available late in the preparation of this report.

4. **Mechanisms of action**, especially those that might produce long-term effects.

5. **Variations in sensitivity and response**, and interactions with the environment and other chemicals.

6. **Studies and experience** as above with analogous chemicals (chiefly organophosphate pesticides).

A prominent theme in many Gulf War discussions is the speculation that some illnesses may result from the combined effects of several drugs and chemicals (Senate, 1994; House, 1997; Haley and Kurt, 1997; Haley, Kurt, and Horn, 1997; Haley, Horn, et al., 1997). Although there has been disagreement about design and conclusions of this hypothesis (Haley et al., 1998a), there is perhaps some experimental support for these concerns (Abou-Donia et al., 1996). These animal studies of high sublethal doses of several chemicals (not agents) have been criticized for using routes of exposure that might not replicate human exposure in the animals used. There is no convincingly predictive, quantitative science available to predict multiple chemical interactions in living organisms. Industrial and environmental exposures are commonly multiple, but the Occupational Safety and Health Administration (OSHA) and the Environmental Protection Agency (EPA) generally regulate chemicals singly. The pharmaceutical industry has an analogous problem because it is not always possible to forecast drug interactions, which is one of the reasons for postmarketing surveillance.

HOW THE REVIEW IS ORGANIZED

The report consists of a brief overview of chemical and biological warfare in Chapter Two, followed by three chapters that discuss the following specific classes of agents:

- skin-damaging agents: lewisite, mustards, and phosgene oxime (Chapter Three)

- toxins: ricin, trichothecenes, and aflatoxin (Chapter Four)

- nerve agents: tabun, sarin, soman, cyclosarin, VX, and thiosarin (Chapter Five).

Chapter Six provides conclusions and recommendations, while additional information can be found in the appendixes. A glossary defines specialized terminology found in the report.

It will be apparent that, despite an extensive amount of information on the many agents, there is a lack of data in specific exposure domains of interest, such as the reported low concentration of 0.01296 mg-min/m^3 for sarin downwind from Khamisiyah (Central Intelligence Agency [CIA], 1997). This level is below what is discussed in most clinical reports and studies.[7]

This report discusses "exposures" and exposure levels. Defining adverse exposure or "no-effect" levels is not straightforward; neither is being certain of the biological effects of chemicals and toxins at low levels. In some cases, natural protective defense mechanisms make low-level exposures innocuous. The American Thoracic Society made a considerable effort to define adverse respiratory health effects rigorously, including standards to judge studies, noting that some "no effect" studies lacked statistical power, giving false negative findings.[8] Some perceived health problems may be false-positive findings.

---

[7]The time-weighted average of exposures for 8 hours that the Surgeon General has approved for workers is 0.0001 mg/m^3 (Watson et al., 1998; DHHS, 1988; MMWR, 1998), a domain below expected physiological responses and below permissible levels for many less-toxic pesticides. (DHHS, 1988, contains the exposure recommendations.)

[8]"Guidelines as to What Constitutes an Adverse Respiratory Health Effect, with Special Reference to Epidemiologic Studies of Air Pollution" (1985).

Chapter Two

OVERVIEW OF CHEMICAL AND BIOLOGICAL WARFARE

A number of books have dealt with the history and more recent developments in the field of chemical and biological weapons (Haber, 1986; Vedder, 1925; SIPRI, 1971; SIPRI, 1973; Harris and Paxman, 1982; Seagrave, 1981; Marrs, Maynard, and Sidell, 1996; Sidell, Takafuji, and Franz, 1997).

Modern chemical warfare began with the extensive use of chemical agents during World War I, initially with German use of industrial chemicals, such as chlorine and phosgene, and later use of agents tailored for military use such as the mustards. Their effects were impressive but not decisive, although Russia suffered enormous casualties from chemicals. All combatants made some use of chemicals. There was considerable research on both agents and protective equipment.

World War II combatants possessed chemical and biological weapons, although the agents were little used, other than Japan's use of such weapons against China early in the war. The Germans did, however, use chemicals in their extermination centers. The reasons for nonuse were complex and went beyond simple mutual deterrence. The views of national political leaders, equipment and training of troops, assimilation of doctrine, perceived tactical or strategic advantage or vulnerability, operational readiness, existence of alternative means, and technical preparedness all were important factors. In several situations during the war, use of chemical or biologicals was very seriously considered, e.g., in the defense of the United Kingdom (UK) against invasion and in dealing with Japanese island defenses (Utgoff, 1998). Research and development activities were intense during the war, with Germany developing nerve agents and with biological warfare programs and weapon development in several other countries (Office of Scientific Research and Development [OSRD], 1946; SIPRI, 1971; SIPRI, 1973).

During the tense Cold War, there was extensive research and development, and both sides deployed weapon systems. Both sides also spent considerable effort on improving defensive systems. During this period, there were sporadic reports of chemical and biological employment in remote regional conflicts

(Crocker, 1984; Cordesman and Wagner, 1991; SIPRI, 1971). In the declining days of the Cold War, some regional powers, such as Iraq, Iran, and Libya, developed and employed chemical and perhaps biological weapons.

Chemical and biological weapons are capable of use across a wide spectrum of warfare, from acts of assassination and small-scale terrorism to various tactical and operational situations, both defensive and offensive, including strategic population attacks. The technical and economic barriers to development and weaponization have decreased.

Although a few chemical agents, such as phosgene, chlorine, and phosgene oxime, may degrade materials (corroding metals, degrading rubber), chemical and biological agents are primarily directed at humans and other living organisms and, unlike nuclear weapons, spare equipment and facilities.

The selection of an agent for use is more complex than a simple judgment of toxicity. Production, stability in storage, persistence, delivery, and dissemination are also important. It is not surprising that Iraq selected some agents that were known but not favored by other countries. For example, the Germans independently discovered lewisite during World War I but chose not to use it because they thought its prompt production of symptoms was a disadvantage. Other countries thought otherwise. It should be kept in mind that military agents often contain stabilizing chemicals that have their own toxicity, but most laboratory research on agent effects is done with chemicals purer than weapon-grade material and thus may not predict all effects of chemical weapons. The objectives of use can affect agent selection, from creating defensive barriers that deny entry to territory and facilities using persistent agents, such as mustards or VX, to supporting attacks with highly toxic but volatile nonpersistent agents, such as sarin.

Agents were once released from pressurized cylinders, but contemporary delivery systems make substantial use of modified conventional bomb and shell systems, although spray tanks and bomblets designed for agent delivery are also used.

Iraqi forces had a variety of delivery systems available: toxin loads for Scud missiles; aircraft using bombs or spray tanks, including unmanned aircraft; and artillery-delivered systems using shells and free rockets. Chemical mines were theorized at the beginning of the war (although no such mines were found after the war). Although Saddam Hussein spoke of binary weapons, no such binary delivery systems have been reported since the war.[1] In general, Iraq's delivery systems were not sophisticated, e.g., Iraq used simple bursters in shells to dis-

---

[1]In a binary weapon, the component chemicals are kept separate, to be combined on launch.

seminate ricin rather than the more efficient bomblets, which the United States had developed during World War II. There would be indications of some technical prowess if the report from 1986 of micronized aerosol systems to deliver mustard were correct (Dunn, 1986; Marshall, 1997; UN, 1984; Zilinskas, 1997; Cordesman and Wagner, 1990).

Although there had been discussions of "dusty" (particulate) agents for some time, Iraq, in the war with Iran, made innovative and effective use of mustard agent adherent to fine silica particles to obtain more rapid and more damaging effects (OSAGWI, 1990; OSAGWI, undated b).

Specialized units appear to have been involved in chemical employment (Cordesman and Wagner, 1990), at least in large-scale operations, but little has been published about Iraqi chemical command and control and doctrine. Descriptions of the weapons U.S. forces destroyed at Khamisiyah indicate that there were no special markings obvious to U.S. forces, raising the possibility that inadvertent use might occur, since the chemical rounds resembled standard munitions.

As improved defensive systems arose, with wide availability of protective masks, chemical weapon designers moved in two directions. One was to develop means of mounting high-concentration attacks with very toxic agents that would be lethal with one or two breaths; even a small leak in a mask would produce dangerous incapacity. Such attacks using sarin might require several hundred pounds of agent on an area the size of a football field. Another means of surprise is the "off target attack," in which a dangerous concentration of agent is established away from the target and is then allowed to drift over the target. Commanders prefer predictable results, and this technique is very sensitive to meteorological conditions (SIPRI, 1973; U.S. Army Command and General Staff College, 1963). Reference books on the use of chemical and biological weapons provide guidelines on downwind hazards for various weights of agent along a width of sector under different weather conditions, although the tables usually show a maximum distance hazard of 100 km for large amounts and inversion conditions. The second direction designers took was to attempt to deliver agents via the skin using either formulations of the agents combined with chemicals to increase skin penetration or designed to have skin-penetrating properties, such as mustards and VX. This in turn has lead to widespread use of protective garments.

It is not widely understood that agents with delayed effects can be very effective. Delayed effects generally cover a period of hours to several days or longer. Delayed toxins are very attractive for assassins, terrorists, and special operations, providing very high toxicity for small weight and permitting escape before the attack is obvious. Botulinum toxin may have been used to kill an SS commander in Czechoslovakia in World War II (Harris and Paxman, 1982; Sidell,

Takafuji, and Franz, 1997). Mustard agents are a further example of efficacy arising from delayed effects. They are not readily detectable by smell[2] or other quick-acting physiological responses or warning properties, so large numbers of personnel may be injured before the danger is recognized. The low lethality of such agents is not necessarily a disadvantage, since care of the disabled is demanding. In World War I, 2 percent of fatalities were mustard casualties (Vedder, 1925).

The use or threat of use of chemical and biological weapons imposes considerable burdens on the defender. It is very difficult to rapidly detect all threats or to recognize all attacks in a complex military environment. Although modern protective equipment is highly effective, it poses very heavy burdens in many circumstances, e.g., heat stress; impaired vision, dexterity, communications, and control; and psychological stress (Taylor and Orlansky, 1993; Carter and Cammermeyer, 1989). The aggregate of these burdens is such that there is an incentive to employ chemicals enough to force an opponent into protective posture, to degrade tactical performance quite independent of any casualties actually produced (Franke, 1967).

Fear and confusion are prevalent in combat. Use or expected use of chemical weapons could further amplify that fear and confusion. During World War II, there were instances of U.S. units on Guadalcanal and in Normandy becoming disorganized at night when gas alarms sounded after troops had discarded their masks. More recently, it appears that fear of a chemical attack appears to have been a factor in flight from urban areas during the Iran-Iraq War, as both sides fired missiles at cities (Cordesman and Wagner, 1990). The high state of training and discipline in U.S. forces appears to have prevented panic during the tense periods of the Gulf War.

The following chapters provide a number of human toxicity estimates, many of which required some extrapolation from animal studies. The Subcommittee on Toxicity Values for Selected Nerve and Vesicant Agents (National Academy of Sciences [NAS], 1997) has pointed out that much of the older literature on these matters was developed to assess the effect of offensive use of such agents. In an offensive operation, the goal is to kill or incapacitate a minimum of 50 percent of the least-sensitive individuals in the target population, which actually results in greater damage when the more-sensitive population is considered. This bias in the older studies results in an understatement of the toxicity of agents and precautions needed to protect personnel.

---

[2]Mustards do have a detectable odor at the level of biological injury, 0.006 mg/m^3 (OSRD, 1946).

Chapter Three

SKIN-DAMAGING AGENTS

The designation of these agents as "skin damaging" gives an incomplete picture of their effects. The several mustards, lewisite, and phosgene oxime have quite different chemistries and mechanisms of action (some of which are poorly understood), but all are capable of eye damage at low levels, pulmonary injury at any level, and notable systemic effects at higher doses. Systemic illness can result from skin absorption alone. It is a maxim in chemical casualty care that, when eye effects occur, pulmonary injury should also be suspected (Rebentisch and Dinkloh, 1980).

Within the context of the Gulf War, typical military level-exposures to these agents would have been readily recognized, particularly when there was so much concern about chemical attacks. At low levels of exposure there may have been some opportunities for very mild cases to go unrecognized in a setting in which eye irritation from sand and other factors was common, as were respiratory symptoms (Korenyi-Both and Juncer, 1997). It seems unlikely that typical vesication (blisters) would have escaped notice, but lesser levels of exposure can resemble sunburn. OSAGWI has located hospital records that can be examined for admissions for blistering. If unit medical records documenting sick-call workloads can be located for the periods before and after hostilities began, it may be possible to compare them to look for a change in the pattern of illness.[1] Hospital experience was also extensive with outpatients, as West (1993) described for the 13th Evacuation Hospital, suggesting other retrievable records.

The agents under consideration vary greatly in the timing of the onset of clinical signs and symptoms: immediately for phosgene oxime, promptly for lewisite (seconds to minutes), and delayed (hours) for mustards.

---

[1]Hines (1993) reports sick call for the First Cavalry Division for November–February, so some records may still exist.

These agents play a variety of military roles, especially to create barriers or deny terrain and facilities (mustards and lewisite), by virtue of their persistence and the ability to create vapor and contact hazards. All can be used in conjunction with other, more toxic agents to enhance their effects, and all are dangerous as vapors, aerosols, or droplets. While these agents are dangerous when ingested, it does not appear that there was much opportunity for food and water contamination during the Gulf War. There are indications that it is possible to disseminate mustards adsorbed on small particles (Dunn, 1986).

Research information is uneven, with little information available on phosgene oxime and only small amounts on the others from the 1960s and 1970s. Modern research techniques have only recently been applied, as a result of concerns about occupational and civilian population exposure risks from demilitarization efforts and recognition of continued use and threats arising from these agents.

LEWISITE

History and Background Information

Lewisite (also known as Agent L), is no longer considered a state-of-the-art chemical warfare agent (Franke, 1967; SIPRI, 1971; SIPRI, 1973) but remains in many countries' stockpiles. Lewisite is relatively simple and inexpensive to produce, making it attractive to less advanced nations beginning chemical warfare programs (Franke, 1967).

Lewisite acts promptly on exposure, persists with moderate potency, and is easily mixed with other chemical agents to augment toxic effects. For example, HL (a mustard-lewisite mixture) is less likely to freeze when dropped from high altitudes. Lewisite can be most effective when mixed with nerve agents. Once absorbed, lewisite induces vomiting, precluding the use of protective masks and making personnel vulnerable to other, more toxic chemicals. Lewisite is a significant threat to unprotected personnel for that reason and also because it causes prompt incapacitation from eye injuries and respiratory irritation, coupled with long-term incapacitation from skin burns, pulmonary injury, and systemic illness (Sidell, Takafuji, and Franz, 1997, pp. 218–220).

Both the United States and Germany synthesized and characterized lewisite during World War I but did not use it during that conflict. The Germans chose not to develop it, apparently because they regarded its prompt irritating effects as a disadvantage, especially contrasted to the delayed and initially unnoticed effects of mustards (Wachtel, 1941). Large munitions expenditures were required to achieve effective concentrations in the field (Pechura and Rall, 1993, pp. 25–29). The United States, Germany, Russia, and Japan built considerable stocks of lewisite during World War II (Franke, 1967; SIPRI, 1971). The Japanese used lewisite against Chinese troops repeatedly before and during World War II, in some cases to impede withdrawing forces (SIPRI, 1971), although the effects are not documented.

Although the use of lewisite was suspected at times during the Iran-Iraq War, it was never proved present in the munitions studied (UN, 1984; Dunn, 1986; Defense Intelligence Agency, 1997) and no elevated levels of arsenic were found in the blood and tissues of Iranian casualties treated in Europe (Heyndrickx, 1984, pp. 90–101).

There is some human exposure experience from accidental exposure to lewisite (Cogan, 1943), human experimentation, and occupational exposures of production workers (although governmental follow-up of these exposures has been criticized for lack of persistence) (Pechura and Rall, 1993). The levels of exposure that resulted from accidents in occupational workers are not known. The accident Cogan (1943) reported involved a group of officers observing a test, who thought they had encountered a riot control agent.

Weaponization

Lewisite is easy to manufacture, and storage stability problems can be overcome. It can be dispersed by aerial spraying, shells, or bombs. Lewisite persists for six to eight hours on the ground in sunny weather. Thickened forms to enhance persistence have been tested. Its decomposition products are toxic, making decontamination difficult. Munitions containing lewisite may contain toxic stabilizers. Lewisite is effective as vapor, aerosol, or liquid.[2]

Detection

There are reports, although they are variable and unreliable, of a characteristic (geraniumlike) odor for lewisite in the range of 0.8 mg/m^3 to more commonly cited 14 to 23 mg/m^3 median detection (OSRD, 1946; Pechura and Rall, 1993, p. 53). Detecting lewisite has not been a high military priority. U.S. forces have detectors for lewisite—paper and kits (M7 and M9A)—and the Fox reconnaissance vehicle is able to detect lewisite with its mass spectrometer system. Other forensic techniques for soil and material analysis exist (e.g., gas chromatography). In biological tissues, increased arsenic levels are a surrogate for lewisite (Haddad and Winchester, 1983).

---

[2]Goldman and Dacre (1989) provided a comprehensive review, and Pechura and Rall (1993) provided an extensive bibliography as an annex.

Chemical and Physical Characteristics

Table 3.1, compiled from Field Manual 3-9 (U.S. Army, 1990), shows the chemical structure of lewisite and some of its important properties. This agent is somewhat volatile, more than mustard but less than water.

Toxicology and Toxicokinetics

Lewisite is a local and pulmonary irritant, a vesicant, and a systemic poison. When ingested with food, it produces severe gastrointestinal irritation. The eyes, respiratory tract, and skin are the most likely sites of exposure when lewisite is used as a chemical warfare agent. The agent is lipophilic and readily penetrates intact skin (Wachtel, 1941; Vedder, 1925; North Atlantic Treaty Organization [NATO], 1973). The approximate lethal dose (LD_{50}, dose expected to kill 50 percent of humans) is 35 to 40 mg/kg, an amount present in 2 ml of liquid agent. However, 1 g on the skin causes severe internal organ injury (NATO, 1973). Lewisite toxicity resembles other trivalent arsenicals that produce peripheral and central neurotoxicity, hepatotoxicity, and epithelial damage.[3] Death may result from fluid loss and hypovolemia secondary to capillary leakage—the so-called "lewisite shock" (Snider et al., 1990; Watson and Griffin, 1992; Sidell, Takafuji, and Franz, 1997, pp. 218–220). The effects noted above are from higher dose exposures.

Early studies of arsenic compounds showed that the toxicity was associated with altered cellular metabolism. The cellular poisoning effects are attributed to the inhibition of cellular enzyme systems (Watson and Griffin, 1992; Pechura and Rall, 1993), especially as a result of arsenic complexing with sulfhydryl groups of proteins and enzymes. This agent affects many sulfur-containing enzymes, including amylase; lipase; cholinesterase; some adenosine triphosphate (ATP) enzymes; creatine phosphokinase; and, of central importance (Snider et al., 1990), the pyruvate oxidase system.

According to the *Textbook of Military Medicine* (Sidell, Takafuji, and Franz, 1997, pp. 218–220), there are two types of mechanisms for these effects:

1. reactions with glutathione leading to loss of protein thiol status, loss of calcium ion homeostasis, oxidative stress, lipid peroxidation, membrane damage, and cell death

2. reactions with sulfhydryl groups on enzymes leading to inhibition of pyruvate dehydrogenase complex, inhibition of glycolysis, loss of ATP, and cell death.

---

[3]Most human experience with trivalent arsenicals is from oral toxicity (Haddad and Winchester, 1983).

Table 3.1

Lewisite: Attributes and Responses

Agent	Lewisite Agent L Dichloro(2-chlorovinyl)arsine
Agent type	Rapid-acting blister casualty agent
Chemical structure	

$$\begin{array}{cc} H & H \\ | & | \\ Cl-C & =C-As \end{array} \diagup \begin{array}{c} Cl \\ \\ Cl \end{array}$$

Physical/chemical properties	
Vapor density	7.1 (compared to air)
Freezing point	18 to 0.1°C (purity- and isomer-dependent)
Boiling point	190°C
Vapor pressure	0.394 mm Hg at 20°C
Volatility	4,480 mg/m3 at 20°C
Decomposition at	>100°C

Hydrolysis rates[a]	Degrades under humid conditions
	    Vapor—rapid
	    Dissolved—rapid

Hydrolysis products	HCl and chlorovinyl arsenous oxide; alkaline hydrolysis destroys blister properties
Toxicity	
Median incapacitating dosage	
Respiratory	Not listed
Skin vapor	>1,500 mg-min/m^3
Eye vapor	<300 mg-min/m^3
Median lethal dosage	
Respiratory	1,200–1,500 mg-min/m^3
Skin liquid	Not listed
Skin vapor	100,000 mg-min/m^3
Symptoms	Immediate stinging to skin, blistering of skin (after 13 hours), respiratory inflammation— plus systemic poisoning
Protection required	Protective impermeable clothing and masks and gloves at all times
Decontamination	Personnel—Washing soda, skin decontamination pads, alkaline soap or detergent and water
First aid	Decontaminate, provide support, British antilewisite (BAL)
Detection method	M256 kit for high concentrations on surfaces or in air; bubbler method for low concentrations

SOURCES: U.S. Army (1990); AD Little (1986, Ch. 2).

[a]Low solubility in water limits hydrolysis.

In vitro studies show that lewisite at 0.3 µg/l stops cell proliferation and inhibits DNA synthesis (Henriksson et al., 1996). Laminin, an adhesion molecule in the basement membrane of the skin, is rich in sulfhydryl groupings, so it is suspected that inhibition of this molecule is the mechanism by which lewisite causes blisters (King et al., 1994). In a rabbit whose skin is exposed to lewisite liquid, absorption of arsenic is very rapid, with the highest levels appearing in the liver, lungs, kidney, spleen, and intestines (Cherkes, 1965). In a more recent rabbit study (Snider et al., 1990), lewisite was widely distributed in the body, with high concentrations (e.g., seven times the blood level) found in liver, lung, and kidneys. Tissue levels actually rose over the course of four days, even as blood levels fell. In the Cherkes (1965) study, arsenic appeared in the urine after a few hours. The kidneys, and to a lesser extent the bile, were the main excretion routes. Although the mechanism of vomiting is not known, arsenic has been shown to bind to, and inactivate, muscarinic receptors (Fonseca et al., 1991).

Exposure-Effect Relationships

Table 3.2 shows incapacitating levels of lewisite. Data from various sources do not agree on irritating and incapacitating effects, and no available information resolves the differences. The tolerance threshold for the irritant effects of lewisite is approximately 0.8 mg/m^3 (Wachtel, 1941). Definite eye and respiratory irritation occurs within 1 minute at concentrations of 10 to 30 mg/m^3. Vapor concentrations sufficient to cause blisters are lethal if inhaled. Unmasked personnel exposed to lewisite vapor would probably not show skin burns because eye and respiratory signs would overcome personnel first. A small amount of liquid on the skin or eyes is hazardous; 0.1 µl in the eye blinded rabbits (AD Little, 1986, Ch. 2; Aponte et al., 1975).

No references discussing interactions with medications or environmental chemicals were located. There are no reports of individuals' developing hypersensitivity to lewisite, as has been seen with mustards. Although arsenic can produce a polyneuropathy, no reports emerged of such peripheral neuropathy in humans or animals following acute lewisite exposure. Arsenic polyneuropathy is more often seen in a setting of chronic exposure (Harrison, 1997).

There is little information regarding chronic and long-term exposures (Watson and Griffin, 1992; Lohs, 1975; Pechura and Rall, 1993). Although there is some information from Japanese munitions workers, occupational exposures from manufacturing have not been well-studied. Judging such exposures is difficult because these workers worked with other arsenicals and mustards, and actual exposure levels were unknown. A 1978 study of Japanese workers (Inada et al., 1978) demonstrated an increased risk of intraepithelial Bowen's squamous cell carcinoma (Pechura and Rall, 1993, p. 99).

Table 3.2

Incapacitating Levels of Lewisite

Exposure	Species	Dose	Comments	Sources
Eye	Human	2.0 mg/m^3	Irritation threshold	Cherkes (1965), Aleksandrov (1969)
	Human	10 to 30 mg/m^3	Definite irritation in 1 min.	Cherkes (1965)
	Human	1 to 5 mg/m^3	Intense irritation	Stade (1964)
	Rabbit	0.1 µl	Liquid; permanent blindness	Aponte et al. (1975)
	Human	10 mg/m^3	Vapor; inflammation and swelling of eye and lids	Franke (1967)
		0.8 mg/m^3	Vapor; limit of tolerance	
	Human	1,500 mg-min/m^3	CT, permanent eye damage	
	Human	<300 mg-min/m^3	Concentration required for incapacitation due to eye irritation	
Skin[a]	Human	0.01 mg/cm^2	Erythema; liquid	Cherkes (1965),
		0.05 to 0.1 mg/cm^2	Erythema; liquid	Franke (1967)
		0.15–0.2 mg/cm^2	Blisters; liquid	Franke (1967)
		10,000 mg/m^3	Blisters; vapor concentration; 15 min	Franke (1967)
		2,000 mg/m^3	Erythema; vapor; 1 hour	Aleksandrov (1969)
		2,800 mg/m^3	Blisters; vapor; 1 hour	Aleksandrov (1969)
		3,340 mg/m^3	Blisters; vapor concentration	Wachtel (1941)
Inhalation	Human	10 to 30 mg/m^3	Vapor—injury to the upper respiratory tract	Aleksandrov (1969)
	Human	50 mg/m^3	Vapor—incapacitation for several weeks	Franke (1967)

SOURCE: Various (AD Little, 1986, Ch. 2).
[a]Erythema/blistering.

Chronic cough and eye irritation can be expected from exposure to lewisite. It is uncertain whether chronic bronchitis or asthma results from lewisite exposure, although reactive airway disease after severe irritations is recognized.

Lohs (1975) warns of the neuropathic capabilities of arsenicals; however, none of the follow-up studies has mentioned neuropathy. There is no indication that chronically occupationally exposed persons develop chronic oral arsenic intoxication with anemia, hyperkeratosis, inflamed mucous membranes, and polyneuropathy (motor and sensory) (Harrison, 1997). Studies of long-term exposure (13 weeks average) of rats to lewisite found no effects on body weight or reproduction with up to five 2-mg/kg doses by gavage per week (Sasser et al., 1996). There was gastric irritation. The no-observed-adverse-effect level was estimated to be between 0.5 and 1mg/kg.

In general, extrapolations from animal studies have served to set exposure standards and estimate human effects, particularly to understand severe intoxication. Low-dose studies have not been found. The Surgeon General's Working Group (Morbidity and Mortality Weekly Report [MMWR], 1988) established the following exposure standards: a time-weighted average level of 0.003 mg/m^3 for 8 hours for workers and 72 hours for the general public (see DHHS, 1988)[4].

Clinical and Pathological Findings

There are few published case reports of human lewisite poisoning. Soviet authors describe clinical findings that may have arisen from accidents but provide no details. Cogan (1943) reported an accidental vapor exposure of several officers who initially thought they had been exposed to "tear gas" and had sustained mild eye injuries. Volunteer studies give a picture of the course of skin injuries. Signs and symptoms of acute lewisite exposure include the rapid onset of irritation to the eyes and mucous membranes of the upper respiratory tract (lachrymation and rhinitis). In more serious cases of vapor intoxication, chest pain, nausea, vomiting, headache, weakness, convulsions, hypothermia, and hypotension occur (Sidell, Takafuji, and Franz, 1997; Karkchiev, 1973; AD Little, 1986, Ch. 2; U.S. Army, 1990; NATO, 1973). Other than serious eye injuries, most acute injuries seem to resolve well.

The pathology literature is largely limited to serious acute exposures (e.g., Vedder, 1925). Laboratory tests of the blood of persons exposed may show hemoconcentration; animal studies suggest elevated liver enzymes, including lactate dehydrogenase (LDH) (King et al., 1992; Sasser et al., 1996). Blood arsenic would be detected at toxic levels. The following subsections describe the effects on specific body sites.

Skin. Exposure of the skin to vapor causes immediate itching or stinging within one minute, followed by erythema over 10 to 30 minutes. Mild exposures resemble a sunburn, with pain decreasing over 24 to 48 hours, sometimes followed by desquamation. More intense exposures, including liquid contact, produce intense stinging and the formation of small vesicles over the next 24 hours, with later enlargement of the vesicles with accumulation of a nontoxic fluid. Gradually, a crust forms, and the lesion dries. The skin shows degenera-

---

[4]That is, the public is permitted one-ninth the worker exposure.

tive, necrotic changes with edema, hemorrhage, and inflammation. The scrotum, axillae, and neck seem most sensitive.

A deep bullous lesion occurs following heavy exposure, worsening over three to four days, with considerable pain. Such lesions take one to two weeks to resolve, a shorter period than with a similar mustard injury.[5] Systemic illness is more likely to occur if such heavy exposures are to the liquid form, with later development of vomiting, pulmonary edema, or shock.

Eye. Immediate eye pain and blepharospasm result from lewisite exposure, followed by conjunctival and lid edema. Within one hour, the lids are closed, and photophobia and headache (perhaps from ciliary spasm) occur. After a few hours, the edema decreases, but corneal opacity and iritis may occur. Severe exposures can produce necrotic injuries of the iris with depigmentation, hypopion, and synechia development. In contrast, very low levels may only involve the conjunctivae. Unlike mustard exposure, there is no latent period.

The pathology of severe eye injuries is not relevant to this review. Mild eye exposures (Cogan, 1943) showed dilated pericorneal vessels, violaceous flush of the ciliary region, and later changes similar to dendritic keratitis in the cornea. A relapsing syndrome (apparent recovery followed by return of keratitis) like that of mustard injury has not been described for lewisite.

Respiratory. Mild respiratory exposures resemble upper respiratory infections, with sneezing, coughing, rhinitis, and mucous membrane erythema, possibly progressing to retrosternal pain, nausea, and malaise. More severe exposures cause lower respiratory effects, with continuous coughing, laryngitis, and aphonia. Crackles and rales may be heard over the lung fields, and mucous and sputum production are abundant. Tracheobronchitis develops more rapidly and is more severe than with mustards. Pneumonia and pulmonary edema may develop on the first day. German authors (see AD Little, 1986, Ch. 2) have described in occupational settings a chronic cough and bronchitis with abundant sputum production that was described as "sweet." There are descriptions of severe pulmonary lesions resulting from serious acute exposure in dogs (Vedder, 1925).

Nervous System. Despite reports of convulsions and coma with severe exposures, neurological findings are inconsistent. Neurologic complications after mild exposures have not been described. Some Soviet authors have reported edema and hemorrhage in the brain, but such findings have not been noted in U.S. studies. No reports of degeneration of peripheral nerves were found.

---

[5]Generally, lewisite injuries respond more favorably than mustard injuries (Wachtel, 1941, Vedder, 1925).

Cardiovascular. In severe intoxication, there may be bradycardia, dyspnea, hypotension, and hemoconcentration. These effects are mediated by vasodilation and increased capillary permeability, which can produce lewisite shock (Watson and Griffin, 1992). Soviet investigators describe patchy subendocardial hemorrhages as characteristic of lewisite toxicity in animals (AD Little, 1986, Ch. 2). Other studies noted dilation of the right side of the heart in severe animal poisoning.

Other Systems. Human ingestion experience is not documented (NAS, 1985), but would be expected to produce severe abdominal pain and bloody diarrhea. Nausea and vomiting occur from respiratory or heavy dermal exposure. Indeed, a Chinese chemical warfare analyst has classified lewisite as a vomiting agent (Fang, 1983). In both people and animals, the vomiting is associated with retching, such that humans might remove protective masks. The retching appears to be distinctive, unlike the more common symptoms of nausea and vomiting (Sidell, Takafuji, and Franz, 1997; Vedder, 1925). In contrast to what might be expected, there is no documentation of liver effects from chronic exposure.

There are no specific musculoskeletal findings, although weakness has been observed. There is little clinical information about effects on bone marrow and the immune and endocrine systems. Renal disorders, although theoretically possible, are not described.

There is no substantial evidence that lewisite is carcinogenic, teratogenic, or mutagenic (Dacre, 1989; Sidell, Takafuji, and Franz, 1997, p. 220).

What to Look for in the Gulf Context

If lewisite exposures occurred during the Gulf War, they must have been relatively mild to have escaped recognition. The setting in which Fox vehicles detected lewisite—near a breaching operation—was a possible situation for lewisite exposure; however, alternative explanations have been given for the readings, mainly that the Fox vehicle's road wheels, which are made of silicone, can off-gas, which results in false lewisite readings (OSAGWI, 1997c). The UN has not reported finding lewisite in the destroyed Iraqi chemicals (UNSCOM, 1991, 1992, 1995).

No clinical cases have been associated with the reports of lewisite detection from Fox vehicles during the Gulf War. The matter has been extensively evaluated, and the reports appear to have been in error, reflecting massive contamination from oil fire products and a misidentification of materials in the system (OSAGWI, 1997c; OSAGWI, 1997e).

It is possible that low-level exposures to lewisite could have resembled common eye irritation and respiratory infections. Clinical association of eye and respiratory symptoms with nausea vomiting and retching might be a clue that lewisite was the cause. Should there be further concern about lewisite exposure in the Gulf, some effort to correlate epidemiological data with tactical events might be useful. It is not likely that lewisite could produce vomiting without eye and skin effects.

If mask filters or other equipment from the war become available, measurements of residual arsenic might document lewisite use. It should be noted that arsenic is present in nature in some soils and waters, so its presence alone would not be solid proof of lewisite use. Since the half-life of arsenic in body tissues is days to weeks, there does not appear to be any merit in measuring arsenic levels in Gulf veterans so long after the possible exposure.

Summary and Conclusions

There is no strong reason to think that U.S. forces experienced a lewisite attack or that lewisite was in the Iraqi arsenal. A real attack would have been hard to overlook. Such an attack would produce blisters, eye injuries, and associated severe vomiting and retching. A small-scale accidental low-level release near U.S. forces could have produced eye and respiratory symptoms that could have been misdiagnosed as routine eye irritation and respiratory infections.

The information on the long-term consequences of lewisite exposure is not extensive. There is no indication that brief low-level exposures are associated with long-term problems. Arsenic can cause polyneuropathy, but there is no documentation of this occurring in humans or animals after acute arsenic-containing lewisite exposure. More chronically exposed munitions workers developed sustained bronchitis but apparently not neuropathy. There is reason to think chronic exposure may predispose to Bowen's squamous cell intraepithelial cancer. There is, however, no indication of the presence of enough lewisite to produce chronic exposures during the Gulf War.

PHOSGENE OXIME

Phosgene oxime (also known as CX, or dichloroform oxime) belongs to a class of chemical warfare agents known as urticants or nettle gases, so named because of their property of intensely irritating the skin immediately after contact. Shortly after skin exposure and initial irritation, erythema, severe itching, hives, and painful blisters that resemble nettle stings develop. The symptoms spread far beyond the region of initial exposure (Franke, 1967). Fatal pulmonary edema has been produced in experimental animals 2 to 24 hours after percutaneous exposure to liquid phosgene oxime. Phosgene oxime is also classified as a vesicant, unlike phosgene, which is a choking agent. Very little is known about the pathophysiology of phosgene oxime intoxication.

Phosgene oxime is an unlikely candidate for a cause of illnesses in Gulf War veterans. UNSCOM has not reported this agent in the Iraqi chemicals they destroyed; the agent is so aggressive that its use would be hard to overlook (UNSCOM, 1991, 1992, 1995). There were indications of Iraqi use of an agent whose effects resembled phosgene oxime against Iran (OSAGWI, 1990), but confirmation is lacking.

History

Phosgene oxime's chemical properties have been known since the late 1920s; researchers Prandtl and Sennewald synthesized it in 1929 (see AD Little, 1986, Ch. 3). Germany, the Soviet Union, and other countries appreciated its military potential, once storage and stability problems were addressed. Major powers stockpiled this agent during World War II, although there is no record of its use (SIPRI, 1971; SIPRI, 1973).

Several German sources (Rebentisch, 1980; Franke, 1967; Hirsch, 1950; Hackman, 1934) indicate that there was interest in the agent, whose immediate incapacitating effects were notable; it was also mixed with lewisite and mustard. Hackman, an advisor on the agent's use, commented that "there are few substances in organic chemistry that exert such a violent effect on the human organism as this compound." However, neither Malatesta et al. (1983) nor Wells and MacFarlan (1938) found the respiratory toxicity in animals to be impressive and judged the vesication responses to the dilute agent to be inferior to mustard. There was initial concern that phosgene oxime, because it attacks rubber, might impair the effectiveness of mask canisters, some of which emitted smoke when exposed to phosgene oxime. Later studies, however, did not support this concern (Goshorn et al., 1956).

No detectors have specifically been configured to detect phosgene oxime, and it was difficult to locate information on its detection. Sidell, Takafuji, and Franz (1997), pp. 220–222, indicated that the M256A1 detector can detect phosgene oxime. This may be a reference to the paper detectors. The authors provided no sensitivity data. However, OSAGWI informed RAND that the M256A1 detector uses the blister test to detect phosgene oxime and responds to levels between 3 and 5 mg/m^3 and that it is possible to program the MM1 detector in the Fox vehicle to detect phosgene oxime.

Weaponization

Phosgene oxime might be delivered by artillery or rockets as a "surprise" agent combined with other chemicals (e.g., smokes or nerve agents) to produce prompt incapacitation and then death in antiarmor or air-defense crews. The pain from phosgene oxime on the face might cause removal of protective masks, while the corrosive effects on the skin might render it more vulnerable to penetration by nerve agents (Franke, 1967; Sidell, Takafuji, and Franz, 1997, pp. 220–222). The extreme irritation and immediate eye injury and later lung injury would also be of military significance (Rebentisch and Dinkloh, 1980; AD Little, 1986, Ch. 3). No information is available about Iraqi views on phosgene oxime (Sidell, Takafuji, and Franz, 1997; U.S. Army, 1990). There is a report that Iraq used a chemical agent on several occasions during the war with Iran, which could not be confirmed. Other reports referred to use of "phosgene," and described eye and skin effects, such as immediate eye irritation, immediate pain, and pallor of spots on exposed skin within 30 seconds, evolving into an open wound within one week. These are all symptoms of exposure to phosgene oxime (OSAGWI, 1990).

Toxicology and Toxicokinetics

Table 3.3 summarizes the structure and physical and chemical properties of phosgene oxime. It may persist in soil for two hours but does not persist on materiel. Water decontaminates it on skin (Sidell, Takafuji, and Franz, 1997, pp. 220–222).

The primary exposure routes for phosgene oxime, when used as a chemical warfare agent, are mucous membranes (eyes, nose, and throat) and the skin. Enough phosgene oxime can be absorbed through the skin to produce systemic poisoning and death, especially if the agent is liquid. The delayed pulmonary toxicity from percutaneous or parenteral exposure is not unique and is similar to effects of phosgene, phorbol, and combustion products.

Mechanisms of Action

While there are many interesting theories about the mechanism of action, recent studies provide no proof. It has not been established whether the toxicity arises from the necrotizing effects of hydrochloric acid liberated during hydrolysis, from the direct effects of the oxime, or from the carbonyl grouping. Delayed pulmonary effects from injection indicate a mechanism other than the direct effects of hydrochloric acid. Taylor (1983) suggested the likelihood that the agent has a bifunctional effect deriving from alkylating and nucleophilic properties. He suggests the alkylating properties might resemble those of mustard. No data on metabolism of phosgene oxime have been found. Sidell, Takafuji, and Franz (1997), pp. 220–222, note that the cellular targets of phosgene oxime are unknown but indicate that there are two main paths of injury:

1. **direct**—involving enzyme inactivation, corrosive injury, and cell death with rapid tissue destruction

2. **indirect**—involving activation of alveolar macrophages, recruitment of neutrophiles, and release of hydrogen peroxide, resulting in delayed tissue injury, such as pulmonary edema.

Exposure-Effect Relationships

Lethal systemic doses of phosgene oxime for humans have not been determined, but estimates are in the range of 30 mg/kg. Other reported human-effect thresholds vary from 1 mg/m^3 for irritation from older German reports (Franke, 1967) to a more recent 3 mg/m^3 for irritation and 1 mg/m^3 for detection (Malatesta et al., 1983). The minimum effective respiratory dosage is estimated to be a CT of 300 mg/m^3, while the lethal dose that kills half the exposed

Table 3.3

Chemical and Physical Properties of Phosgene Oxime

Agent	Phosgene oxime CX Dichloroformoxime
Chemical structure	

Molecular weight	113.94
Physical state (20°c)	Yellowish-brown liquid (munitions-grade) or colorless, crystalline solid (pure). When cooled, pure solid turns pink on long standing; less pure material gives light yellow slurry.
Vapor density (compared to air)	3.9
Liquid density (g/cc)	Not found
Boiling point (°c, 760 mm hg)	129° (decomposes)
Melting point (°C)	35–40° (pure)
Vapor pressure (mm hg)	13 at 40°C
Volatility (mg/m^3)	1,800 at 20°C; 76,000 at 40°C (evaporates readily)
Viscosity (cp at 20°C)	Not found
Surface tension (dynes/cm at 20°C)	Not found
Solubility	Readily soluble in water; very soluble in organic solvents
Decomposition temperature (°C)	<128
Odor	Disagreeable, prickling odor

SOURCE: AD Little (1986, Ch. 3), U.S. Army (1990).

population (LCT$_{50}$) is 3,200 (which is about twice the LCT$_{50}$ of mustard) (Sidell, Takafuji, and Franz, 1997, pp. 220–222; U.S. Army 1990; AD Little, 1986, Ch. 3).[6]

Human responses vary with increasing phosgene oxime skin concentrations. There was slight irritation from a 1-percent solution after 24 hours (Wells and MacFarlan, 1938). In one subject, intense itching and a raised red nodule developed, surprisingly, 11 days after such an application. Malatesta et al. (1983) found moderate erythema in four of six volunteers after exposure to a 1.5 percent solution, and three of six exposed to a 2-percent solution developed intense erythema and itching with vesicles a few hours later. All subjects exposed to a 3-percent phosgene oxime solution developed intense erythema and vesicles. A 70-percent liquid exposure produced an intense reaction, with skin damage (McAdams and Joffe, 1955). No information about sustained low-dose exposures, as might have occurred in munitions production, has been found; neither have other reports of delayed reactions.

There is no information about drug and environmental chemical interactions with phosgene oxime. McAdams and Joffe (1955) found that methenamine pretreatment, which was used in U.S. Army munitions plants to protect workers from phosgene, did offer some protection.

Clinical and Pathological Findings

No standard descriptions are available, and symptoms vary depending on the route, form (vapor or liquid), and dose of exposure. In the case of vapor, immediate eye and respiratory irritation are expected, with coughing, throat pain, increased lachrymation, keratitis, and impaired vision (Franke, 1967). Systemic effects, including headache and anxiety, may occur later. Hypersensitivity reactions to mustard agents have been described (Daughters et al., 1973); because phosgene oxime has alkylating properties and is able to bind to proteins, it is theoretically possible that it could serve as a hapten in creating some autoimmunity. There are no definitive laboratory studies of phosgene oxime, although some experimental data are available (Mol and Wolthuis, 1987). The effects of phosgene oxime, especially on the skin, resemble those of strong acids. Its effects are greatest on the first capillary bed encountered, e.g., cutaneous or intravenous exposures cause pulmonary edema, while portal-vein injection causes liver necrosis but spares the lung (McAdams and Joffe, 1955; Sidell, Takafuji, and Franz, 1997, pp. 220–222).

Skin. There is immediate severe itching and pain after exposure to higher concentrations of liquid phosgene oxime, lasting 30 minutes to three hours (Hirsch,

---

[6]CT is measured in milligrams per minute per cubic meter. Appendix A explains CT, LCT, etc., dosages.

1950; Franke, 1967; AD Little, 1986, Ch. 3). A pale translucent area surrounded by erythema may develop at the site of contact, with hives forming in about 10 minutes. As the itching spreads, a rash may also appear in unexposed areas, suggestive of the action of substance P, a mediator that acts locally and on dorsal root ganglia. Pain lasts three to four hours but may recur for several days if the affected area is moistened or irritated. Subsequently, the skin lesion forms an eschar that may be deep, pitted, and slow to heal (Franke, 1967; Malatesta et al., 1983; McAdams and Joffe, 1955; Joffe, et al., 1954; Wende, 1977). Secondary infections are common, and complete healing may take one to two months.

Histologically, phosgene oxime lesions show a through-and-through injury extending into underlying panniculus and muscle with a polymorphonuclear infiltrate at the margins. Congestion and hemorrhage accompany thrombosis in small arteries and veins.

Eye. The eye effects appear similar to those of lewisite, with pain, tearing, conjunctivitis and keratitis. There is no information about the longer-term course of these injuries. Alexandrov, a Soviet scientist, has stated that phosgene oxime can cause blindness at low levels but has not been explicit about quantities and does not provide histological data (AD Little, 1986, Ch. 3).

Respiratory. Death in animals requires high concentrations, even though respiratory irritation occurs at lower levels. Tachypnea, dyspnea, and cyanosis would be expected to occur if pulmonary edema arises. Aerosol exposures produce necrotizing bronchiolitis and pulmonary edema, with pulmonary vein thrombosis (Petersen, 1965). Although phosgene oxime skin lesions are prone to secondary infections, it has not been documented that pulmonary infectious complications are common. Rats exposed to sublethal doses of phosgene were predisposed to increased severity of influenza (Ehrlich and Burleson, 1991).

Long-Term Effects. There are no long-term respiratory injury data, although pulmonary fibrosis could develop, as it does with some alkylating agents, such as bleomycin. Information about long-term eye and skin effects is also lacking. If concern about possible Gulf War exposure increases, the German government may be able to provide information from studies of exposures of World War II munitions workers (Lohs, 1975). It seems possible that phosgene oxime, like mustard, might induce hypersensitivity, perhaps by serving as a hapten linked to proteins encountered. There is one reported case of a delayed skin response to phosgene oxime (Wells and MacFarlan, 1938).

What to Look for in the Gulf Context

Had phosgene oxime exposures from proximate weapon release occurred, there should have been reports of severe eye and respiratory irritation with dermal stinging and itching. The respiratory symptoms would resolve fairly rapidly, but eye and skin problems would last longer. Long-term pulmonary problems from mild exposures are unlikely. Although late effects from symptomatic exposures cannot be ruled out, had pulmonary edema occurred from any Gulf War exposure, it would not have escaped attention. There do not appear to have been any false-positive phosgene oxime reports during the war. Liquid or droplet exposures would have produced painful, slow-healing lesions, which patients and caregivers would recall, although the effects of the mildest exposures might seem nonspecific. Here again, it is not possible to exclude long-term effects entirely. Thus, it might be useful to create a picture of the dermatological problems seen in troops during and after the Gulf War (and not just those for phosgene oxime).

Although there were unverified reports of the use phosgene oxime several times during the Iran-Iraq War (OSAGWI, 1990), no events during the Gulf War raised serious questions about its use. Its presence was suspected in one instance, at a girls' school in Kuwait after the war, but later disproven. The school had been used by Iraqi forces that left a tank of liquid behind. Fumes that came from the tank were investigated and liquid from the tank wet the protective ensemble of a coalition officer, who sustained a prompt and painful burning injury of his skin. This caused phosgene oxime to be suspected. It was later shown that the liquid was some kind of nitric acid, a missile propellant, and the injury was an acid burn (OSAGWI, 1998a).

Summary, Conclusions, and Recommendations

Exposure to phosgene oxime liquid, vapor, or aerosols would be expected to produce immediate eye and respiratory irritation and skin pain. Typical skin burns would require attention and would heal slowly. The literature does not suggest profound central nervous system problems. Phosgene oxime has not been well studied, and its mechanisms of action are not understood. No information about low-level and chronic effects exists, but it is not possible to rule out delayed effects. Phosgene oxime is highly reactive and volatile, so it is unlikely to produce persistent environmental hazards or to survive long-distance environmental transportation from remote release. It is nonpersistent (Franke, 1967). There is no information proving Iraqi phosgene oxime possession, and the experiences recounted in congressional testimony and elsewhere are not consistent with phosgene oxime exposure.

If phosgene oxime continues to be a threat agent, more research will be needed to determine its mechanisms of action and to improve prevention and therapy, particularly if reasons to suspect low-level sustained exposures in Gulf War personnel emerge. Inquiries should then be made about the health and experiences of production workers in countries that have produced military amounts of phosgene oxime.

MUSTARDS

The mustard agents are a family of sulfur-, nitrogen-, and oxygen-based compounds with similar chemical and biological effects (OSRD, 1946; Franke, 1967; U.S. Army, 1990). This review focuses on sulfur mustard (H), or Levinstein mustard, the compound Iraqi forces were most likely to have used, although the more stable distilled mustard (HD) may have been available.

Other potent sulfur-based mustards (Q and T) have been found in small amounts in Iraqi mustard from weapons used in Iran (UN, 1984). These agents have also been placed in U.S. chemical weapons. Agent T is a more potent vesicant than H and is more stable, with a lower freezing point. Agent T has been incorporated into U.S. agent HT (HD+T) and is two to three times as toxic as H. However, it has a lower vapor pressure than H, making it inefficient as a vapor (U.S. Army, 1990; Franke, 1967; Karakchiev, 1973; UN, 1984). Agent Q is a potent vesicant and lung-injuring agent (more so than H) but has a very low vapor pressure, so it is not much of a respiratory threat except in aerosol form.

Nitrogen mustard is poorly soluble in water but highly soluble in organic solvents. This agent (as Mustargen®) is used in cancer chemotherapy for a variety of conditions, including Hodgkin's lymphoma (PDR, 1998).

Mustards produce slow-healing injuries to the eyes, respiratory tract, and the skin. They have potentially lethal systemic effects and produce late long-term effects after substantial exposures (Vedder, 1925; Papirmeister et al., 1991; U.S. Department of Health and Human Services, 1992; Wachtel, 1941; Watson and Griffin, 1992; Smith and Dunn, 1991; Smith et al., 1995, Dacre and Goldman, 1996; Sidell, Takafuji, and Franz, 1997, pp. 198–217).

History

Sulfur mustard (see Table 3.4) was synthesized before World War I and was known to be toxic (Wachtel, 1941). It was effectively used in World War I, first by the Germans and later by the Allies. Mustards had low lethality (1 to 6 percent) but produced incapacitating eye, respiratory, and skin injuries, disabling thousands for short or long periods. Mustards were persistent; hard to detect; and, because of the skin injuries, dangerous even to troops wearing protective masks. Psychologically, they precipitated exhaustion, chronic anxiety, and poor morale (Vedder, 1925). These agents accounted for 10 percent of all man-days lost by U.S. forces in France and for 77 percent of the British chemical casualties (Vedder, 1925; Gilchrist, 1928).

Table 3.4

Chemical and Physical Properties of Sulfur Mustard

Agent	Sulfur mustard
	Hs
	Bis-(2-chloroethyl) sulfide
	Yperite
	Levinstein mustard
	Lost
	Senfgas
Chemical structure	

$$S \Big\langle \begin{array}{l} CH_2CH_2Cl \\ CH_2CH_2Cl \end{array}$$

Molecular weight	159.08
Physical state (20°C)	Oily, colorless (pure) to yellowish dark-brown (munitions-grade) liquid
Vapor density (compared to air)	5.4–5.5 (hovers near ground, settles in depressions)
Liquid density (g/cm^3)	1.262–1.2741 at 20°C
Boiling point (°C, 760 mm Hg)	227.8 (decomposition calculated at 216°C)
Freezing point (°C)	13–14.4
Vapor pressure (mm Hg at 20°C)	0.06–0.11
Volatility (mg/m^3 at 20°C)	610 (liquid); 625
Viscosity (cp at 20°C)	4.59
Surface tension (dynes/cm at 20°C)	42.8
Solubility	Slightly soluble in water (0.7–0.92 g/l at 22°C); miscible in most organic solvents
Decomposition temperature (°C)	149–177
Odor	Almost odorless in pure state at typical field concentrations; horseradish, garlic, or mustardlike odor at higher concentrations

SOURCES: U.S. Army (1990), Vedder (1925), Wachtel (1941), Karakchiev (1973), Franke (1967), Dacre and Goldman (1996).

In World War II, all major combatants produced mustard, and much of what is known of long-term effects comes from studies of World War II munitions workers. Research exposing large numbers of troops was performed (Pechura and Rall, 1993). Although mustards were not operationally used during the war, one large release resulted from a German air attack on Bari, Italy. The 16 ships sunk during the attack included a U.S. freighter carrying 100 tons of mustard. Several thousand mustard casualties occurred, including many deaths. Several ships burned, and some mustard may have been spread by smoke from the oil fires, since casualties occurred in ships offshore (Infield, 1971; Dacre and Goldman, 1996).

Iraqi forces used mustards against Iranian forces beginning in 1984 and continuing through the war (Cordesman and Wagner, 1990; UN, 1984). Some Iranian casualties were cared for in western European medical centers, resulting in many clinical reports (Heyndrickx, 1984). Most Iranian chemical casualties were caused by mustard.

A novel feature of Iraq's use of mustard against Iran included mustard that was adhered to fine (0.1 to 10 µm) silica particles, in a mixture of 65 percent mustard and 35 percent silica. This combination produced more-serious respiratory injuries than other forms of mustard and a different form of skin injury, with symptoms beginning in 15 minutes to one hour (as opposed to four to eight hours). A fine rash with multiple small dots was produced, progressing to vesication with darkened skin and peeling of the epidermis after several days (OSAGWI, undated a). Before the Gulf War, it was uncertain whether U.S. systems would be able to detect dusty mustard or nitrogen mustard and whether such particles could penetrate protective clothing (U.S. Army XVIII Corps, 1998). Coalition forces apparently did not encounter this agent, and it is not mentioned in the UNSCOM reports of 1991, 1992, or 1995. We were unable to locate reports of laboratory studies of the effects of mustard in this form.

Weaponization

Mustard is attractive for military use because

1. Its potency is fairly high (five times that of phosgene).
2. It is able to inflict casualties despite use of respiratory protection.
3. Detection by odor is unreliable, although toxic levels can be noted (Smith, Hurst, et al., 1995)
4. It causes delayed effects, producing no signs or symptoms until irreversible injury is inflicted.
5. It causes prolonged disability.
6. It is stable in storage and persistent in the environment.
7. It is easy and inexpensive to produce.
8. It is difficult to decontaminate.
9. It penetrates many materials.
10. It mixes well with other chemical agents.
11. It can be used in vapor form (denser than air).
12. It can be used in aerosol form, permitting large-area and off-target attacks.
13. It can be used in liquid form, permitting long-term denial of terrain, facilities, and equipment.

Mustard is readily delivered by mortar rounds, artillery, free rockets, aerial bombs, aerosol spray tanks, and liquid spray tanks. Its tendency to freeze with aerial delivery can be reduced by mixing with lewisite or nerve agents or other solvents. In artillery rounds, effective amounts can be delivered using explosive charges equal to ordinary rounds, thus concealing the use of chemicals (OSRD, 1946). Iraq used aircraft and artillery to deliver mustard during its war with Iran.

The press mentioned that Iraq might have intended to contaminate oil-well fires and smoke with chemicals (OSAGWI, 1998; Spektor, 1998). High temperatures destroy mustards, but the Bari experience suggests toxic smokes are possible (Franke, 1967; Wachtel, 1941; Vedder, 1925; OSRD, 1946; SIPRI, 1971; U.S. Army, 1990; Infield, 1971).

Operationally, mustard is usually a defensive agent, creating barriers against attacking forces and complicating their operations by requiring protective systems. After the build-up of coalition forces, the situation favored Iraqi defensive use of mustards (SIPRI, 1971; SIPRI, 1973).

Gulf Relevance

When coalition forces deployed to the Gulf in 1990, there was concern that Iraq might use mustard agents. No large-scale use was encountered, but there were scattered reports of detection alarms, and at least one U.S. soldier developed skin lesions typical of mustard after being in an Iraqi bunker (OSAGWI, 1997d).[7] During the air war, at least two targets containing mustard (and sarin) were hit—both in remote areas west of Baghdad (Muhammadiyat and Al Muthanna). Iraq declared to the UN that 200 mustard-filled and 12 sarin-filled bombs were destroyed at Muhammadiyat. Only 5 percent of Iraqi chemical stores appear to have been destroyed by bombing. CIA calculations of agent dispersal from these attacks indicate that they did not yield significant concentrations of agents in the vicinity of U.S. forces, which were some 400 km away (CIA, 1996). Artillery shells containing mustard were present at Khamisiyah. They apparently escaped destruction by U.S. demolitions (OSAGWI, 1997a).

Low-level exposures might have produced mild and nonspecific responses. However, releases sufficient to have a biological effect on many personnel would lead to some inequality in exposures, such that some typical lesions would be recognized. The extensive human experience with mustards has not produced large numbers of cases with high similarities to illnesses in Gulf War veterans, but some less-well-studied neurobehavioral and skin problems are

---

[7]According to an interview in *Army Times*, this soldier is experiencing long-term health problems; he is quoted as having problems with memory and concentration which began after his return to the United States (Funk, 1997).

discussed later. There is controversy about detector reports that cannot be resolved here.

Detection

Humans can detect the odor of mustard (or associated chemicals), although unreliably. The smell is described as resembling garlic or mustard—differing from the geranium smell associated with lewisite (Sidell, Takafuji, and Franz, 1997, p. 198). Field items that are part of the M256A1 detection kit can colormetrically detect mustards (e.g., M8 paper). The UK's Chemical Agent Monitor (CAM) detects mustard using an ion mobility spectrometer, and the Fox vehicle has a mass spectrometer (note that there are concerns about detection of dusty agent). Other laboratory techniques may be used including gas chromatography and flame photometry.

The detection and monitoring of exposure to mustards and other alkylating agents have been well studied. Gas chromatography and mass spectroscopy can demonstrate the presence of mustard adducts in DNA at the level of 10 picomoles (Ludlum and Austin-Ritchie, 1994). Immunochemical (monoclonal) and mass spectroscopy can now detect sulfur mustard adducts (Noort et al., 1996). Other tissue detection of mustards and alkylating agents is based on adducts with hemoglobin and was used to confirm nonterminal valine adducts of hemoglobin in red blood cells from Iranian casualties (Ehrenberg and Osterman-Golkar, 1980; Hoffman, 1998).

Thiodiglycol, a chemical resulting from sulfur mustard hydrolysis (see next section), can be detected in the urine and indicates exposure. Tests for thiodiglycol have been positive in Iranian casualties and in laboratory accident cases (OSAGWI, 1997d). In the one U.S. Gulf mustard casualty (OSAGWI, 1997d; Sidell, Takafuji, and Franz, 1997), there is uncertainty. One early urine test was reported as positive, but a repeat study at a U.S. laboratory did not confirm. The small size of the injury would make detection difficult (OSAGWI, 1997d).

Discussions with AFIP indicate it has registries of tissue from the Gulf period and material from fatalities in the United States after return. It should be possible to detect evidence of mustard in blood and tissues taken within a few months after suspected exposures.

The structure of nitrogen mustard (Figure 3.1) resembles that of sulfur mustard. There are some other nitrogen-based mustards. The one shown in Figure 3.1 is still used in cancer therapy.

Sulfur mustard, when it hydrolyzes in the water of biological fluids, produces hydrochloric acid and thiodiglycol, the latter of which can be detected in fluids and urine and is relatively nontoxic (Figure 3.2). Chlorination is effective in destroying mustard but the reaction is highly exothermic (Lohs, 1975).

RAND *MR1018_5-3.1*

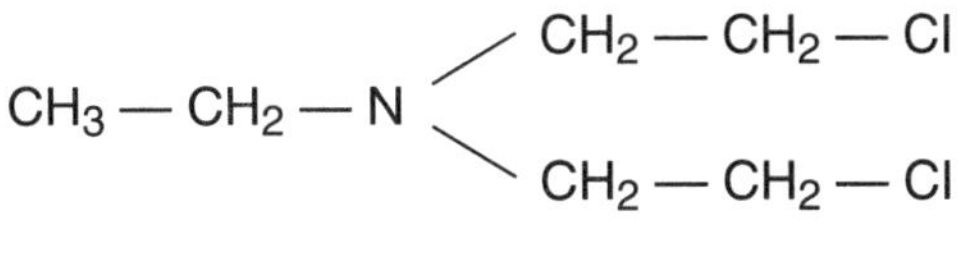

$$CH_3 — CH_2 — N \Big\langle \begin{matrix} CH_2 — CH_2 — Cl \\ CH_2 — CH_2 — Cl \end{matrix}$$

Figure 3.1—Structure of Nitrogen Mustard

RAND *MR1018_5-3.2*

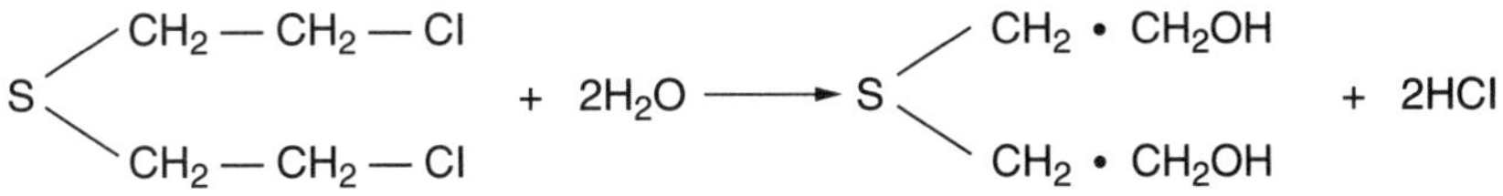

$$S \Big\langle \begin{matrix} CH_2 — CH_2 — Cl \\ CH_2 — CH_2 — Cl \end{matrix} \quad + \quad 2H_2O \quad \longrightarrow \quad S \Big\langle \begin{matrix} CH_2 \cdot CH_2OH \\ CH_2 \cdot CH_2OH \end{matrix} \quad + \quad 2HCl$$

Figure 3.2—Hydrolysis of Sulfur Mustard

Mechanism of Action

There is a large body of literature on the biochemical interactions of mustards, stimulated in part by interest in their application to cancer chemotherapy. Public health considerations arising from demilitarization have focused on lower-level effects and longer-term consequences, in an effort to establish safety standards (U.S. Department of Health and Human Services, 1992).

Although clinical manifestations of mustard injury are slow to appear, the initiating events occur rapidly. It appears that mustard is actively transported across the cell membrane using a system involved in choline transport.[8] Mustards probably are not metabolized in the usual sense by enzymatic degradation. Instead, they form highly reactive chemical species that alkylate macromolecules, most importantly DNA in the cell nucleus. Rapidly dividing cells are most sensitive to these effects, accounting for the similarities between mustard and radiation injuries, with mustards being characterized as radiomimetic agents. Although dividing cells are sensitive, mustards at significant concentrations kill cells whether dividing or not.

Mustards produce several forms of highly reactive compounds. Among these are carbonium ions, which react readily with nucleophilic entities within the cell. The two side chains in mustard favor the insertion of alkyl groups into other molecules (alkylation), which is the most important factor in the biologi-

---

[8]Some resistant cell lines do not transport mustards well (Goldenberg et al., 1970; AD Little, 1986, Ch. 2).

cal effects of these agents (Karakchiev, 1973; Dacre and Goldman, 1996; Papirmeister et al., 1985).

Nucleophilic guanine moieties of the DNA helix permit alkylation and subsequent cross-linking of the strands, impairing the ability of the DNA to divide and be "read" for translation by RNA. Mustard-resistant bacteria have the ability to repair damage by excising the cross links, but mammalian cells cannot do this. Mustards cause cell death through chromatin condensation and energy loss following DNA breakage, loss of cell membrane integrity, or perturbation of cytoskeletal organization (Smith et al., 1995). Induction of programmed cell death, or apoptosis, has also been demonstrated (Hinshaw et al., 1996). The longer-term consequences of DNA alkylation are reflected in mustards' mutagenicity and carcinogenicity (Brookes, 1990).

The stage in the cell cycle at which division occurs (G stage) is the most sensitive for mustard effects, while the S-stage cells seem more resistant. Tissues with high cell turnover (e.g., bone marrow, intestinal epithelial cells, and some skin elements) are especially sensitive to mustards because a higher percentage of cells is dividing (Meyn and Murray, 1984).

The main effects of DNA alkylation and reactions with glutathione set in motion a cascade of effects that includes depletion of cell energy by activation of DNA repair mechanisms (Watson and Griffin, 1992; Papirmeister et al., 1985, 1991). Cell membranes may be directly or secondarily affected by glutathione depletion, with alterations of cytokine activity (Smith et al., 1995; Dannenberg et al., 1985; Gross et al., 1985; Papirmeister et al., 1985). Although not all mechanisms have been established conclusively, Figure 3.3 shows the putative multiple mechanisms for tissue damage from mustards.

The mustards also directly bind to biological materials other than DNA (e.g., cell membranes, proteins). Mustards react with the active portions of enzymes, such as hexokinase, pyruvate oxidase, creatine kinase, ATPase, and acetylcholinesterase (AChE), with subsequent loss of enzyme function (Karakchiev, 1973; OSRD, 1946; Vojvodic et al., 1985; Krustanov, 1962). Dacre and Goldman (1996) summarized several reports of irreversible inhibition of AChE by mustard.

Krustanov (1962) showed that, in rabbits, 10 mg/kg of mustard on the skin lowered serum cholinesterase by 33 percent, an amount similar to 0.4 mg/kg of tabun subcutaneous.

Another alkylating agent, cytoxan, inhibits AChE in clinically significant ways; anesthesiologists must be warned if succinylcholine is planned within ten days of using cytoxan [PDR, 1998].

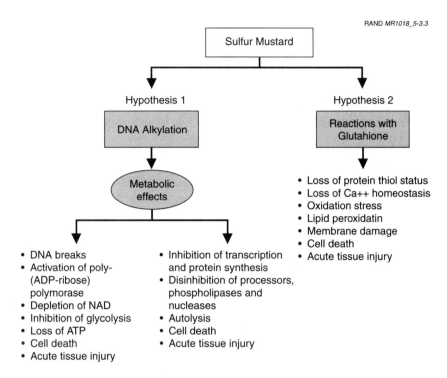

RAND *MR1018_5-3.3*

SOURCE: Reprinted with permission from Sidell, Takafuji, and Franz (1997), p. 202.

Figure 3.3—Sulfur Mustard's Putative Tissue-Damaging Mechanisms

Metabolism and Distribution

Until recently the common view has been that mustards were not metabolized by enzymatic processes, although they did hydrolyze in biological tissues (see below) (Sidell, Takafuji, and Franz, 1997). Their effects accumulated as a result of binding to critical structures.

An enzyme, thioethermethyl transferase (TGMTase), was identified in mice in 1986 and has now been shown via recombinant methods to be present at least in human livers. The enzyme methylates and thereby inactivates the S atom on mustard agents. It may provide some endogenous protection from mustard agents, although quantitative data are not available (Hoffman, 1998).

As noted previously, sulfur mustard hydrolyzes to thiodiglycol and hydrochloric acid. The high reactivity of mustards causes binding to sulfhydryl groups, which serve to detoxify the agents, as in the case of glutathione systems. Studies in a variety of species, including humans, have shown conjugates with glutathione in the urine, reflecting alkylation, rather than enzymatic action. Other products were thiodiglycol, conjugates of thiodiglycol with glutathione, and conjugates of bis-beta-chloroethylsulfone with glutathione or cysteine (Dacre and Goldman 1996).

Radioactively labeled mustard given intravenously to rabbits disappeared rapidly from the circulation, with much of the label appearing in urine and bile within 20 minutes, with a small remainder widely distributed, especially to liver, kidney, and lungs. How much of this represents metabolism by TGMTase, conjugation with glutathione, or hydrolysis is not known. Findings from intravenous administration to cancer patients were similar, with immediate disappearance of 90 percent of the label from blood and only a small amount residing on plasma proteins (Dacre and Goldman, 1996).

Because they are lipophilic, mustards readily penetrate the skin. Liquids or saturated vapor are absorbed at a rate of 1 to 4 $\mu g/cm^2/min$, indicating the importance of the total area of exposure (Papirmeister, 1991; Dacre and Goldman 1996). It takes about 10 minutes for mustard to penetrate the skin, with 12 percent being fixed in the skin and 88 percent disappearing rapidly from the circulation (Dacre and Goldman 1996). No technical studies of dusty mustard on the skin appear to be available. The rapid development of symptoms raises the possibility that the silica particles are capable of penetrating the stratum corneum of the skin, which ordinarily delays the passage of chemicals.

Although mustard exposure appears to have neurological consequences, the detailed distribution to the brain has apparently not been reported thus far. Vojvodic et al. (1985) did not find decreases in AChE in the brains of animals exposed to mustard. Lipophilic materials generally are well distributed to the brain. Scremin et al. (Scremin, Shih, and Corcoran, 1991; Scremin and Jenden, 1996) have noted that regional blood flow to the brain reflects regional brain activity, with the probability that lipophilic agents would be preferentially distributed to neurologically and metabolically active sites in the brain.

This raises the possibility that brain activity at time of exposure might significantly influence distribution of lipophilic agents to the brain, such as mustards and nerve agents.

Effects of Exposure and Exposure Limits

Table 3.5 summarizes the quantitative aspects of the exposure-effects relationships for various regions of exposure (Lethal figures for humans are estimates). In general, there is little information about sustained low levels of exposure. McNamara et al. (1975) report no mortality, but tumor prevalence increased in four animal species exposed to 0.1 mg/m^3 for a year. Dacre and Goldman (1996) give a no-effect exposure level for rats of 0.1 mg/kg, taken orally for 90

Table 3.5

Effects of Exposure to Mustards (H or HD)

Area	Dose[a]	Effect[b]	Time of Effect Onset	Sources
Eyes	<5	None		McNamara et al. (1975)
	12	Irritation, reddening	Hours to days	Karakchiev (1973), Dacre and Goldman (1996)
	30–70; 50–100	Conjunctivitis, tearing, photophobia	4–12 hours	AD Little (1986), Wachtel (1941), McNamara et al. (1975)
	100–200	ICT_{50} (est.), corneal edema, lid edema, corneal ulceration	3–12 hours	U.S. Army (1990), Wachtel (1941), OSRD (1946)
Respiratory	33–70	Irritation of nasal mucosa	12 hours–2 days	Wachtel (1941), OSRD (1946)
	100	Severe effects		NAS (1997)
	150	ICT_{50}, sneezing, lachrymation, nose bleed, sore throat		U.S. Army (1990)
	133–600	Tracheobronchitis, cough, pseudomembrane, fever	4–6 hours	OSRD (1946)
	390–900	Serious lung injury, pulmonary edema, pneumonia	4–6 hours	Wachtel (1941)
	900	Revised LCT_{50}		NAS (1997)
	1,500	LCT_{50}, respiratory failure, delayed death	4–6 hours	U.S. Army (1990)
Skin (vapor)	15–150	Erythema, threshold effect	Hours to days	AD Little (1986)
	25–50	Erythema, threshold effect	Hours to days	NAS (1997)
	75–300	Skin injury	Hours, days	AD Little (1986), OSRD (1946)
	450	Injury with large blisters	Hours	Vedder (1925), OSRD (1946)
	500	Severe effects (<200 hot temp)		NAS (1997)
	600	Sustained vomiting		Wachtel (1941)
	1,000–2,000	Incapacitating skin injury	Hours	U.S. Army (1990)
	5,000	Revised LCT_{50}		NAS (1997)
	10,000	LCT_{50}	3 hours	U.S. Army (1990)

Table 3.5—Continued

Area	Dose[a]	Effect[b]	Time of Effect Onset	Sources
Skin (liquid)	610 mg[c]	ED$_{50}$, severe effects[d]		NAS (1997)
	1,400 mg[c]	LD$_{50}$		SIPRI (1973).
	4,000–7,000 mg[c]	LD$_{50}$		SIPRI (1973), U.S. Army (1990)
	60 mg/cm^2	Lethal dose (est.)		NATO (1983)
Miscellaneous	480	Impaired military efficiency		Wachtel (1941)

[a]CT (in mg·min/m^3) unless specified otherwise.

[b]Vapor or aerosol.

[c]For a 70 kg person.

[d]ED stands for "effective dose."

NOTE: There are considerable variations in the data that the reviewer cannot readily explain. They may reflect differences in experimental design, extrapolations from animal studies, temperature, and individual variations. Eye and respiratory systems have similar sensitivities, but eye effects have shorter latency (Somani, 1992, p. 54).

days. Troops on World War I battlefields endured sustained exposure at times, but the levels are unknown, as is also the case for occupational exposures from that period. The judgment of International Agency for Research on Cancer that mustard is a carcinogen seems well founded on the basis of animal research and human epidemiology studies.

Exposure standards are as follows: For H, HD, and HT, the concentration limit for workers is 0.003 mg-min/m^3 over eight hours (MMWR, 1988). For the general public, the limit established by the Army Surgeon General Working Group (MMWR, 1988) is 0.0001 mg-min/m^3 over 72 hours (Watson and Griffin, 1992).[9] The Environmental Protection Agency–recommended maximum levels of mustard in drinking water are 28 µg/liter for 5-liter daily intake and 9.3 µg/liter for 15-liter daily intake.

Unlike contact with lewisite, phosgene oxime, and riot-control agents, contact with mustards produces no immediate signs or symptoms. The subsections below review the delayed effects by organ. It should be kept in mind throughout the following that there are substantial differences among persons in their responses to mustards. Racial differences in sensitivity to mustards exist; dark-skinned people are more resistant (Vedder, 1925; Haldane, 1925). Other studies show up to a 100-fold difference in sensitivity (Hassett, 1963). Glutathione, which is important in mustard detoxification, has circadian variations in cellular levels and may be depleted by oxidative stress, medications, smoking, and ethanol.

The following excerpt provides a compelling overall picture of clinical mustard injury as observed in World War I mustard casualties:

> On exposure to the vapor or to a finely atomized spray of mustard, nothing is noticed at first except the faint though characteristic smell. After the lapse of several hours, usually four to six, the first symptoms appear. The systemic symptoms are intellectual dullness or stupidity, headache, oppression in the region of the stomach, nausea or vomiting, malaise and great languor and exhaustion. In many cases these symptoms may not be noticed, and the local symptoms first attract attention. The eyes begin to smart and water. There is a feeling of pressure or often of a foreign body, and photophobia, and when examined the conjunctiva is found to be reddened. The nose also runs with thin mucous as from a severe cold in the head, and sneezing is frequent. The throat feels dry and burning, the voice becomes hoarse, and a dry harsh cough develops. Inflammation of the skin now shows itself as a dusky red erythema of the face and neck which look as though they had been sunburned, but are

---

[9]There are considerable variations in the data, which reflect differences in experimental design, extrapolations from animal studies, temperature, and individual differences. Increased ambient temperature and sweating can increase agent effects. Eye and respiratory systems have similar sensitivities, but eye effects generally have less latency (Somani, 1992, p. 54). The reverse cannot explain all the variances.

almost painless. The inner surfaces of the thighs, the genitals, the buttocks, the armpits, and other covered portions of the body are similarly affected. Mustard affects more severely those parts of the body where the skin is tender and well supplied with sweat glands. Itching and burning of the skin may be spontaneous, or first noticed as the result of washing. Even these mild symptoms may be sufficiently irritating to cause sleeplessness. At the end of 24 hours, a typical appearance is presented. The conjunctivitis has steadily increased in intensity, the vessels are deeply injected, and one of the main items of distress is caused by the pain in the eyes which may be very intense. The patient lies virtually blinded, with tears oozing from between bulging edematous eyelids, over his reddened and slightly blistered face, while there is a constant nasal discharge, and continuous harsh, hoarse coughing. Frontal headache is often associated with pain in the eyes and photophobia and blepharospasm is always marked. During the second day the burned areas of the skin generally develop into vesicles, and the scrotum and penis and other badly burned areas become swollen, edematous and painful to the touch. Bronchitis now sets in with abundant expectoration of mucus, in which there may later be found large actual sloughs from the inflamed tracheal lining. The temperature, pulse rate and respiration rate are all increased. (Vedder, 1925.)

These symptoms increase in intensity for several days if the case has been severely burned. On the other hand cases that have been only slightly poisoned may never proceed to the blister stage. Note that more recent literature often overlooks the mental and performance effects.

Eyes. The eyes were involved in some 85 percent of U.S. World War I mustard casualties (Gilchrist, 1928). One would have expected widespread "outbreaks" of conjunctivitis had there been extensive low-level exposures in the Gulf. Inflammation is one of the earliest symptoms of mustard exposure, varying from mild conjunctivitis, with lachrymation resembling that from a foreign body in the eye, and photophobia up to very severe injury. A severe keratitis with clouding and edema of the cornea is common, and there may be corneal ulceration (although this is rare) and superficial erosion. Loss of eye contents is rare (where corneal damage is so severe that it ruptures and vitreous contents leak out) (Vedder, 1925; McNamara et al., 1975). Subconjunctival hemorrhages have been reported in Iranian patients (Momeni and Aminjavaheri, 1994). As mentioned above, these symptoms manifest hours after initial exposure, but symptoms evolved more quickly following subsequent exposures (Otto, 1946). In uncomplicated cases, swelling and photophobia decrease after several days, and corneal clouding clears after several weeks. Blindness rarely results (Vedder, 1925). A delayed keratopathy with corneal erosions has been described 8 to 40 years after World War I acute exposures (Dacre and Goldman, 1996), but this effect appears to have been limited to persons with severe initial injuries involving cornea and conjunctivae (Sidell, Takafuji, and Franz, 1997, pp. 210–211).

Lohs (1975) describes chronic conjunctivitis and other delayed eye effects in World War II munitions plant workers. Dacre and Goldman (1996) reviewed Huntsville Arsenal reports of chronic conjunctivitis in mustard workers, whose symptoms cleared with short absences from work. Workers at Edgewood Arsenal were found to have decreased corneal sensitivity.

Respiratory. Respiratory injuries were the main cause of death in 75 percent of the 6,980 U.S. World War I mustard casualties analyzed (Gilchrist, 1928). Respiratory symptoms are expected for persons not wearing protective masks. Early symptoms (and symptoms from mild exposures that do not progress) include sneezing, nasal and throat irritation, and a loss of taste and smell within 12 hours (Vedder, 1925; Dacre and Goldman, 1996; Wachtel, 1941). The loss of taste and smell might be useful in retrospectively reviewing Gulf-associated medical records for evidence of mustard exposure.

More severe exposures produce laryngitis, aphonia, and incapacitating bronchitis, with severe constant coughing that worsens at night. A secondary pneumonia may occur within 36 to 48 hours. Difficulty swallowing begins on day 2 or 3 and lasts four to six days, and there may be a burning sensation in the pharynx and chest lasting several weeks. There is thick mucus and diphtheric-type pseudomembrane formation in the trachea and bronchi, with dyspnea and hypoxia in severe cases. Fever is common (Vedder, 1925; Wachtel, 1941; Dacre and Goldman, 1996).

Very severe exposures have the most complications, with bronchopneumonia due to *Staphylococcus, Streptococcus,* and *Pseudomonas.* X-rays show cellular infiltration and hypoxia and are consistent with adult respiratory-distress syndrome. Lung abscesses and tuberculosis activation have been reported. Persistent bronchiectasis also occurs (Vedder, 1925; Somani, 1992, pp. 55–57; Pauser et al., 1984; Sohrabpour, 1984; Colardyn and De Bersaques, 1984). Shedding of columnar cells has been seen in experimental animals and humans, along with disorganization of cells and atrophy of the tracheal and bronchial epithelium (Dacre and Goldman, 1996; Calvet et al., 1994).

Exposed munitions workers experienced a number of respiratory problems from their more sustained exposures, including chronic bronchitis, emphysema, and some bronchiectasis, and many were placed on disability (Dacre and Goldman, 1996). The high prevalence of chronic bronchitis and heavy smoking complicated the evaluation of chronic bronchitis, emphysema, asthma, and cancer following World War I exposures (Pechura and Rall, 1993). Epidemiologic studies in the UK and the United States did not find compelling evidence of a role for mustards in chronic pulmonary disease after acute World War I exposures (Dacre and Goldman 1996). Studies of Japanese munitions workers definitely show increased laryngeal and lung cancer among those exposed to mustards (Tokuoka et al., 1986; Yamakido et al., 1996). Late long-term obstructive and restrictive disease is expected from mustards, as when the pulmonary fibrosis complicates the use of other alkylating drugs (Rall and Pechura, 1993). There is some controversy on these matters, especially on the long-term hazards of exposure without sign of acute injury (Rall and Pechura, 1993; Bullman and Kang, 1994).

Skin. Although mustard is classed as a skin-damaging agent, the skin effects are neither the most common nor the most serious, but they can still be formidable. Also, the skin can be an important absorption pathway for the agent to produce system toxicity. Because they are lipophilic, the mustards readily penetrate the skin. Liquid or saturated vapor is absorbed at 1 to 4 $\mu g/cm^2/min$, indicating the importance of the total area exposed in determining toxicity. Labeled mustard penetrates the skin in 10 minutes (with 12 percent fixing in the skin, and 88 percent going into the circulation) (Papirmeister, 1991; Dacre and Goldman, 1996). Mustard vapor is absorbed more readily from the skin and lungs than are mustard aerosols. A concentration of mustard vapor as low as 1 mg/m^3 of air over the course of a day impairs the military efficiency of exposed troops (Wachtel, 1941).

A 10-μg droplet of mustard on the skin is sufficient to cause vesication. Of this, about 80 percent evaporates and about 10 percent enters the circulation, leaving only about 1 μg to produce the vesicle. The amount of mustard in a teaspoon, about 7 g, spread over 25 percent of body surface area is sufficient to cause death (Sidell, Takafuji, and Franz, 1997, p. 201).

Mustard does not produce skin injuries uniformly. The face, scrotum, and anal regions are frequently involved, while the hands are often spared. Figure 3.4 shows the anatomic frequency of involvement for nearly 7,000 World War I U.S. casualties. Data from Iran are similar (Momeni et al., 1992; Momeni and Aminjavaheri, 1994).

Warm, moist skin is more vulnerable to mustard injury, as the high prevalence of scrotal, anal, and axillary injuries indicates, so mustards are a greater threat during warm weather (Gilchrist, 1928). World War II studies in tropical areas showed increased vulnerability and delays in onset of 7 to 12 days (Dacre and Goldman, 1996).

Mild cases (estimated exposure 1 mg/m^3 for perhaps one hour) may show only erythema resembling a sunburn. Many mustard skin lesions result in hyperpigmentation, but that is not commonly mentioned for the mildest cases (Vedder, 1925; Requena et al., 1988; Helm and Weger, 1980). Groin erythema might further suggest possible low-level mustard exposure. There is a report of Stevens-Johnson syndrome with bullae and mucosal lesions following clinical use of nitrogen mustard (Newman et al., 1997).

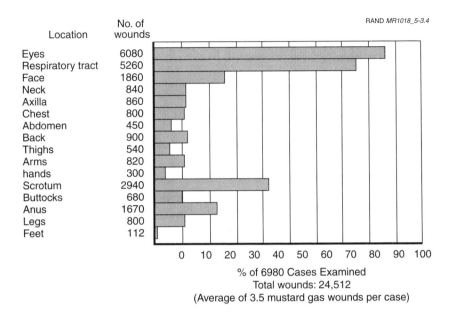

SOURCE: Reprinted with permission from Vedder (1925).

Figure 3.4—Anatomical Distribution of World War I Mustard Injuries

Lesion resolution is prolonged. Papirmeister et al. (1991) give 22 to 29 days, collated from multiple experimental sources; most World War I casualties were hospitalized for 65 days (Smith and Dunn, 1991). These lesions resemble a medical condition called toxic epidermal necrolysis that has a 20-percent mortality rate. Secondary skin infections are problematic. The most severe cases may have marked fluid losses, hypovolemia, renal failure, and difficulty in retaining body heat. Large mustard injuries are associated with systemic illness, catabolism, poor appetite, depression, and secondary infections (Requena et al., 1988; Vedder, 1925).[10]

Resolving lesions are strikingly hyperpigmented (Requena et al., 1988). Intense burning during recovery, which is unresponsive to opioids but responsive to carbamazepine, has been described (Newman-Taylor and Morris, 1991). There is little scarring from these lesions, perhaps since the basal cell layer of the skin is the main location of injury, and there is little deep injury. Histologically, basophils are prominent, and serum enters the lesion carrying mediators and modulators of tissue injury (Dannenberg et al., 1985). Biopsies of human casualties at the erythema stage showed inter- and intracellular edema and

---

[10]Despite more significant systemic injury, mustard cases do not seem to have a higher incidence of mortality than cases of toxic epidermal necrolysis.

nuclear pyknosis, edema of the upper dermis and lymphocyte infiltration of the dermis. Later biopsies of bullous lesions showed perivascular infiltration by neutrophils and lymphocytes, with leukocytic infiltration of the dermis (Momeni et al., 1992).

Momeni et al. (1992) found 92 percent of 525 Iranian mustard casualties had skin lesions; 79 percent had erythema; 55 percent bullae; and 20 percent had pigmentation. Of note were findings of urticaria in 5 percent and purpura in 1.2 percent—conditions that had not previously been described in mustard cases.

Exposed German and Japanese mustard workers have multiple skin tumors (e.g., basal cell carcinoma, Bowen's carcinoma, and squamous cell carcinoma). World War I veterans did not apparently experience an increased prevalence of skin cancer; however, the U.S. Department of Veterans Affairs recognizes skin cancers arising from mustard application in its veterans as service related (Pechura and Rall, 1993).

Nervous System. Nervous system toxicity is evident in animals given high doses of H, especially intravenously, with a resulting cholinergic picture of hypersalivation, hypotension, bradycardia, and marked skeletal muscle weakness that begins superiorly and descends (OSRD, 1946; Krustanov, 1962; Dacre and Goldman, 1996). Atropine has some protective effects in animal models (Vojvodic et al., 1985). Krustanov (1962) showed that sublethal skin doses of mustard in rabbits sharply lower serum cholinesterase. Dacre and Goldman (1996) summarized a fatal human exposure to ingested mustard (suicide) with a similar clinical picture; pathological changes occurred in the brain, spinal cord, sympathetic ganglia, cerebellum, and olivary nuclei.

Neuromuscular. Neurological effects are subtly present at all levels of exposure but are primarily recognized with massive percutaneous or systemic poisoning. Symptoms include nausea, vomiting, nystagmus, reflex disturbances, decreased motor activity, apathy, disturbed consciousness, anxiety, excitement, insomnia, and depression and can proceed to seizures, coma, and death (Rebentisch and Dinkloh 1980; Momeni et al., 1992). Chronically exposed workers have impaired concentration, altered autonomic function, depression, and decreased vitality and libido and are hypersensitive to stimuli (Lohs, 1975).

In light of concern about neurological impairments in Gulf veterans, it is notable that Vedder (1925) repeatedly commented on lethargy and dulled thinking in milder mustard cases; in severe patients, he observed that "the picture is one of a serious disturbance of the central nervous system." Overall, the picture resembles cholinergic overactivity, and mustards can impair AChE, although the significance of this is uncertain. To date, the neurological mechanisms of mustard injury have received little attention. No data emerged from the literature that suggest that subtle neurological effects occur in persons who did not manifest more definite eye, respiratory, or skin injury.

The occurrence of post-traumatic stress disorder (PTSD) in World War II veterans involved in mustard experiments is somewhat surprising (Schnurr et al., 1996). However, in a November 1997 address to the Association of Military Surgeons, Dr. Horvath of the VA reported a very high prevalence of PTSD in veterans so exposed. Cholinergic mechanisms are involved in memory, and it is possible that the agent itself in contributing to this disorder. Although the anticholinesterase-exposed experimental subjects the NAS-NRC Committee on Toxicology (NAS, 1985) followed up on did not have indications of increased mental disorders, the stress of mustard exposures may have been greater, with obvious skin injuries and in some cases very unpleasant scrotal injuries (NAS, 1997). Subjects exposed to other agents have not reported PTSD (NAS, 1985).

Little attention has been paid to the muscle effects of mustards. Humans and animals exposed to high levels develop weakness, seizures, tremors, hypothermia, and increased creatine phosphokinase (Dacre and Goldman, 1996).

Cardiovascular. Intoxicated Bari-disaster patients manifested gradual shock and cardiovascular collapse that was unresponsive to fluid replacement (Infield, 1971; Dacre and Goldman, 1996). Circulatory collapse in some Iranian cases has been reported. Patients with large skin burns have hypovolemia, hemoconcentration, initial bradycardia with later tachycardia, and peripheral edema.

Hematologic and Lymphatic. Hematological effects include, at higher doses, bone-marrow depression, marked leukopenia, thrombocytopenia, and anemia. With milder exposures, white cell counts initially rise and then fall. The systemic effects of mustard include injury of immune cells in the skin and lymphatic system, with impaired resistance to infection and secondary *Staphylococcus*, *Streptococcus*, and *Pseudomonas* infections (Momeni et al., 1992). Casualties have low white counts similar to those of chemotherapy patients (Pauser et al., 1984).

Gastrointestinal. Intoxication is rapid and severe by this route. Mustard ingestion produces nausea, vomiting, abdominal pain, diarrhea, and later gastrointestinal bleeding with intestinal necrosis (Vedder, 1925). During World War I, constipation was a more common problem. The prevalence of gastrointestinal bleeding in Iranian casualties was low (10 percent) (Momeni et al., 1992). Systemic signs and symptoms with nausea and vomiting are common (as they are in radiation injuries), possibly representing an effect on the central nervous system rather than on the gastrointestinal tract, with loss of appetite, weakness, lethargy, and apathy.

Immune System. Mustards are immunogenic, perhaps by acting as haptens with proteins to which they bind. Persons with prior mustard exposure develop signs and symptoms at lower exposure levels than those with initial exposure. Contact sensitization to nitrogen mustards with urticaria and anaphylactic reactions is known (Daughters et al., 1973; Grunnet, 1976; Sanchez-Yus and Suarez, 1977).

Other Organ Systems. Mustards do not appear to have serious direct renal effects, although acute tubular necrosis can follow shock and hypotension. In experimental animals, low levels of mustard produce adrenal hypertrophy (Dacre and Goldman, 1996). Patients with substantial mustard injuries have changes in levels of thyroid hormones, thyroid stimulating hormone, cortisol, and adrenocorticotropic hormone (ACTH) that are similar to those of burn victims, but these patients show a steady fall in cortisol levels despite high ACTH levels (Azizi et al., 1993).

Reproductive and Teratogenic Effects. Mustards inhibit spermatozoa production in animals for about four weeks (Dacre and Goldman, 1996). There do not appear to be similar effects on the ovary. Pregnant rats subjected to low levels of mustard did not show an increase of fetal mortality (McNamara et al., 1975). (See also the Iranian reports discussed in the next subsection.)

Chronic and Late Systemic and Miscellaneous Effects. Mustard workers (Lohs, 1975; Yamakido, 1996; Rall and Pechura, 1993; Dacre and Goldman, 1996) are in poorer health than their peers, with increased depression, chronic bronchitis, nervousness, infection, and autonomic disorders. Skin lesions can recur at sites of prior injury. They appear to have more eye difficulties and a higher prevalence of skin and respiratory tract cancer. It seems well established that mustards are mutagens and carcinogens (Brookes, 1990; U.S. Department of Health and Human Services, 1992).

Late effects from acute exposure have been published, mostly from the Iranian experience, although the analyses sometimes lack detailed rigor. These include:

1. cleft lip and palate (of 79 such defects per 21,000 live births, 30 were associated with mustard exposure) (Taher, 1992)[11]

2. lung and skin problems, decreased libido (Pour-Jafari and Moushtaghi, 1992)

3. change in the ratio of male to female births (Pour-Jafari, 1994)

4. increased congenital malformations (258 in mustard-exposed versus 33 in controls per 1,000) (Pour-Jafari, 1994)[12]

---

[11]Taher did not report on the total number of mothers exposed to mustards.

[12]But the contribution of other nutritional and environmental factors could not be excluded.

5. cough, fatigue and persistent headaches (Deneauve-Lockhart et al., 1992)[13]

6. decreased health perceptions and increased PTSD among U.S. men who had participated in mustard tests (Schnurr et al., 1996).

What to Look for in the Gulf Context

The Iraqis had considerable amounts of mustard, but there is only one probable case of mustard injury among U.S. troops. It is hard to know what to make of later press reports of an interview with that soldier who reported memory and cognitive problems. Such persisting problems were not described after World War I or reported by Iranians. It should be noted that mustards can affect the central nervous system in poorly understood ways. Although mustard effects should be included in considering the cause of the soldier's memory and cognitive problems, it is an anomalous event in the history of mustard exposures, and many other causes also need consideration (e.g., stress response), and there also may be possible medical reasons for memory loss.

Theoretically some mild mustard vapor exposures could be overlooked, because their symptoms—eye irritation, runny nose, sore throat, cough, malaise, and sunburn—like erythema—could be diagnosed as more-common disorders. As for other agents whose lower-dose effects can be misinterpreted, it is hard to visualize a situation in which a low-dose exposure of many persons and of such uniformity could occur that no definite typical clinical signs would develop. The soldier with probable mustard injury was rapidly and effectively identified as a possible mustard case. This review does not provide guidance about a role of mustard in complex interactions with other chemicals and drugs, except for speculative comments about cholinergic effects of mustards enhancing the effects of other cholinergic agents such as cholinesterase inhibitors (e.g., pyridostigmine bromide (PB), organophosphate pesticides, or nerve agents).[14] Other stresses, such as smoking or ethanol, may lower glutathione levels and enhance the effects of mustards.

Summary

Exposure to mustard has not been known to result in symptoms that correspond to those seen in Gulf War veterans. The protracted symptoms of the one

---

[13]This is an isolated report of a 39-year-old French mechanical-shovel operator who exposed some mustard gas cylinders, which apparently were leaking. He developed eye irritation and laryngeal irritation, followed by nausea and dizziness several hours after exposure to the cylinders. The next day, he developed a fever and vesicles on his fingers and trunk. Two months later, he still had the complaints above.

[14]Chapter Five mentions animal research showing increased toxicity from combinations of nerve agents and mustards in Bulgarian research (Krustanov, 1962), while Vojvodic et al. (1985) has shown some protection of mustard-exposed animals by atropine.

probable casualty from mustard are atypical, unexpected, and not understood. Behavioral, cognitive, and performance consequences of low-level mustard exposures have not been comprehensively studied. At high and sustained doses, mustards produce chronic and serious delayed effects, but these effects are not expected from brief, low-level exposures. Mustards are mutagens and carcinogens, but the risk from brief lower exposures is apparently small. It may be possible to test archived tissues from the Gulf War to detect mustard that has interacted with DNA. The tests, although fairly well established, are not yet routine, and consultation with AFIP is advisable if they may seem useful for analyzing hypotheses about illnesses in Gulf War veterans. The loss of taste and smell characteristic of low-level mustard exposure might help differentiate mustard exposures from nonspecific respiratory infections and irritation.

Hypothesis and Analysis

Some mustard effects seem to be cholinergic, perhaps as a result of inhibiting AChE, and might increase the effects of other cholinergic chemicals in the environment, e.g., PB, organophosphate pesticides, or nerve agents. The previously noted wide variation in individual responses to mustards should be kept in mind. Although the finding of impaired memory (in one solder) is unexpected, one cannot totally exclude mustard from contributing to cognitive problems. However, other veterans of the Gulf War with no evident mustard exposure have similar symptoms.

The high prevalence and long persistence of PTSD in World War II veterans exposed in studies (generally small, localized exposures with injuries that were not massive) remains an enigma. The simplest hypothesis is that the tests were extremely stressful (more so than in the experience of the nerve agent volunteers). Some properties of mustards might affect brain function. It has not been determined whether mustards (as is the case for several cholinergic agents) induce the expression of proto-oncogene (transcription factors) c-fos in the brain (Kaufer et al., 1998).

Chapter Four

TOXINS

Toxins are natural poisons that include the most toxic substances known. Toxins are sometimes classified as chemical warfare agents and sometimes as biological warfare agents (SIPRI, 1972; Franke, 1976). Bacteria, fungi, dinoflagellates, algae, plants, and animals (e.g., corals, snails, frogs, arachnids, and snakes) produce toxins (U.S. Army, 1990; SIPRI, 1971; SIPRI, 1973; Raskova, 1971; Gill, 1982). Table 4.1 (SIPRI, 1973) compares the relative toxicity of chemicals and toxins, listed in order of toxic magnitude. As the table shows, sarin, a nerve agent, is set at 1,000 (an arbitrary scale), and many toxins are at the upper ranks of toxicity.

Human use of toxins has been both constructive and destructive. Toxins have been used to develop drugs, such as digitalis and physostigmine; as research probes to "dissect out" mechanisms of biological action (kainic acid, ryanodine); and to treat neurological disorders (botulinum toxin) and cancer (ricin). They also may be used for assassination and in warfare.

Toxins have been used periodically in warfare. The Moors may have used aconitine in warfare in the 14th century. It was perhaps used earlier in India and China. Aconitine was studied in World Wars I and II and tested in bullets (SIPRI, 1971; SIPRI, 1973). During World War II, toxins were produced and reached weapon status in several countries, perhaps with limited use in sabotage and special operations. Table 4.2 compares the lethality of some toxins and chemical agents in mice.

Although most countries signed treaties in the 1970s and 1980s prohibiting the use of biologic and toxin weapons, indications of toxin use were reported in Laos, Cambodia, and Afghanistan and were alleged during the Iran-Iraq War (Seagrave, 1981; Heyndrickx, 1984; House, 1982). Rapid development in the biological sciences has enabled the production of toxins outside their organisms of origin, e.g., placing the genetic information of the toxin in *E. coli* for expression (Gill, 1982).

Table 4.1

Relative Lethalities of Selected Natural and Synthetic Poisons

Relative Lethality[a] (Sarin = 1,000)	Synthetic Poisons[a]	Natural Poisons[b]	
		Name	Source
10^{-4} to 10^{-3}		Botulinum toxin type A, α fraction	Botulinum toxin type A
10^{-3} to 10^{-2}		Botulinum toxin type A, crystalline	*Clostridium botulinum* bacteria
		Tetanus toxin, crystalline	*Clostridium tetani* bacteria
10^{-2} to 10^{-1}		Botulinum toxin type A, amorphous	*Clostridium botulinum* bacteria
10^{-1} to 10		Palytoxin	*Palythoa* zoanthid coelenterates
1 to 10			
10 to 10^2	Homocholine Tammelin-ester (3-trimethylammoniopropyl methylphosphonofluoridate iodide)	Ricin, crystalline	Castor beans, the seeds of *Ricinis communis*
	Dioxin (2,3,7,8-tetrachlorodibene-*p*-dioxin)	C-alkaloid E	Calabash-curare arrow poison
	35 SN⁺ (O-ethyl S-2-trimethylammonioethyl methylphosphonothiolate iodide)	Saxitoxin	*Gonyaulax catanella* dinoflagellate marine algae
		Tetrodotoxin	Puffer fishes and certain salamanders
		Atelopidtoxin	*Atelopus zeteki*, a Panamanian arrow-poison frog
		Abrin, crystalline	Jequirity beans, the seeds of *Abrus precatorius*
		Indian cobra neurotoxin	Indian cobra venom
10^2 to 10^3	Ethylthioethyl-metasystox (OO-dimethyl S-2-(S'-ethylthioethylsulphonio)ethyl phosphorothiolate bromide)	Ricin, amorphous	Castor beans, the seeds of *Ricinis communis*
	Seleno VE (O-ethyl Se-2-diethylaminoethyl ethylphosphonoselenolate)	Kokór arrow poison	*Phyllobates aurotaenia*, a Colombian frog
	HC 3 (4,4'-*bis*(NN-dimethyl-N-2-hydroxyethylammonioacetyl)biphenyl dibromide)		

Table 4.1—Continued

Relative Lethality[a] (Sarin = 1,000)	Synthetic Poisons[a]	Natural Poisons[b] Name	Source
	VX (O-ethyl S-2 diisopropylaminoethyl methylphosphor o-thiolate)	Russell's viper venom	*Vipera russelli*
	Ro 3-0422 (3-(diethylphosphoryl)-1-methylquinolinium methosulphate)		
	TL 1236 (2-methyl-5-trimethylammoniophenyl N-methylcarbamate chloride)	Israeli scorpion venom	*Leiurus quinquestriatus*
	Gd-42 (O-ethyl S-2-(S'S'-methylethylsulphonio)ethyl methylphosphonothiolate methosulphate)		
	DCMQ (5-NN-dimethylcarbamoyl-1-methylquinolinium bromide)	α-Aminitin	*Amanita phalloides*, the death cap mushroom
	Phospholine (OO-diethyl S-2-trimethylammonioethyl phosphorothiolate iodide)		
	3152 CT (1-(3'-trimethylammoniophenoxy)-3-(-(3'-trimetriy-lammoniophenoxy-5'-NN-dimethylcarbamoyl)propane diiodide)	Indian cobra venom	*Naja naja*
	Soman (1,2,2-trimethylpropyl methylphosphonofluoridate)	Brown widow spider venom	*Latrodectus geometricus*
1,000	**Sarin (isopropyl methylphosphonofluoridate)**	d-Tubocurarine	Tube-curare arrow poison
10^3 to 10^4	Tabun (ethyl NN-dimethylphosphoroamidocyanidate)	Aconitine	Roots of monkshood, *Aconitum napellus*
	Armin (O-ethyl O-4-nitrophenyl ethylphosphonate)	Physostigmine	Calabar bean, the seeds of *Physostigma venenosum*

Table 4.1—Continued

Relative Lethality[a] (Sarin = 1,000)	Synthetic Poisons[a]	Natural Poisons[b]	
		Name	Source
	Gd-7 (O-ethyl S-2-ethylthioethyl methylphosphonothiolate)	North American scorpion venom	*Centruroides sculpturatus*
	Methyl fluoroacetate	Strychnine	*Stryhnos nuxvomica* bark or seeds
		Black widow spider venom	*Latrodectus mactans mactans*
		Ouabain	*Strophanthus gratus* seeds
10^4 to 10^5	Hydrogen cyanide	Nicotine	*Nicotiana* tobacco plants
	Cadmium oxide	Western diamondback rattlesnake venom	*Crotalus atrox*
	Mustard gas (*bis*(2-chloroethyl) sulphide)		
	Parathion (OO-diethyl O-4 nitrophenyl phosphorothionate)		
	Lewisite (2-chlorovinyldichloroarsine)		
	Phosgene oxime		
	Arsine		
10^5 to 10^6	Cyanogen chloride	Bee venom	The honey bee *Apis mellifera*
	Chlorine		
	White arsenic		

SOURCE: SIPRI (1973).

[a]The "relative lethality" was determined as follows: Reported LD_{50} figures for the following combinations of route of administration and experimental animal were assembled from the cited literature: intravenous, mouse; subcutaneous, mouse; intravenous, rat; subcutaneous, rat; intravenous, guinea pig; intravenous, cat; intravenous, rabbit. Within each set, each agent's LD_{50} was converted into a lethality index relative to sarin, assigning a reference value of 1,000 to the sarin LD_{50} concerned. For example, the subcutaneous, mouse index for batrachotoxin is taken as 10 because its subcutaneous, mouse LD_{50} and that of sarin were around 0.002 and 0.2 mg/kg, respectively. In this table, the agents are ranked according to their lowest lethality index. When the animal parenteral LD_{50} was unavailable, the respiratory LCT_{50} was used instead, except for white arsenic, for which an oral LD_{50} was used. The respiratory LD_{50} of sarin in man is estimated to be about 1,000 µg.

[b]The venoms of *Vipera russelli*, *Leiurus quinquestriatus*, and *Latrodectus geometricus* appear to be, respectively, the most poisonous snake, scorpion, and spider venoms known.

Table 4.2

Comparative Lethality of Some Toxins and
Chemical Agents in Mice

Agent	LD$_{50}$ (μg/kg)[a]	Molecular Weight	Source
Botulinum toxin	0.001	150,000	Bacterium
Ricin	3	64,000	Plant
VX	15	267	Chemical agent
Soman	64	182	Chemical agent
Sarin	100	140	Chemical agent
Aconitine	100	647	Plant
T-2 toxin	1,210	466	Fungal toxin
Aflatoxin[b]			

SOURCE: Sidell, Takafuji, and Franz (1997), p. 609.

[a]Interperitoneal or intravenous.

[b]Franz did not report aflatoxin. The reviewer did not locate mouse toxicity data for this toxin.

Toxins have also been associated with public health and agricultural problems, primarily contamination of food (botulinum, mycotoxins), and, more recently, health problems arising from airborne contamination (Steyn, 1995; Coulombe, 1993; Hendry and Cole, 1993; DiPaolo et al., 1994; Ueno, 1983; Wang, Hatch, et al., 1996).

The diverse toxins available for military use span a wide range of effects, from immediate lethality to delayed illness and incapacity. Some toxins are highly stable, making them suitable for long-term storage in weapons and as persisting environmental hazards. They offer high potency, and many can be produced with modest technology investments. Toxins can be used as "strategic" weapons, as indicated in a 1970 World Health Organization (WHO) study, which indicated enormous casualties in urban settings from toxin use and chemicals (WHO, 1970).

Toxins are also quite suitable for tactical employment (U.S. Army, 1990). They may be distributed as aerosols, liquids, or powders, with attacks capable of covering tens to hundreds of square kilometers, and can be delivered by air- or ground-bursting munitions, aircraft spray tanks, or ground-based aerosol generators (U.S. Army, 1990). There are no volatile toxins (Sidell, Takafuji, and Franz, 1997, p. 609). According to Zilinskas (1997), an American arms control specialist who worked with UNSCOM inspecting Iraqi chemical and biological facilities, Iraq possessed the relevant systems and made a great effort to weaponize toxins.

Although the eye and respiratory systems are thought to be the primary routes of toxin exposure, skin and gastrointestinal exposures are also possible (Adams, 1989). Thus, sabotage might concentrate on food, water, and ventilation systems. Toxins have also been used in bullets and in other projectiles (SIPRI, 1973). Some toxins are capable of sustained surface contamination and may also represent a secondary aerosol hazard as soil is disturbed (Adams, 1989).

In general, toxin attacks are difficult to recognize. Most toxins are odorless, and their aerosols are not visible. Their potency and diversity have, to date, precluded the deployment of specific detector systems, although there are military systems that can detect aerosol clouds. Technology, such as microencapsulation, has the potential of altering delivery systems to permit skin intoxications, tailoring particle sizes, and making agents more resistant to environmental degradation (U.S. Army, 1990). Because the body has a limited number of ways to respond to chemicals and toxins, clinical recognition and diagnosis may not readily distinguish among different agents. It is not easy to demonstrate toxins in biological tissues or the environment, which may account for some of the controversy about their suspected use (Heyndrickx, 1984; Watson, Mirocha, and Hayes, 1984).

The defensive preparations coalition forces made (IOM, 1996; DSB, 1994) anticipated Iraq's postwar admission that it had developed and deployed biological weapons, including toxins, prior to the Gulf War (Marshall, 1997; PAC, 1996b; Zilinskas, 1997). The Iraqis had deployed botulinum toxin, the most toxic material known, in weapons, and Heyndrickx (1984) suspected that they also possessed and used trichothecene mycotoxins. Ricin had been the subject of advanced military research and development since World War I, and considerable unclassified public information about the development of weapons with ricin was available after World War II (OSRD, 1946; SIPRI, 1973, WHO, 1970). Thus, its properties were well known to the Iraqis. In addition, castor beans, ricin's basic source, are inexpensive and readily available.

Recent reports that aflatoxins (of which aflatoxin B_1 [AFB_1] is a hepatoxic material and suspected carcinogen) were produced and deployed in Scud warheads were surprising because this family of toxins had not generally been considered to be militarily useful (Marshall, 1997; Zilinskas, 1997; U.S. Army, 1990; SIPRI 1971).

Since the Gulf War, the occurrence of delayed and poorly understood illnesses in Gulf War veterans has raised the question of whether unrecognized toxin exposure may have played a role in such illnesses, either from clandestine use or from "fallout" from coalition attacks on Iraqi biological facilities (Riegle and D'Amato, 1994; GAO, 1997). Three toxins are reviewed in detail below: ricin (a plant toxin) and the trichothecenes and aflatoxins (two families of mycotoxins).[1]

_____

[1]As noted earlier, anthrax and botulinum toxin are covered in Hilborne and Golomb (2000).

RICIN

Ricin, also known as Agent W, is the toxic protein derived from the castor bean plant. Ricin's properties have been known since ancient times, and it has a long history of accidental and intentional intoxication (Klain and Jaeger, 1990). Ricin was studied as a possible weapon in World War I, and the United States, Canada, and the United Kingdom developed it as a weapon during World War II (OSRD, 1946). Recent scientific interest in ricin stems from its possible use in cancer therapy, as a probe to study protein metabolism, and as a selective tool in neurophysiology research (Wellner, Hewetson, and Poli, 1995; de la Cruz et al., 1995). Ricin achieved some notoriety when it was used in a sophisticated pellet to kill the Bulgarian political dissident Georgi Markov in London and to injure another dissident in Paris (Klain and Jaeger, 1990). There is little information about the long-term consequences of ricin exposure, but its patterns of acute toxicity have been characterized (OSRD, 1946), as described below.

Weaponization

Ricin is easily extracted from the cultivated plant *Ricinus communis.* The World War II effort led to refined ricin in a crystalline form, although it was the amorphous form that was used in high-explosive bombs and shells and in more specialized delivery systems, such as plastic containers and cluster bombs. Attaining effective particle sizes with ricin powder is difficult, and use of the material in water or suspended in glycerol or carbon tetrachloride is more effective (OSRD, 1946; Franke, 1976). Because, as a protein, ricin degrades in the environment, it can also serve as a research surrogate for other agents of biological origin (OSRD, 1946; SIPRI, 1973).[2] World War II studies, conducted on unpurified material, found ricin to be 7 to 40 times as toxic as phosgene, and postwar comparisons found it to be comparable in toxicity to the nerve agents (Franke, 1976; OSRD, 1946; WHO, 1970).

The agent is difficult to detect. It is fairly stable in clear, dry weather, persisting in the soil or environment for up to three days. (U.S. Army, 1990; Sanches et al., 1993).[3]

Evidence from the Gulf War indicated that Iraq had previously developed and tested weapons containing ricin (Zilinskas, 1997). The reported delivery system—artillery shells with bursters—was not very sophisticated, compared to

---

[2]OSRD (1946) says that "Ricin was recognized as a prototype of toxic protein materials of bacterial origin which were known to have even greater toxicity but which were less conveniently prepared and handled." (The reviewer assumes that the microbial toxin was botulinum toxin.)

[3]This favorable weather may not have always occurred during the air and ground war period of the Gulf War.

World War II U.S. delivery systems (OSRD, 1946). There was no evidence that ricin was actually used in the Iran-Iraq conflict or in the Gulf War.

Detection

No military detectors have been deployed for ricin to date. During World War II, guinea pigs hypersensitized to ricin, so that they would develop anaphylaxis, were used to detect aerosols and assess persistence (OSRD, 1946). Efforts were made at that time to use hemaglutination to detect microgram amounts, but results were nonspecific. An anti-ricin precipitation reaction was also used.

More recently, competitive radioimmunoassays have been used in a chemotherapy project to detect ricin in the 50 to 100 pg/ml range. Several enzyme-linked immunoadsorbent assay (ELISA) systems are able to detect ricin in tissues, and immunocytochemical tests exist but are not highly sensitive (Wellner, Hewetson, and Poli, 1995). It appears possible, based on animal studies, to detect ricin aerosol exposures using ELISA techniques on material from oro-nasal swabs up to 24 hours after exposure (Franz and Jaax, 1997).

Regardless of the mechanism used, ricin cannot be detected long after it is used, because, as a protein, it degrades in the environment. Persistence for up to three days in dry weather was found in World War II studies (OSRD, 1946).

Physical and Chemical Characteristics

Ricin in dry form, depending on its purity, is either an amorphous solid or crystalline material. It is soluble in water and weak acid and forms stable suspensions in glycerol or carbon tetrachloride. It has no odor (OSRD, 1946; U.S. Army, 1990).

Ricin is a protein composed of two globular polypeptide chains linked by a disulfide bridge, with the enzymatically active A chain folding into a cleft in the globular B chain, which is responsible for adhesion to and transportation into the cell. The molecular weight is about 64,000. Chemicals that break the disulfide bond inactivate the toxin (Sanches et al., 1993).

Toxicology and Toxicokinetics

A great deal is known about the cellular and molecular mechanisms by which ricin interrupts protein synthesis within the cell. Basically, ricin inhibits protein synthesis by inactivating ribosomal RNA (Wellner, Hewetson, and Poli, 1995). Ricin's A subunit possesses the enzymatic biological activity, while the B unit is involved in binding the toxin to the cell surface receptors (galactose) and subsequent transport into the cell. After entry, the A unit in the cytosol inhibits protein synthesis by inactivating ribosomal RNA. The detailed mechanisms of binding, transport, and RNA inhibition have been studied in great detail (Sandvig and Van Deurs, 1996; Simpson et al., 1996; Morino et al., 1995; Li, Frankel, and Ramakrishnan, 1992). Inhibition of protein synthesis in eukaryotes is caused by ricin's cleaving of an adenosine ribose bond in messenger RNA (Wellner, Hewetson, and Poli, 1995).

A single molecule in a cell can cause that cell to die. Ricin intoxication may induce "programmed cell death" (apoptosis), as noted in cultured pulmonary endothelial cells and in lymphatic tissues of poisoned rats (Leek et al., 1990; Hughes and Lindsay, 1996).

What remains unclear is how ricin causes injury and death in complex organisms (Wellner, Hewetson, and Poli, 1995; Klain and Jaeger, 1990). However, because mice can be protected from an intravenous ricin challenge by intracerebral anti-ricin antibodies, and because alterations of blood-brain barrier permeability increase ricin toxicity, the "lethal" target tissue is probably the central nervous system (Foxwell et al., 1985). This is not certain because studies of distribution in tissue seldom mention the brain, and it may be difficult to find ricin there anyway because a mouse can be killed by administration of only a picomole.

Exposure-Effect Relationships. The sensitivity of various animal species to ricin varies over a hundredfold range (Franz and Jaax, 1997). Toxicity and time of death vary considerably depending on the route of exposure, as exemplified by studies in mice: The inhalation LD_{50} is 3 to 5 μg/kg (absorbed dose), with death at 60 hours; the subcutaneous LD_{50} is 24 μg/kg, with death at 100 hours; and the oral LD_{50} is 20 mg/kg, with death at 85 hours (Franz and Jaax, 1997, p. 633).

Ricin can produce severe to fatal injury by contact with eyes or by ingestion, inhalation, or parenteral routes. Little has been reported, however, regarding dermal toxicity or chronic effects. According to the OSRD, dermal toxicity was not an issue for the U.S. researchers and production workers during World War II. Although ricin poisoning is noted for delayed onset of symptoms, larger doses produce a more rapid onset (OSRD, 1946; Balint, 1993).

Table 4.3 summarizes some selected exposure-effect data by route of exposure. No chronic exposure data are available, although ricin is immunogenic. Some World War II workers probably experienced brief allergic respiratory reactions (OSRD, 1946). The rapid development of immunity apparently protected World War II workers from major toxicity, in the same way that immunity thwarts chemotherapy with ricin. It has been shown in animals that when the immune system is impaired by T-cell depletion and ricin is repeatedly administered at sublethal levels (50 ng weekly for five weeks), deaths occur in 35 to 46 days. This indicates that an irreversible injury has occurred, perhaps to the heart or

Table 4.3

Exposure Effects of Ricin

	Dose	Species	Effect	Reference
Ocular	0.5 µg (particle)	Rabbit	Conjunctivitis for one week	OSRD (1946), p. 189
	1.5 mg (particle)	Rabbit	Serious eye injury	OSRD (1946), p. 189
Respiratory LCT_{50}	24 mg-min/m^3	Dog	Lethal pneumonia	OSRD (1946), p 188
	100 mg-min/m^3	Monkey	Lethal pneumonia	OSRD (1946) p. 188; Franz and Jaax (1997)
	30–70 mg-min/m^3 (est.)	Human	Lethal pneumonia	Franke (1976), OSRD (1946)
Pareneral	0.5–0.75 µg/kg	Human	Mild illness	Fodstad et al. (1984)
	0.1–0.3 µg/kg (est.)	Mouse, injected	LD_{50}	U.S. Army, (1990), pp. 73, 83, and 105; Gill (1982), p. 83
	30.27 µg/kg	Monkey	LD_{50}	Balint (1993)

brain, and demonstrates that cumulative toxicity can occur (Foxwell et al., 1985).[4]

The acute clinical picture varies by route of exposure. The most well-documented human experience with ricin concerns the ingestion of castor beans (Klain and Jaeger, 1990, reviewed 314 cases). There are fewer data on human exposures via other routes. Mild systemic illness (i.e., delayed onset of a "flulike" syndrome, with malaise, fatigue, muscle pain, and some nausea and vomiting) occurred in humans receiving 0.5 to 0.75 µg/kg of ricin intravenously as part of Phase I cancer chemotherapy trials. Onset of symptoms was in four to six hours and lasted two to four days. Muscle cramps, fatigue, and weakness were prominent problems (summarized by Wellner, Hewetson, and Poli, 1995; Fodstad et al., 1984). Similar systemic signs and symptoms occurred in World War II workers with mild exposures (OSRD, 1946; see "Respiratory System," below). Laboratory findings are nonspecific.

The fever ricin produces in mammals is consistent, predictable, and dose-related. Linear dose-response curves for several species have been developed (Balint, 1993). The suspected cause of the fever is release of endogenous (leukocyte) pyrogens.

---

[4]This raises the possibility of cumulative toxicity from sustained low-level exposures in immune-compromised humans. The U.S. personnel in the Gulf region are presumed to have been immuno-competent.

No data exist regarding mutagenic and teratogenic effects of ricin (Klain and Jaeger, 1990). However, in one case, a pregnant woman was poisoned with ricin, which suggested teratogenic effects.

Two cases of injection in humans are worth mentioning in some detail. In the first, severe headache and fever followed an intentional intramuscular injection of a castor bean extract (approximately 150 mg of ricin [2 mg/kg]) (Fine et al., 1992). After ten hours, the patient's pulse and blood pressure were elevated; he had a white count of 18,000/mm^3 (above normal) and a low sedimentation rate. Serum amylase and transaminases were slightly elevated, and bilirubin was also high, but creatine kinase was not, suggesting liver injury as the source of the enzyme elevation. The patient remained febrile for eight days without renal problems and was discharged home asymptomatic on day 10. The patient initially received supportive therapy with intravenous fluids and antibiotics.

The second case is the well-known 1978 murder of Georgi Markov by ricin (Klain and Jaeger, 1990). The toxin was contained in a pellet shot into the victim's thigh with an umbrella. At the time of the encounter, the patient noted only a stinging sensation. Later studies indicated the pellet contained 500 µg of ricin. After five hours, Markov complained of weakness. The next day, he developed fever and vomiting and had trouble speaking. When admitted to the hospital, he was hot and ill, with a fast, regular pulse. Lymph glands in his groin were swollen. The patient and staff had no idea he had been attacked. Markov's white blood cell count was 10,600/mm^3 (normal). On the third day, his blood pressure fell; his pulse rose to 160/min; and he was cold, sweaty, and dizzy. The white blood cell count rose to 26,300/mm^3 (quite elevated, with granulocytes predominating) and he was given plasma expanders. The following day, he became anuric, and acute tubular necrosis was suspected. Vomiting with hematemesis worsened. His white blood cell count rose to 32,200/mm^3, and he developed heart block, became confused, and died. Only at autopsy was the pellet discovered. Other autopsy findings included pulmonary edema, liver fatty change, and hemorrhage in the intestine (with necrosis) and in the lymph nodes, adrenals, pancreas, and heart. Another patient recovered from a similar attack after hospitalization for 12 days, the pellet in this case having released less toxin (Franz and Jaax, 1997; Klain and Jaeger, 1990).

Eye. No reports of human eye exposures or injuries were found (neither have eye signs been noted in systemic exposures) (Franz and Jaax, 1997; Klain and Jaeger, 1990). Animal studies report conjunctivitis lasting one week after ocular introduction of 0.5 µg of ricin and corneal lesions with keratitis lasting 11 days after exposure to 1.5 µg (OSRD, 1946). Ricin is potent enough to produce lethal illness via the eye (OSRD, 1946). Presumably, any systemic illness resulting from eye exposure would be associated with very intense conjunctivitis and corneal injury, including erythema, exudate, and corneal clouding.

Respiratory System. World War II animal studies indicated that the amounts of ricin for lethality were roughly the same for systemic or respiratory exposures (OSRD, 1946). Respiratory exposures produce effects confined to the respiratory tract, with modest systemic toxicity and lethality explicable by pulmonary failure (Franz and Jaax, 1997; Wilhelmson and Pitt, 1996). After exposing mice to aerosolized ricin, Doebler et al. (1995) found significant concentrations in the lungs and gastrointestinal tract, with only low tissue levels elsewhere; however, concentrations in the central nervous system were not assessed. No reports of serious human respiratory exposures were found. However, animals and humans exposed via other routes have experienced pulmonary congestion and edema. Only animal data exist concerning the pathology resulting from respiratory exposure. Studies in the UK and the United States have indicated that lesions were confined to the lungs, with intra-alveolar edema, acute alveolitis, and diffuse necrosis of epithelial linings (Griffiths et al., 1994; OSRD, 1946). Sublethal exposure in rats (a CT of 16.5 mg-min/m^3) sacrificed at 30 hours showed increased pulmonary water and albumin. Bronchoalveolar lavage showed leukocytosis, and there was a mild inflammatory response with minimal alveolar damage (Kokes et al., 1994). Rhesus monkeys exposed to lethal ricin aerosols in doses ranging from 21 to 42 µg/kg developed respiratory distress at 36 to 48 hours (Wilhelmsen and Pitt, 1996).[5] Pulmonary findings ranged from limited focal lesions to coalescing fibrinopurulent pneumonia, diffuse airway inflammation and necrosis, diffuse alveolar flooding, and peribronchial edema. All monkeys had purulent tracheitis, fibrinopurulent pleuritis, and purulent mediastinal lymphadenitis. There was no systemic lymphadenopathy. No bacterial role was identified. All monkeys died or were sacrificed. Activation and infiltration by leukocytes may play a role in the injury resulting from inhaled ricin (Assad et al., 1996).

World War II workers manifested two different clinical syndromes from presumptive low-level respiratory exposures (OSRD, 1946). First, among laboratory workers, the reaction resembled that of people hypersensitized to a foreign protein, with rapid onset of sneezing, coughing, and symptoms reminiscent of severe asthma. The reactions lasted less than one hour and were probably due to workers' becoming sensitized to ricin during work. One would not expect this syndrome in the Gulf War setting because prior ricin exposure was unlikely. The second syndrome arose in persons who inhaled low doses of ricin. Four to eight hours after exposure, there were fever, coughing, dyspnea, chest tightness, inflammation and burning of the trachea, aching joints, and nausea. Several hours later, profuse sweating occurred, usually coinciding with symptom

---

[5]The animals were exposed to 1.2 µm particles in an aerosol of 128–353 mg-min/m^3 (10 min) with absorbed dose calculated from respiratory parameters and impinger measurements.

abatement (OSRD, 1946). No follow-up or sustained observations were reported.

Gastrointestinal System. Ricin is less potent when delivered orally, although this route has produced the greatest human experience with the toxin (Franz and Jaax, 1997; Klain and Jaeger, 1990). Ishiguro et al. (1992) has shown that, in rats, active ricin is absorbed from the small bowel by blood and lymphatics, with the highest subsequent concentrations in the liver and spleen. Human oral exposures chiefly follow ingestion of castor beans (Klain and Jaeger, 1990). Symptom onset is often delayed but can range from hours to several days. The illness spectrum ranges from mild cases of weakness and prostration to, more commonly, nausea, vomiting, diarrhea, abdominal pain, and bleeding. Severe dehydration may occur, as can other constitutional symptoms, including fever, tachycardia, muscle cramps, dyspnea, lethargy, and confusion. In fatal cases, sudden collapse with hypotension and seizures can occur. Renal failure and evidence of hepatotoxicity are variable. The main findings are usually gastrointestinal (OSRD, 1946; Wellner, Hewetson, and Poli, 1995; Klain and Jaeger, 1990).

Autopsy studies of lethal castor bean poisonings show erosions and ulceration of stomach and small bowel with hemorrhagic inflammation of the stomach (Klain and Jaeger, 1990). Remote hemorrhage and necrosis of lymphatic tissues are common, but renal congestion and cerebral edema vary.

Exposure via other routes also produces gastrointestinal injury, especially in the liver, although histologic findings vary. Markov's autopsy findings include gastrointestinal necrosis and hemorrhage, with hepatic fatty change (Klain and Jaeger, 1990).

Dermal. Ricin does not have impressive dermal toxicity. It was not a clinical occupational-medicine problem with laboratory or production workers during U.S. World War II (OSRD, 1946), and animal research of that period did not report dermal toxicity. OSRD reports mentioned British observations that injection of ricin intradermally produced local inflammation and systemic effects similar to those of mild respiratory exposures (described above). It is unlikely that ricin in the Gulf operational environment could have produced dermal injury, and it would not explain later dermatological problems in Gulf veterans, based on World War II reports.

Nervous System. A prominent nonfocal neurological finding in serious ricin intoxications is the seizures noted in humans and animals (Klain and Jaeger, 1990; OSRD, 1946). Originally, hypoglycemia was suspected as the cause, but detailed studies indicate otherwise. The mechanism by which ricin induces seizures remains unknown, although experimental evidence exists for a central-nervous-system mechanism for ricin toxicity (Foxwell et al., 1985). Further, personal communication from USAMRIID indicates that, in mice, rats and sub-human primates exposed to 5 to 10 LD_{50} of aerosolized ricin, no toxin-related lesions were seen in the brain or other nervous tissue. This conforms to some of the institute's published data, which show main pathologic findings from inhaled ricin are confined to the lungs.

Concerns about neuropathy following the Gulf War (Haley, Horn, et al., 1997—none of whose group had seizures) led to a special effort to find information about ricin's distribution to the brain and nervous system. Neurological disease, including neuropathy, has not been documented as a consequence of ricin exposure. However, it is known that, if introduced into the nervous system, ricin is extremely toxic and that axons can transport ricin into nerve cell bodies (De la Cruz et al., 1995). There is also some evidence from studies of rats that ricin can alter the "blood-nerve barrier" (Bouldin et al., 1990).

Intracerebral injection of ricin in young rats produces hydrocephalus. Periventricular cortical necrosis occurs, with typical features of neuronal degeneration, such as displaced nuclei and mitochondrial swelling and disintegration (Kaur and Ling, 1993). Brain hemorrhage and cerebral edema have been reported in human ricin poisoning cases (Klain and Jaeger, 1990).

Musculoskeletal. Clinically, muscle cramps and weakness are a common, early finding in ricin toxicity by all routes (OSRD, 1946; Klain and Jaeger, 1990; Fodstad et al., 1984). Some studies (e.g., Doebler et al., 1995) indicate substantial distribution of ricin to muscle tissue after parenteral administration, but the work of Fodstad et al. (1984) showed little distribution to muscle and suggested that some secondary mechanism was involved. There appear to be no reports demonstrating musculoskeletal pathology.

Other. Clinical evidence of cardiac injury with ricin includes reported cases of heart block, prolonged Q-T intervals on an electrocardiogram, and arrhythmias (Klain and Jaeger, 1990). Autopsy reports describe myocardial softening and necrosis and diffuse myocardial and systemic hemorrhage, raising the possibility of a selective effect on blood vessels (Klain and Jaeger, 1990).

Christiansen et al. (1994) conducted experiments with rabbits with intravenous doses of 44 µg/kg and a sublethal toxic dose one-half that (22µg/kg).[6] The higher dose produced significant systolic and diastolic blood pressure declines, while the lower dose did not produce a significant change in blood pressure. Heart rates (EKGs) were not significantly affected in either group. The study concluded that hypotension was peripheral in origin, not cardiac.

---

[6]The larger dose here is the minimum lethal dose, the lowest amount that killed rabbits in LD_{50} tests—48 hours of LD50 0.54 µm/kg.

There is no indication of bone marrow injury. Splenic hyperplasia occurs in animals given sublethal doses of ricin, while necrosis is seen in lethal exposures (OSRD, 1946; Klain and Jaeger, 1990). The specific mechanism causing hemorrhage is unknown, and no platelet abnormalities have been found following ricin exposure.

Swollen kidneys, renal failure, acute tubular necrosis, and acute renal failure have been reported (Klain and Jaeger, 1990; OSRD, 1946; Wellner, Hewetson, and Poli, 1995). Some of the renal findings may be due to hypovolemia and hypotension.

Combined Effects. Little information exists regarding the combined effects of ricin and medications or environmental factors. If stress or pretreatments are shown to alter the blood-brain barrier, they could increase sensitivity to ricin, based on Foxwell et al. (1985). For example, in mice, toxicity increased when ricin was administered with mannitol, which impairs the blood-brain barrier (Foxwell et al., 1985). Friedman et al. (1996) has demonstrated in animals that severe stress makes the blood-brain barrier more permeable.

Prevention and Treatment

No immunizations or treatments are available as yet for human use. Care is supportive. Active and passive immunizations show promise experimentally (Griffiths et al., 1995; Franz and Jaax, 1997). Drug therapy is in the very early stages of laboratory efforts (Franz and Jaax, 1997).

What to Look for in the Gulf Context

Ricin ingestion causes weakness, abdominal pain, and bloody diarrhea. However, there were few opportunities for food or water contamination in the Gulf. Thus, if any military exposures to ricin happened during the Gulf War, they would more likely have occurred via ocular, dermal, and respiratory routes. One would expect conjunctivitis (based on animal studies) and signs of persistent respiratory irritation from low-level exposures to ricin, generally followed by malaise, arthralgia, muscle aches, and a low fever, although these symptoms are not specific to ricin. One would not expect consequences from dermal exposure to ricin unless the agent gained entry through small cuts and abrasions. Muscle cramps and weakness are a distinctive finding common in low-level exposures (Fodstad et al., 1984).

There is no particular reason to think the 3rd Armored Cavalry regiment had any exposure to ricin or chemical agents, but its records give some idea of the background of illness in the region and the prevalence of illnesses that can also be produced by low levels of agents. Carefully collected medical data from this regiment during in the Gulf War showed increased respiratory illness rates before the start of the air war. There was no increase in eye complaints, and there were few cases of fever of unknown origin (Wasserman et al., 1997). Examination of other unit records would be helpful.

Because ricin is immunogenic, individuals occupationally exposed to low levels during World War II may have developed ricin hypersensitivity, indicative of the presence of antibodies to ricin. Antibodies to ricin definitely developed in cancer patients given the agent intravenously (Fodstad et al., 1984). It might similarly be possible to document antibodies to ricin in persons who served in the Gulf. Although Fodstad's is not a routine study, his technique could be replicated.

At present, however, there is no evidence that ricin exposure occurred in the Gulf or that long-term illness is a consequence of low-level exposure. If such evidence is ever uncovered, it may be possible to test for exposure through antibody determinations in exposed persons. Although ricin should degrade in the environment over time, if canisters or filters from the Gulf War can be located, it might be valuable to examine them using antibody techniques to look for evidence of ricin.

Summary and Conclusions

Ricin is a potent plant toxin with delayed onset of effects and an aerosol toxicity equivalent to soman and sarin. It cannot be detected in the field and can persist in dry weather for up to three days but will environmentally degrade because of moisture, heat, light, and oxygen.

Ricin use had progressed to the point of unsophisticated weapon status in Iraq, but there is no evidence that it was used in the Gulf War against U.S. forces. Of the toxins of concern, ricin was probably the least stable and unlikely to withstand explosions and lengthy atmospheric transport to Saudi Arabia from releases in Iraq.

During the war, there were no mass outbreaks of the conjunctivitis and respiratory disease that ricin can cause, and such conditions are not specific to ricin in any case. Little is known about late long-term effects from clinically significant exposures; chronic low-level exposures have not been studied. An effort to follow up World War II workers and documented human poisonings would be helpful.

Some of the nonspecific general signs and symptoms of low-dose ricin exposure may resemble features of illnesses in Gulf War veterans, particularly muscle aches, sweating, and respiratory difficulties. Follow-up studies are lacking, so no evidence of ricin-induced recurrent or persistent illness after low-dose exposures was found.

Ricin is highly immunogenic. If reason to suspect ricin exposure of Gulf War patients increases, it may be useful to look for antibodies to ricin. Lacking information about the prevalence of such antibodies in the general population, suitable controls would be needed.

Neurological disease, including neuropathy, has not been documented as a consequence of ricin toxicity, although ricin is neurotoxic and can produce axonal degeneration. There are indications that neural factors are important in lethality and that ricin may alter the permeability of blood-neural barriers. Increased permeability of the blood-brain barrier enhances ricin toxicity. Further study of neural mechanisms in ricin toxicity should be pursued.

There is a remote possibility (based on an animal study by Foxwell et al., 1985) that cumulative toxicity from sustained subclinical ricin exposures could occur in immune-compromised subjects. The possibility that there were many such persons in the Gulf population seems very small.

Ricin should not be in the forefront of Gulf concerns, but other small countries and terrorists could turn to it as an inexpensive weapon, and thus further research on its mechanisms of action and treatment is warranted. The following areas in particular deserve more attention: the longer-term effects of ricin exposure, blood-brain barrier modulation of toxicity, neural mechanisms of ricin-related illness, and effects of ricin on disease resistance.

TRICHOTHECENE MYCOTOXINS

Trichothecene mycotoxins are produced by fungi (e.g., *Fusaria, Trichoderma, Myrothecium, Stachybotrys*); 60 are known. These were originally isolated as possible antifungal microbials or as antiplant agents. Analysis of trichothecene (and aflatoxin) exposures is complicated by their natural occurrence: Their presence alone does not prove a biological attack.

Iraq has admitted to possessing trichothecene mycotoxins and testing them in animals and has been accused of using them against Iran (UNSCOM, 1991, 1992, 1995; Zilinskas, 1997; Heyndrickx, 1984). The report of Iraqi possession of trichothecenes followed a considerable period of interest, attention, and controversy about their use in Southeast Asia (between 1974 and 1981, against Lao and Khmer populations by communist forces) and in Afghanistan (by Soviet forces) (Crocker, 1984; Haig, 1982; Schultz, 1982; Seagrave, 1981). Wannemacher and Wiener (1997), concluded that the Soviets and their clients have used trichothecenes, and the authors present a detailed review of the history of the subject and associated controversy. There may have been shortcomings in the epidemiological approaches (Hu et al., 1989). There were also many difficulties and inconsistencies in agent sampling, transport, and analysis.

These toxins, until discovered in Southeast Asian attack environments, had not been on the usual lists of potential toxin weapons (SIPRI, 1973). Analysts recognized that the toxins could produce the injuries encountered (Watson, Mirocha, and Hayes, 1984). Subsequent research identified properties of military significance, e.g., skin injury from nanogram amounts; eye injuries from micrograms; and serious central nervous system, respiratory, gastrointestinal, and hematological toxicity via multiple routes of exposure (Watson, Mirocha, and Hayes, 1984; Bunner et al., 1985; and Wannemacher and Wiener, 1997).

History

These mycotoxins have been poisoning people and animals for a long time. They grow well at low temperatures and frequently contaminate grain and other foodstuffs. They have been implicated in foodborne illnesses on several continents (Ueno et al., 1984). A large disease outbreak in the Soviet Union during World War II, which involved thousands and had high mortality, was eventually traced to the consumption of grain contaminated by *Fusaria* molds, which had been left in the fields over the winter. The disease, alimentary toxic aleukia, resembled a severe radiation injury with nausea, vomiting, diarrhea, leukopenia, hemorrhagic diathesis, and sepsis.

These toxins are also hazardous via other routes. Domestic animals and farmers manifested skin and respiratory irritation and systemic malaise from exposure to contaminated dusts and hay. Human illnesses have arisen from trichothecene mycotoxin contamination of houses and ventilation systems, resulting in so-called "sick building" syndrome (Croft et al., 1986; Jarvis, 1985; Smoragiewicz et al., 1993). One family so exposed was affected with nonspecific symptoms whose cause was not identified for months (*Myrothecium* and *Stachybotrys* were identified). For a time, several trichothecene mycotoxins were tested as anticancer agents in clinical trials (Thigpen et al., 1981; Bukowski et al., 1982; Yap et al., 1979; Diggs et al., 1978; Murphy et al., 1978; Goodwin et al., 1981). Some laboratory accidents have added to experience with human exposure (Wannemacher and Wiener, 1997). In addition, there is considerable information on the effects of trichothecene mycotoxins on economically important animals (Ueno et al., 1984).

Reports of communist attacks on Lao tribal people, and later on the Khmer, began in 1974 with aircraft and helicopter delivery of colored smokes, dusts, and droplets. People near these attacks had signs and symptoms that did not resemble known chemical warfare agents. Later similar attacks were reported in Cambodia and Afghanistan. Symptoms included vomiting, dizziness, seizures, hematemesis, respiratory distress, hypotension, and blisters. Survivors were ill for a long time with rashes, joint pains, fatigue, and memory problems (Haig, 1982; Schultz, 1982; Crossland and Townsend, 1984).

Investigative teams in refugee camps were puzzled, identifying a toxic epidermolysis without other expected findings from known chemical agents (House, 1979), but intelligence analysts recognized the similarities to trichothecene intoxication. Later, clinical examinations, autopsies, laboratory tests, and tissue samples showed trichothecene mycotoxins (and a propylene-glycol carrier) together with tissue damage compatible with trichothecene effects (Crocker, 1984; Watson, Mirocha, and Hayes, 1984; Rosen and Rosen, 1982; Stahl et al., 1985).

Chinese analysts attributed a higher toxicity to trichothecene mycotoxins than to nerve agents. They alleged that, between 1975 and 1982, 6,000 Laotians; 1,000 Cambodians; and 3,000 Afghans had died from attacks with what came to be known as "yellow rain" (Fang, 1983).

During the Iran-Iraq War, especially in the fighting around Majoon Island, colored smokes and powders were used against Iranian forces, perhaps reflecting combinations of agents. Although controversial in the scientific community, Heyndrickx (1984) found trichothecene mycotoxins in Iranian casualties who appeared to have sustained mustard injuries. Although other laboratories did not confirm these findings from the same material, Professor Heyndrickx argued that biological tissues had degraded the toxin over time.[7]

It is not known if, during the Gulf War, any of the Iraqi chemical and biological facilities hit by Allied fire contained trichothecenes. Trichothecenes are very resistant to environmental degradation and resist heat below 500°F; hence, the production of effects after long-distance transport following explosive release is possible but unlikely because the chemical would be very diffuse by that time (U.S. Army, 1990; Wannemacher and Wiener, 1997; Trusal, 1985). However, no events described during the war closely correspond to known acute effects of trichothecene syndromes. Lethal effects require substantial doses (milligrams), but eye and skin irritation can occur at much lower levels (U.S. Army, 1990; Wannemacher and Wiener, 1997; Coulombe, 1993), raising the remote possibility that low-level exposures might have been misinterpreted as being due to some other cause.

Weaponization

Production using contemporary fermentation methods similar to those of brewing and antibiotic production is easy and inexpensive, and conventional bioreactors can readily produce tons of these agents (Wannemacher and Wiener, 1997). AD Little (1986, Ch. 4) described the conditions defining pro-

---

[7]The professor also observed chemical casualties in Iran, and his treatment recommendations were a subject of controversy in 1997 and 1998 letters in *Lancet*.

duction. The large-scale production of *Fusaria* and trichothecenes for civil purposes in the former Soviet Union indicates the ease of large-scale production for other purposes (Buck et al., 1983). Formulations of T-2—one of the most potent trichothecenes—might also include polyethylene glycol, sodium lauryl sulfate, or dimethylsulfoxide (DMSO). These materials facilitate dispersal and handling of the toxin, possibly enhancing toxicity. Trichothecenes do not degrade to nontoxicity when exposed in the natural environment (for weeks at least) and are stable when stored. They can be delivered by mortars, artillery, free rockets, aerial bombs, and surface or aerial sprayers (Wannemacher and Wiener, 1997). Iraq possessed all the systems previously used to deliver trichothecenes.

T-2 is a skin-damaging agent of great potency (Bunner et al., 1985)—several hundred times more potent than mustards or lewisite (Wannemacher and Wiener, 1997). It is able to injure the eye in microgram amounts, which again indicates that it is more potent than mustards.

Toxicity by inhalation is comparable to mustards. NAS (1983) estimated that LC_{50} exposures of aerosols of 1 mg/m^3 or surface contamination or LD_{50} of 1 g/m^2 could readily be attained.

Trichothecenes readily result in vomiting, rather promptly at low concentrations, which might compromise the ability of exposed troops to use protective respirators. Other symptoms, including mild incapacitation, follow. Operationally, the persistence of trichothecenes makes them a threat even to military forces with protective equipment; Soviet troops in Afghanistan avoided operating in areas where these toxins were used (Fang, 1983). There are some indications that trichothecenes may have been used in combination with other agents in Southeast Asia and Afghanistan (Fang, 1983; Schultz, 1982).

Chemical and Physical Properties

The trichothecenes are classed as sesquiterpenes (Ueno, 1983). The members of this family of toxins vary depending on their side groups and include T-2, HT-2, nivalenol, deoxynivalenol, anguidine, diacetyoxyscirpenol (DAS), and crotocin.[8] When the toxins are extracted from fungal cultures, a yellow greasy residue remains. Had the various reported Asian attacks involved a crude extract containing some of that residue, the result might have been the yellow rain reported. The toxins are stable in air and light for weeks and can withstand

---

[8]Many other tricothecene toxins, such as verrucarin A, roridin A, satratoxin H, have greater intravenous and intraperitoneal toxicity in the mouse (Wannemacher and Wiener, 1997), but this review touches on them only occasionally (e.g., Croft, Jarvis, and Yatawara, 1986).

heat; a temperature of 500°F is required to destroy T-2 (Trusal, 1985; Wannemacher and Wiener, 1997).

These toxins can be inactivated with 3- to 5-percent hypochlorite solutions (Wannemacher and Wiener, 1997). The toxins are relatively insoluble in water but are soluble in acetone, chloroform, DMSO, glycols, ethanol, and other organic solvents. They have a peppery odor and negligible vapor pressure.

Figure 4.1 shows the general structure of trichothecene toxins. The olefinic bond at position 9-10 and the epoxide group at position 12-13 are important in the chemical and biological reactions of these agents.

Detection

No military field detection systems currently deployed can detect tricho-thecenes, although laboratory techniques (e.g., antibody-ELISA, gas chro-matography or mass spectroscopy, and thin-layer chromatography coupled to fluorimetry) have been used. Biological detection systems using animals are neither specific nor easy (Fontelo et al., 1983; Mirocha et al., 1984; Thompson and Wannemacher, 1984; Rosen and Rosen, 1982; NAS, 1983). Wannemacher and Wiener (1997), reviewing confirmatory procedures, indicated that mass spectroscopy is the procedure of choice, requiring little specimen "cleanup" and enabling detection of one part per billion (ppb) of toxin. More-complex systems being evolved may detect 0.1 ppb.

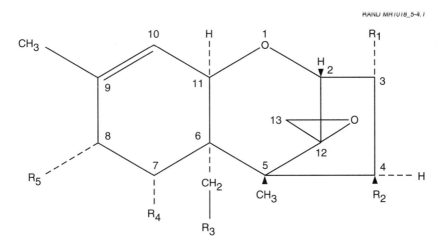

SOURCE: AD Little (1986, Ch. 4).

Figure 4.1—General Structure of Trichothecene Toxins

Toxicology and Toxicokinetics

Mechanisms of Action. The many mechanisms by which trichothecenes produce toxicity are varied, and their relative importance in producing illness is not fully understood (Coulombe, 1993). They include the following:

- inhibition of protein synthesis, thought to be the most important effect (Ueno, 1983; Ueno et al., 1984; Tutelyan and Kravchenko, 1981)

- inhibition of DNA synthesis (Thompson and Wannemacher, 1984), which might contribute to their radiomimetic properties

- impairment of ribosome function (NAS, 1983; Coulombe, 1993; Tutelyan and Kravchenko, 1981)

- inhibition of mitochondrial protein synthesis (Pace et al., 1985)

- induction of reparable single strand breaks in DNA

- immunosuppression, allowing secondary and opportunistic bacterial infections and possibly delayed hypersensitivity (Ueno, 1983; Yarom et al., 1984; Jagadeesan et al., 1982).

Trichothecenes react readily with thiol groups and, at low concentrations, inhibit thiol enzymes (e.g., creatine kinase, lactate dehydrogenase) (Tutelyan and Kravchenko, 1981; Ueno et al., 1984). They can be incorporated into lipid or protein elements of cell membranes. Tissue culture studies show alteration of membrane function (Coulombe, 1993; Pfeifer and Irons, 1985). Sulfhydryl effects in cell membranes are important in cell-to-cell interactions in the immune system. T-2 toxin induces cell membrane injury with hemolysis, apparently via a free-radical mechanism (Segal et al., 1983; Coulombe, 1993).

Metabolism may be more important in detoxification than in producing toxicity. Unlike the aflatoxins that require metabolic activation, the trichothecenes are directly toxic without activation, as their prompt effects on the gastrointestinal mucosa with epithelial cell necrosis suggest (Busby and Wogan, 1979).

T-2 and other trichothecene toxins are deacetylated in the liver. Metabolites are also toxic but less so than T-2 (Ueno et al., 1984). Carboxyesterases (-SH serine esterases) in liver microsomes hydrolyze T-2 to the less potent HT-2. These enzymes may be clinically important. Inhibition of this enzyme by paraoxon (an organophosphate pesticide) in subclinical doses increases the toxicity of T-2 in mice (Johnsen et al., 1986). Other potent inhibitors of this enzyme are tri-o-cresyl phosphate (TOCP, an organophosphate), eserine (a carbamate), and diisopropyl fluorophosphate (DFP, a weak organophosphate nerve agent) (OSRD, 1946). These all inhibit hydrolysis of T-2 (Johnsen et al., 1986). This raises the strong possibility that similar compounds, such as PB; low levels of nerve agent; or other carbamate or organophosphate insecticides might enhance the toxicity of T-2 or other trichothecenes at low levels.

Exposure-Effect Relationships.   T-2 toxin and other trichothecenes are absorbed slowly (12 to 24 hours) via the intact skin but rapidly through abraded skin. DMSO or similar penetrants can increase the rate of absorption, but even then the systemic toxicity appears slowly (Bunner et al., 1985; Schiefer, 1984; Kemppainen et al., 1986a, 1986b; Solberg et al., 1990).

The rapid appearance of symptoms after respiratory exposure in humans, along with the results of animal inhalation studies, indicates rapid absorption and high retention of aerosolized T-2 toxin, with the respiratory tree retaining small amounts (Creasia et al., 1987).[9] Tritium-labeled agent and immunoperoxidase studies have also been used to follow the distribution and disposition of T-2 toxin (Pace et al., 1985, Lee et al., 1984). Intramuscularly injected agent is distributed to liver, kidney, lung, and other tissues within 30 minutes. The plasma concentration has a biphasic course, with half-lives of 1.8 and 50 hours for the two phases. T-2 toxin and metabolites concentrate in bile with evidence of enterohepatic circulation. The liver and kidney are the main organs for detoxification. Oral intoxication showed T-2 toxin in the gastrointestinal tract and kidneys, but not in the liver, reflecting rapid hepatic metabolism. The brain showed a rapid uptake to levels higher than plasma but below many other tissues, with a rapid fall to levels similar to plasma in six hours. One would expect trichothecenes to enter the brain readily, since they are lipophilic (Wang, Wilson, and Fitzpatrick, 1992).

Table 4.4 gives effects for various acute exposure levels and pathways. Effects accumulate with repeated exposures. It has been shown, for example, that the effects of sustained low doses can accumulate to the clinical picture associated with alimentary toxic aleukia (Mayer 1953a, 1953 b; Lutsky et al., 1978). Or they can yield the more diffuse problems that Croft et al.(1986) and Jarvis (1985) reported: a case of ongoing illness for several years in a family of five, with recurring respiratory illness, flu syndromes, sore throats, diarrhea, cough, headaches, fatigue, and episodes of alopecia. One man had leg pains. Eventually, trichothecenes were identified in air ducts and ceiling material in the family's house. Material extracted from these areas was toxic to rats and mice. Croft cited other reports by Forgacs (1972) of toxin exposures producing similar symptoms with central nervous system and neuropsychiatric manifestations.[10]

Respiratory is high and comparable to parenteral injections. Oral and dermal lethal toxicities are lower but produce similar systemic effects (Creasia et al.,

---

[9]The LD_{50} was 0.24 mg/kg for young adult mice and 0.94 mg/kg for mature mice. For mice, inhalation was 10 times more toxic than systemic administration and 20 times more toxic than dermal administration.

[10]As noted earlier, the toxins were tricothecenes other than the main ones covered in this review, e.g., verrucarin A, B; satratoxin H, and trichoverrin A, B.

Table 4.4

Effects of Varied Trichothecene (T-2) Exposures

	Dose	Effect	Source
Skin Exposures	5–50 ng in liquid	Minimal erythema dose (guinea pig, rat)	Ueno (1983), Wannemacher et al. (1983)
	209 ng/cm^2 in liquid	Minimal erythema dose (monkey)	Wannemacher et al. (1983), Bunner et al. (1983)
	1 μg/cm^2	Irritation (guinea pig, rabbit)	Fairhurst et al. (1987)
	2 μg	Vesication, skin injury	Bunner (1983)
	0.25 mg/kg	Severe illness, diarrhea (monkey)	Bunner et al. (1983)
	1.5 mg/kg in DMSO	LD$_{50}$ (rat; mean time to death, 19 hr.)	Wannemacher et al. (1983)
	4.2 mg/kg in methanol	LD$_{50}$ (guinea pigs; mean time to death 190 hr.)	Wannemacher et al. (1983)
Eye	1 μg	Detectable corneal injury	USAMRIID (1983)
	>2 μg	Severe corneal injury, conjunctivitis	Bunner (1983)
Respiratory[a]	0.24 mg/kg (absorbed)	Mouse LD$_{50}$	Creasia et al. (1987)
	0.05 mg/kg (absorbed)	Rat LD$_{50}$	Bunner et al. (1985)
	0.6–2.0 mg/kg (absorbed)	Guinea pig LD$_{50}$	Wannemacher and Wieser (1997, p. 661)
	5,479 mg-min/m^3	Guinea pig LD$_{50}$	AD Little (1986)
	200–1,800 mg-min/m^3	Estimated LCT$_{50}$	Calculated from U.S. Army (1990)
Systemic Toxicity	500 μg/kg	Estimated human LD$_{50}$	U.S. Army (1990)
	470 μg/kg intramuscular	Rat LD$_{50}$	Bunner et al. (1985)
	1.17 mg/kg	Rat LD$_{50}$	Bunner et al. (1985)
	650 μg/kg intramuscular	Monkey LD$_{20}$	Cosgriff et al. (1986)
	790 μg/kg intravenous	Monkey LD$_{50}$	AD Little (1986)
	850 μg/kg intramuscular	Rat LD$_{50}$	Chan and Gentry (1984)
	111 mg/kg intramuscular	Rabbit LD$_{50}$	Chan and Gentry (1984)

Table 4.4—Continued

	Dose	Effect	Source
Oral Toxicity	0.1–0.2 mg/kg	Swine, emesis	Busby and Wogan (1979)
	0.1–1.0 mg/kg	Swine, diarrhea	Ueno (1983a)
	2.29 mg/kg	Rat LD_{50}	Bunner et al. (1985)
	3.06 mg/kg	Guinea pig LD_{50}	AD Little (1986)
	1.0 mg/kg[b]	Male monkey LD_{100}	Rukimi, Prasad, and Rao (1980)
	1 5 mg/kg	Estimated human LD_{50}	Calculated from U.S. Army (1990)

[a]No primate data were located.

[b]Per day for 15 days

1987; Bonomi et al., 1995; Wannemacher et al., 1993; Schiefer and Hancock, 1984).[11] For less-than-lethal dosages and for all routes of administration, sequelae of leukopenia, thrombocytopenia, bleeding tendency, weakness, diarrhea, dyspnea, recurrent infections, vomiting, anorexia, and weight loss are expected. Other sequelae of acute exposures include prolonged rashes, joint pains and fatigue (Schultz, 1982), fever, chills, hypotension, confusion, somnolence, seizures, memory loss, hallucinations, and burning erythema (Belt et al., 1979; Murphy et al., 1978; Yap, et al., 1979; Diggs et al., 1978; Bukowski et al., 1982; Thigpen et al., 1981; Crossland and Townsend, 1984).

Pathology and Pathophysiology

The clinical manifestations of trichothecene intoxication are derived from several sources. They are summarized here prior to more detailed treatment of individual organ systems.

Known effects from evidence other than the yellow rain attacks are nausea, vomiting, seizures, central nervous system dysfunction, chills, fever, hypothermia, hypotension, epithelial necrosis, myelosuppression, and gastroenteritis with hematemesis and melena (bloody vomiting and stools). In the yellow rain attacks, the Hmong victims were probably exposed by several routes, including dermal, respiratory, and oral (the last from swallowing larger particles trapped in upper airways and returned to the oropharynx by ciliary action (Wannemacher and Wiener, 1997). Vomiting was induced and lasted several days. There was a feeling of intense heat, itching and burning of the skin, dizziness, tachycardia, chest pain, headache, and decreased vision. Within hours, victims reported intense eye pain, red eyes, bleeding gums, and hematemesis. Trembling was common, and some patients had seizures. Severe itching ensued with the formation of small hard blisters, some of which were hemorrhagic, occasionally progressing to large bullae. Abdominal pain and bloody diarrhea continued (Watson, Mirocha, and Hayes, 1984).

Khmer yellow rain casualties had similar acute symptoms (Crossland and Townsend, 1984) with the following longer-term effects: intermittent weakness, anorexia, reduced memory and ability to concentrate, intermittent diarrhea, impotence, increased fatigue, cough and dyspnea, increased susceptibility to infection, and suspected increases in fetal abnormalities and spontaneous abortions (Haig, 1982; Schultz, 1982; Watson, Mirocha, and Hayes, 1984; Stahl et al., 1985; Crossland and Townsend, 1984). It must be noted that the Hmong cases with memory loss that Crossland described were not evaluated for the presence of toxins. These persons had undergone a harrowing experience,

---

[11]Note the NAS (1983) LD_{50} estimates under "Weaponization," above.

having been attacked, seen kinfolk die, fled, and become refugees. Severe apathy, confusion, and depression are common in survivors of natural or man-made disasters.

A limited autopsy was performed on a Kampuchean man injured in a toxic attack in February 1982, who died a month later having initially showed signs of recovery, then developing fever, jaundice, heoptysis, and anariax coma. Malaria was ruled out. The heart tissues showed interstitial myocardial hemorrhage and acute myocarditis, while the lungs showed only pulmonary edema. There was diffuse hepatitis with micronodular cirrhosis, as well as acute renal tubular necrosis. Tissues showed T-2 toxin in amounts ranging from 6.8 to 80 ppb, but there is little information with which to interpret the findings. The pathologist considered them to be compatible with mycotoxin poisoning (Stahl, Green, and Farnum, 1985).

Four stages were identified in the early Soviet *Fusaria* consumption incidents (a chronic oral exposure) (Mayer 1953a, 1953b):

- **Stage 1** begins within a few hours and lasts three to nine days. It consists of mild inflammation of the mouth and gastrointestinal tract, gastroenteritis, nausea, vomiting and diarrhea.

- **Stage 2** is a quiet period of two weeks or more with few symptoms even while contaminated grain was still being ingested. There were laboratory abnormalities in some patients, but most appeared well.

- **Stage 3** reveals the results of bone marrow aplasia with hemorrhagic diathesis, oral mucosal necrosis, and multiple infections.

- **Stage 4** is a period of convalescence requiring several months after ingestion stopped.

Grain elevator workers are in a complex environment with dusts, plant products, and trichothecenes. They frequently experience coughing, breathlessness, wheezing, fever, and dermatitis (Kemppainen et al., 1986b); similar problems occur in "sick" buildings (Hendy and Cole, 1993; Jarvis, 1985).

Respiratory. Rats, mice, and guinea pigs die rapidly from large respiratory exposures (1 to 12 hours) but show little sign of pulmonary injury, unlike direct effects on gastrointestinal mucosa (Creasia et al., 1987; Wannemacher and Wiener, 1997; Bunner et al., 1985). At low levels of respiratory exposure, coughing and upper respiratory irritation occur. Higher exposures produce pulmonary edema, collapse, hypoxia, and death within a few hours, or more indolent symptoms with later pulmonary hemorrhage, hypotension and shock, edema, or infections (Rukmini, Prasad, and Rao, 1980; Lutsky et al., 1978; Bunner, 1983; Bunner et al. 1985). Fifty Hmong survivors reported the following: smell of gunpowder or pepper (14 percent), rhinorrhea (28 percent), nasal itching (14 percent), sore throat (40 percent), aphonia (26 percent), cough (60 percent), dyspnea (52 percent), severe chest pain (52 percent), and hemoptysis (18 percent). Systemic signs (vomiting, tachycardia, hypotension, etc.) follow. Oral or intravenous exposures result in pulmonary edema, hemorrhage, consolidation, and secondary pulmonary infection.

Toxicity by the respiratory route may be influenced by the material used to suspend the toxin (Creasia et al., 1987). Fibrinous exudate may be seen, and pulmonary fibrosis was a late complication in some of the trichothecene cancer trials (Goodwin et al., 1981). In contrast to inhaled ricin, where effects are confined to the lungs, respiratory exposure produces much less pulmonary change and pronounced systemic toxicity.

Eyes. Conjunctivitis begins several hours after exposure, although the mechanism of the immediate visual disturbances is unclear. Corneal changes begin at 12 hours, with the peak effect in 24 to 48 hours. Blurred vision continues, with recovery from mild injuries in three to seven days. Hmong yellow rain victims reported eye pain and burning (68 percent), blurred vision (58 percent), and tearing (47 percent). Eyelid edema and scleral inflammation are associated with more-intense exposures. Corneal thinning can follow toxin exposure, with irregularities lasting up to six months (Bunner, 1983).

Skin. The skin responds to nanogram amounts of toxin with edema and inflammation. T-2 administered with DMSO to animals produced almost no local reaction (Bunner et al., 1985), but the systemic effects were substantial, although delayed, and cutaneous LD_{50}s were elevated, compared to application without DMSO. Dermal application can produce the same effects as oral administration: bone marrow, thymus, and lymphatic changes and gastrointestinal effects (Schiefer, 1984; Wannemacher et al., 1983).

In T-2 laboratory accidents, vesication has not been a problem. Despite decontamination, a burning sensation developed from 4 to 24 hours in the contact area, followed by numbness. In cancer trials, erythema, burning stomatitis, and alopecia were common (Schiefer and Hancock, 1984; Murphy et al., 1978; Bukowski et al., 1982; Diggs et al., 1978; Belt et al., 1979; Yap et al., 1979; Thigpen et al., 1981; Goodwin et al., 1981). Hmong survivors reported persistent burning sensations, with tingling, itching, and pain lasting several hours. Some numbness lasted two days to several months in some victims. Scattered erythema was noted after a few hours, but only 23 percent reported blisters. In some cases, large hemorrhagic bullae occurred, with underlying necrosis. Necrotic areas sloughed easily when corpses were moved (Wannemacher and Wiener, 1997). Sequelae include secondary infections, hyperpigmentation, and recurrent rashes.

Gastrointestinal. T-2 and other trichothecenes readily injure the rapidly dividing cells of the gastrointestinal tract. Tissue responses include edema, cytolysis, and sloughing, with loss of gastric epithelium and villus tips (Lee et al., 1984; Rukmini, Prasad, and Rao, 1980). The trichothecene DAS given intravenously showed marked gastrointestinal tract necrosis (Coppock et al., 1985) and pancreatic damage resulting in hyperglycemia. Some jaundice was seen in yellow rain victims. The liver is involved in detoxification, but liver failure is rare (Lutsky et al., 1978). Liver enzymes and amylase rise initially but return to normal in three to seven days (Bunner et al., 1985). As a later consequence, the bowel may become less resistant to bacterial penetration, which can increase susceptibility to infection (Lutsky et al., 1978).

Nervous System. The central nervous system effects are striking. Animals and humans exposed via the respiratory route show early central nervous system signs and symptoms. Symptoms reported from cutaneous exposures—burning pain followed by numbness—suggest that these toxins may directly affect the peripheral nerves.

The early and sustained vomiting suggests direct central nervous system effects involving chemotactic and vomiting centers. Hallucinations are a distinctive feature of trichothecene intoxications. Headaches, drowsiness, anxiety, confusion, and seizures occur, but their mechanisms have not been studied (Yap et al., 1979; Thigpen et al., 1981; Bukowski et al., 1982).

There are few autopsy reports. DAS-poisoned swine showed cerebral hemorrhages (Coppock et al., 1985), while other animal studies showed meningeal bleeding and scattered petechial hemorrhages (Ueno et al., 1984). Experimental studies show alterations in levels of hydroxyindoleacetic acid and seratonin in the brain, with regional norepinephrine increases. Trichothecenes make the blood-brain barrier permeable to mannitol, although not dextran (Wang, Wilson, and Fitzpatrick, 1992). Intracerebral administration of T-2 decreased learning in mice, and intraperitoneal administration disturbed both learning ability and memory (Umeuchi et al., 1996).

The descriptions of chemotherapy patients (Thigpen et al., 1981; Yap et al., 1979), home exposures (Croft et al., 1986), and yellow rain cases (Watson, Mirocha, and Hayes, 1984; Crossland and Townsend, 1984) convey a picture of neurotoxicity, with somnolence, confusion, tremors, depression, weakness, malaise, and memory problems (some of which resemble findings in some Gulf veterans). In the cases just cited, however, symptoms appeared promptly, and there were other conspicuous indications of exposure.

Cardiovascular, Lymphatic, Hematologic. Hmong yellow rain victims reported chest pain, sometimes crushing, along with weakness. Animals poisoned with T-2 develop tachycardia and later bradycardia. Hypotension occurs early and may persist for several days, sometimes proceeding to shock. Hypotension and orthostatic hypotension were common in chemotherapy patients (7 to 40 percent) (Yap et al., 1979; Thigpen et al., 1981; Murphy et al., 1978; Bukowski et al., 1982). Mucous membranes are bright red, reflecting vasodilation. Commonly, hemorrhagic foci are found throughout the myocardium (Ueno et al., 1984; Stahl et al., 1985), and the electrocardiogram may show a prolonged P-R interval and prolongation of the QRS and QT intervals, reflecting conduction system abnormalities and increased risk of arrhythmias.

Beginning with the alimentary toxic aleukia diagnoses, bone marrow and lymphatic system injury has been a consistent finding (Mayer 1953a, 1953b; Ueno et al., 1984). Cell culture studies show stem cells to be sensitive to T-2 toxin. Mycotoxins produce profound alterations in hemostasis, as noted in yellow-rain cases and documented by primate studies (Cosgriff et al., 1986). Prothrombin and activated partial thromboplastin times are increased early in intoxication from decreased coagulation factors. Lethal hemorrhage risk is greater because T-2 inhibits platelet aggregation (Yarom et al., 1984).

Other. There are clinical signs of muscle involvement. The Hmong complained of weakness, fatigability, tremors, and cramps. Animals show flaccid weakness after T-2 poisoning. The early elevation of serum creatine kinase could reflect muscle or cardiac injury, or both. Isoenzyme studies have not been reported (Bunner, 1983).

Impaired immunity and infection resistance is another effect of these toxins. The ability of leukocytes to kill bacteria is impaired (Yarom et al., 1984); immunoglobulin levels are depressed; and cell-mediated immunity is suppressed (Jagadeesan et al., 1982; Schiefer, 1984; Ueno et al., 1984).

Renal output decreases after T-2 intoxication, and the toxin is found in substantial amounts in the kidney. Observed tubular necrosis could be related to hypotension and liver disorders.

The endocrine effects of T-2 and other trichothecenes are not prominent. Adrenal cortical necrosis from T-2 exposure has been reported in rats (Thurman et al., 1986). Decreased spermatozoa production has been seen in several species.

Interactions. The literature on trichothecene interactions is limited. Combining aflatoxins and trichothecenes may increase toxicity (Schultz, 1982; U.S. Army, 1990). No reports emerged of studies examining combined inhalation exposures. There were indications of synergism in feeding studies of chickens (Huff et al., 1988). (However, a study of DAS and aflatoxin in lambs did not show any enhanced toxicity from combined oral exposures of these toxins (Harvey et al., 1995). There is a strong possibility that the severity of trichothecenes could be potentiated by exposure even to low levels of organophosphate pesticides, carbamate pesticides or pretreatments, or low levels of nerve agent, through inhibition of carboxyesterases involved in detoxification (Johnson and Read, 1987). Drugs inducing the increase of detoxifying enzymes, such as epoxide hydrolase or cytochrome P450, may favorably interact to decrease toxin severity. Such drugs as phenobarbital, metoclopramide, metochlopramide carbamazepine, metyrapone, and clofibrate have shown beneficial effects in animal models (Fricke, 1993; Wannemacher and Wiener, 1997).

What to Look for in the Gulf Context

Because of the high sensitivity of the skin and eyes to trichothecenes, injuries to these organs should be looked for in unit medical records. Conjunctivitis, erythema, burning skin, and blurred vision were followed by nausea, vomiting, and diarrhea might increase suspicion of trichothecene exposure.[12]

Summary and Recommendations

The trichothecenes are credible biological warfare toxins for some purposes. However, there is no proof or even a strong indication of their use against U.S. forces in the Gulf. With more concentrated exposure, hematological changes, seizures and other serious sequelae might have been expected.

Current information arises from clinically recognized exposures or laboratory research. Trichothecenes have multiple toxic effects with potential long-term consequences, such as central nervous system injury, immune suppression, and prolonged disability. The sequelae noted in the Hmong, e.g., long-term memory problems; the animal memory studies; and the story of the household exposure may resemble some features of the illnesses in Gulf War veterans, but the expected hematological alterations have not been reported among Gulf War patients. Furthermore, the Hmong effects resulted from substantial exposures with major short-term consequences. Little is known about the behavioral effects of sustained low-level exposures. The extreme sensitivity of the skin and eyes to T-2 and other trichothecenes makes it unlikely that delayed systemic illnesses in Gulf veterans represent a late effect of exposure to toxin "fallout." One would have expected an "epidemic" of painful dermatitis and conjunctivitis, as well as a number of other symptoms, which would have drawn attention to the exposure.

As in other cases, the AFIP should be consulted. The tests for trichothecenes are not routine, but have been used enough to be considered more than exper-

---

[12]However, troops dermally exposed to trichothecenes in DMSO might only have systemic symptoms, since little agent might remain in the skin after enhancement of transport by the solvent.

imental. The AFIP might be consulted about the possibility of detecting tricho-thecene metabolites in tissue specimens obtained from the Gulf and im-mediately after. If used protective mask filters from the war period become available, it might be possible to analyze them for the presence of tricho-thecenes, which are very stable molecules. Had trichothecenes been used, it is possible that their toxicity might have been increased by interactions with nerve agents or PB, although this has not been studied explicitly.

AFLATOXINS

This family of related toxins is produced by the molds *Aspergillus flavus* and *A. parasiticus*, which commonly contaminate food grains before and after harvest. Their toxicity was recognized in the 1960s, and it was later appreciated that they are a significant health problem for domestic animals and humans. The toxins are stable and survive cooking. Attention has focused on chronic exposure and illness from oral intake, although there have also been acute effects (Steyn, 1995; Coulombe, 1993; Bonomi et al., 1995). This review concentrates on AFB_1, the most toxic of the aflatoxin family, although the actual mixture Iraq weaponized is unknown. Aflatoxins show delayed acute toxicity (eight hours to several days) because most require metabolic activation (Daniels et al., 1990). However, most interest in aflatoxins arises from their carcinogenicity. They are implicated in the genesis of hepatocellular carcinoma, which is prevalent in tropical regions (Nigam et al., 1994, Groopman et al., 1996).

Aflatoxins do not appear to have attracted much of the military interest in tox-ins (SIPRI, 1973).[13] It was thus surprising when, after the War, Iraq informed the UN that it had produced aflatoxins and several trichothecene toxins (PAC, 1996a, 1996b; Zilinskas, 1997). Aflatoxins have, however, been mentioned as possibly enhancing the toxicity of trichothecene mycotoxins after the latter were recognized as military agents (U.S. Army, 1990; Schultz, 1982). Still, Iraq's placing aflatoxins in long-range missiles has surprised and puzzled analysts. Zilinskas (1997) offers three hypotheses:

1. The Iraqis discovered that aflatoxin possessed previously unknown proper-ties useful in biological warfare.

2. The long-term potential for carcinogenesis was used to terrorize civilian populations.[14]

---

[13]Aflatoxins are not discussed in the extensive coverage of biological warfare and toxins in Sidell, Takafuji, and Franz (1997).

[14]During the Iran-Iraq War, fear of chemical warheads was a factor in the terror urban missile attacks inspired (Cordesman and Wagner, 1990).

3. Because aflatoxin is easy to produce, it was produced and deployed to meet toxin production quotas set by higher authorities.

This report examines the first and second hypotheses.

Although concerns about human exposure have focused on carcinogenic risks, acute aflatoxin toxicity has been recognized, primarily from oral exposure but also via the respiratory route (e.g., aflatoxin-contaminated grain dust) (Hendry and Cole, 1993; Zarba et al., 1992; Massey, 1996; Baxter et al., 1981, Autrup et al., 1993). Respiratory exposure would have been the most likely route in the Gulf. The available information indicates that the food and water supplies of U.S. forces in the Gulf theater were diverse but secure and did not present an opportunity for long-distance attack. Dermal exposure producing systemic toxicity from aflatoxins has not been described. Animal studies suggest that respiratory exposure is more toxic than oral exposure (Northup et al., 1995).

There is uncertainty about human clinical manifestations of low-dose respiratory exposure to aflatoxin, although both acute and chronic illnesses are expected. The symptom onset is delayed, and there is evidence of cumulative effects.

Although many humans are exposed to aflatoxin in food, gastrointestinal symptoms predominate; neuropathy, rashes, memory problems, and joint pain are not commonly reported. Aflatoxins do impair resistance to infection experimentally (Jakab et al., 1994; Raisuddin et al., 1993), although determining their role in increasing human infectious diseases has been difficult (Allen et al., 1992; Denning et al., 1995).

Weaponization

Information about military deployment of aflatoxin is apparently confined to the Iraqi experience, although the sources for this report were limited to the unclassified literature. Zilinskas (1997) was a member of the UNSCOM team that had access to Iraq and analyzed that country's biological warfare program, including toxin activity. It is evident that much of what the Iraqis chose to discuss could not be verified independently (Zilinskas, 1997).

Iraq began evaluating biological weapons in the late 1970s but began an earnest program in 1985. By April of 1991, Iraqi scientists had investigated the biological potential of five bacterial strains, one fungal strain, five viruses, and four toxins, while also developing two harmless bacteria for testing purposes. Major centers of development were Muthanna State Establishment (also the center of chemical weapon development) and Salman Pak, which became the biological warfare center, with production occurring at the Al Hakam Single Cell Protein plant. Virus research was conducted at an animal disease research station at Al Manal (Zilinskas, 1997).

Substantial efforts went toward weaponizing aflatoxin, botulinum, ricin, and perhaps trichothecenes. Generally, the Iraqis manufactured crude solutions of toxins. Iraq developed a method of producing aflatoxin using cultured rice as a growth medium. UNSCOM was told that some 2,200 liters of aflatoxin were produced at Salman Pak. Some toxin was stored after weapons were filled.

The weapons filled with biologicals (at Al Muthanna) included 250- and 400-pound bombs (60 to 85 liters of toxin solution) (Zilinskas, 1997). An unknown number of 122 mm rockets were filled with aflatoxin as were some ten Scud warheads (Zilinskas, 1997). The UN inspectors were told that tests were made using toxin-filled and stimulant-filled 122-mm rockets, but as far as they knew such weapons were not deployed. Iraqi munitions used a simple burster charge to open the walls and disseminate the agent. The Iraqis also possessed several hundred Italian-made pesticide dispensers suitable for biological dissemination by aircraft or land vehicle. A MiG aircraft was modified for unmanned operation and fitted with a 2,200-liter tank to disseminate chemicals or toxins. It must be understood that UNSCOM has not independently verified most information Iraq provided pertaining to toxins.

The amount of toxin needed to produce severe illness or death (2 to 4 mg/kg) via oral routes is greater than for many military toxins. This level of toxicity places it in the second order of toxicity classification on a six-category scale, in which 1 indicates "extremely toxic" ($LD_{50} \leq 1$ mg/kg), 2 indicates "highly toxic" (1–50 mg/kg), and 6 indicates "harmless" (Proctor and Hughes, 1978). Such chemicals as lewisite, DFP, and the organophosphate pesticides parathion and isosustox fall in this category (SIPRI, 1973). The uncertain late cancer effects provide an implausible military motivation for use.

Although Zilinskas (1997) was not certain about what military effects would result from use of aflatoxins, they are capable of producing death, seizures, respiratory injury, nausea, vomiting, and liver failure, which would be militarily significant (Chao et al., 1991; Northup et al., 1995; Jakab et al., 1994; Bourgeois, 1971a, 1971b). Inhaled aflatoxins in microgram amounts are highly immuno-suppressive (Jakab et al., 1994) (milligrams would be needed for humans), but this effect would not provide the predictable effects weapon developers favor (use in conjunction with an infectious agent might be an exception).

In sum, the Iraqis were well informed about the effects of biological weapons and admitted conducting extensive field trials. A variety of fairly unsophisti-cated delivery means existed, as well as toxin stocks not placed in weapons. No information is available about bombing results on known biological warfare facilities. There is no indication that Iraq employed biologicals during the war, and there is no information about forward deployment of toxins in the theater. However, no detection system was deployed; no such system is available for aflatoxin, although there are mechanisms for detecting aflatoxin in the laboratory (Autrup et al., 1993; Harrison and Garner, 1991; Wang, 1996; Groopman et al., 1996; Ross et al., 1992). GAO (1997) suggested that aflatoxin exposure arising from U.S. attacks on chemical storage sites might have contributed to illnesses in Gulf War veterans but did not provide evidence to support the hypotheses.

The toxin is stable in the environment, is resistant to heat, and would be active after atmospheric transport from an attacked Iraqi depot. However, it is questionable how much significant toxicity would result after atmospheric dilution.

Chemical Characteristics

Figure 4.2 shows the chemical structures of eight of the 17 aflatoxins. The top four—B_1, B_2, G, and G_2,—are the four most commonly mentioned. All occur naturally. The "B" and "G" designations of these toxins relate to the fluorescence color in ultraviolet light (blue or green) while the subscripts refer to chromatographic mobility.

Mechanisms of Action

The concern about aflatoxin producing cancer in humans and animals has produced an extensive literature on the metabolism of aflatoxin and the biochemical reactions of the metabolites (Steyn, 1995; Coulombe et al., 1991, McLean and Dutton, 1995; Tutelyan and Kravchenko, 1981). Active metabolites act on several cell structures (e.g., mitochondria, lysosomes, endoplasmic reticulum), but the cancer concern has focused attention on the effects on the nucleus and DNA.

Activated AFB_1 attacks nucleic acids with the formation of adducts that can act like point mutations, damaging DNA and impairing RNA and protein synthesis (McLean and Dutton, 1995). Proteins, including receptors and those with important intracellular functions, may also be nonspecifically but irreversibly bound by toxins, producing diverse loss of function (e.g., enzyme inactivation) (Tutelyan and Kravchenko, 1981).

Acute mycotoxin injury inhibits cellular energy production. The aflatoxins act on the electron transport system, interfering with the cytochrome system (Tutelyan and Kravchenko, 1981), depleting ATP, inhibiting ATPase, and causing mitochondrial swelling (Sajan et al., 1995). The effect of aflatoxin on the electron transport system may not require activation of the toxin. Recent studies draw attention to mitochondrial disease and injury, producing liver failure

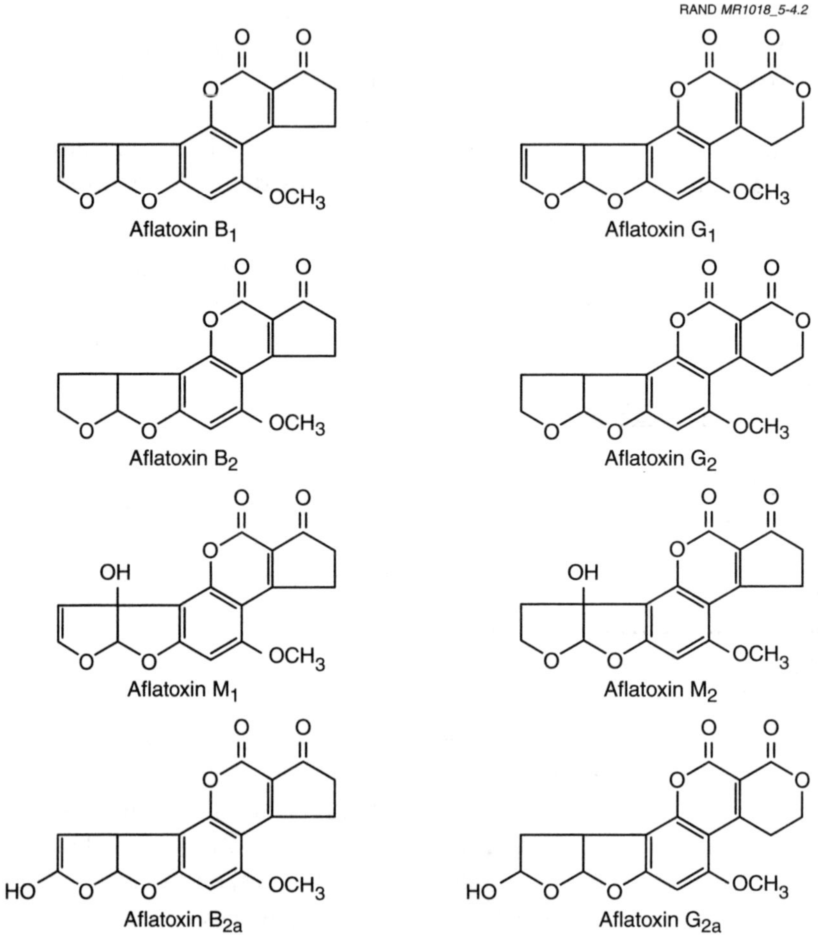

RAND MR1018_5-4.2

Aflatoxin B$_1$

Aflatoxin G$_1$

Aflatoxin B$_2$

Aflatoxin G$_2$

Aflatoxin M$_1$

Aflatoxin M$_2$

Aflatoxin B$_{2a}$

Aflatoxin G$_{2a}$

SOURCE: Reprinted with permission from McLean and Dutton (1995).

Figure 4.2—Chemical Structures of Several Aflatoxins

and associated disorders (e.g., Reyes syndrome), with brain and liver injury (Schafer and Sorrel, 1997). Carbohydrate and lipid metabolism are impaired, and hepatic glycogen stores are depleted, with a secondary rise in blood sugar. Lipids accumulate in the liver and fatty oxidation decreases, perhaps secondary to mitochondrial injury. These effects occur at levels lower than those producing RNA and growth effects (McLean and Dutton, 1995; Tutelyan and Kravchenko, 1981; Verma and Choudhary, 1995).

Activation. Metabolic activation is required to produce toxicity from AFB$_1$. After crossing the cell membrane, the molecule is activated by microsomal mixed-function oxidases involving the cytochrome P450 enzymes and nicotin-amide adenine dinucleotide phosphate reductase (NADPH) and oxygen. The active and toxic AFB_1 8,9-epoxide (Figure 4.3) is the result. This active molecule has a short half-life and binds to DNA and other structures in the endoplasmic reticulum. Other NADPH reactions can reversibly produce aflatoxicol, which can serve as a sink or source of AFB_1 in the cell. The microsomal monoxygenase system may transform AFB_1 into more polar molecules, such as AFM_1, Q_1, or P_1, which can be eliminated by liver cells (McLean and Dutton, 1995). The situation is complex, and there are other concepts of toxicity involving more indirect mechanisms associated with membrane actions involving lipid peroxidases and aldehydes (Shen et al., 1994; Tutelyan and Kravchenko, 1981); see Figure 4.4.

Detoxification. Aflatoxins are also detoxified by mechanisms that deal with xenobiotics—leading to conjugation with glucuronic acid, sulfates, or glutathione. The major route for AFB_1 detoxification is conjugation of the epoxide with glutathione (through glutathione S transferase) and subsequent excretion in bile (McLean and Dutton, 1995). This means that toxicity may vary depending on intracellular glutathione stores in various tissues, which can vary considerably with circadian effects or depletion by other factors—diet, smoking, alcohol, and medications (Tsutsumi and Miyazaki, 1994). Other aflatoxins appear to be primarily eliminated via glucuronide or sulfate conjugation. Various species differences in sensitivity to aflatoxins may reflect differences in detoxification mechanisms (McLean and Dutton, 1995).

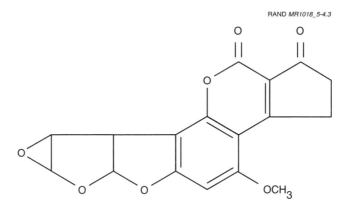

RAND *MR1018_5-4.3*

Figure 4.3—Activated AFB₁ Molecule

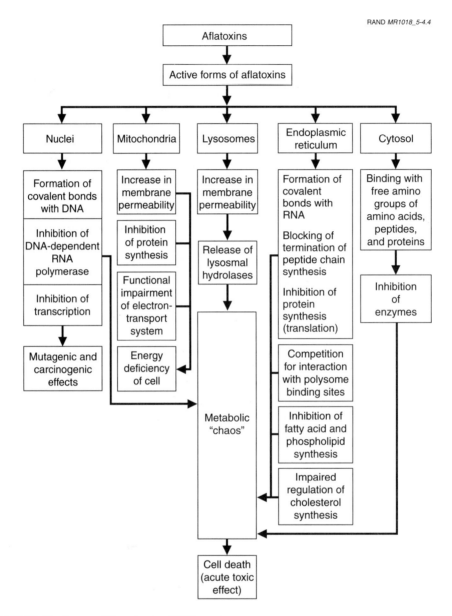

SOURCE: Tutelyan and Kravchenko (1981).

Figure 4.4—Mechanism of Effects of Aflatoxins on Cell

Exposure-Effect Relationships and Clinical Manifestations

Gastrointestinal. In Southeast Asia, intoxication occurs from ingestion of food, chiefly rice and noodles, that has been contaminated by the fungus. Outbreaks of illness attributed to oral intoxication by aflatoxin (Bourgeois et al., 1971b) have been reported in humans. Some 40 cases in Thai children were character-ized by abrupt onset of coma or convulsions, fever, respiratory distress, vomit-ing, and death within 72 hours. Serum transaminases were elevated; pro-thrombin times were prolonged; and blood sugars were lowered. Pathology findings showed neuronolysis; cerebral edema; fatty infiltrations of liver, kid-ney, and heart; and lysis of lymphatic tissues (Chao et al., 1991; Chao, 1992).

In monkeys, a Reyes-like syndrome develops, with fatty degeneration of the liver (and encephalopathy) (Bourgeois et al., 1971a). Young monkeys were given 0, 1.5, 4.5, 13.5, or 40.5 mg/kg of AFB_1 orally. Doses of 1.5 mg/kg were not fatal, and no unusual clinical signs were noted. Deaths began at 4.5 mg/kg, with others sick. All animals at higher levels died. Cough, vomiting, diarrhea, and coma were the key clinical findings. Laboratory findings were similar to those in the Thai children. Pathology was similar but also showed bile duct hyperplasia.

A well-studied outbreak occurred in Malaysia in 1988, with severe illness occurring in several towns that was eventually traced to noodles prepared from aflatoxin-contaminated grain. The noodles were also discovered to be contam-inated with boric acid used as bleach. It took an average of eight hours (a range of 3 to 16 hours) from eating the noodles to the onset of symptoms. The illness began with vomiting (in 100 percent of cases), followed by seizures (82.4 per-cent), hematemesis (82.4 percent), fever (17 percent), diarrhea (23 percent), and abdominal pain. Liver and renal failure ensued, as did coma and respiratory failure. The outbreak killed 13 children, and another 45 persons had milder symptoms. The mortality rate was high, despite supportive modern medical care (Chao et al., 1991; Lye et al., 1995; Chao, 1992; Harrison and Garner, 1991). The estimated lethal amount was 2 mg/kg (Harrison and Garner, 1991).[15]

High doses result in multiple injuries. Those the Malay children sustained included gastric erosions, although these may have been related to the boric acid simultaneously ingested (Chao et al., 1991). Chao et al. made some effort to distinguish between the effects of aflatoxin and those of boric acid. They noted the patients lacked the "boiled lobster" skin changes of heavy boric acid poisoning but believed that the diarrhea, renal problems, and metabolic acido-sis probably reflected boric acid effects. Overall, the researchers considered the toxicity to be primarily an effect of the aflatoxin. The most common findings in human and animal poisoning is liver injury (Lye 1991; Fernandez, Ramos, et al., 1995; Fernandez, Verde, et al., 1995), including macrovesicular steatosis (also a finding in Reyes syndrome), bile duct metaplasia, and centrilobular coagulative necrosis (Chao et al., 1991). AFB_1 metabolizing enzymes are present in intesti-

---

[15]As noted previously, this falls in the "highly toxic" category described by Proctor and Hughes (1978)—less toxic than most nerve agents but in the same category as lewisite and parathion.

nal epithelial cells, which can sustain mild injury from low-dose AFB_1 ingestion, impairing nutritional intake in animals (Guengerich et al., 1996). No follow-up reports are available to reveal what sequelae, if any, occurred in the survivors of acute exposures.

Northup et al. (1995) indicate that the oral LD_{50} for guinea pigs is 1 mg/kg for AFB_1.

Respiratory. No estimates for an acute human lethal or incapacitating respiratory dose are available. There are also no descriptions of acute human or other primate respiratory exposures. The human lung does possess the enzymes necessary to activate AFB_1 (Massey, 1996). At high levels of exposure, enough aflatoxin might be absorbed to produce the serious systemic illness seen in Malay children, with seizures, vomiting, coma, hepatorenal failure, and death. At low levels of exposure, there might be few obvious acute effects or only mild respiratory symptoms. However, there is some indication in animal studies that acute respiratory effects are possible at doses much lower than those required for dangerous oral intoxication (Cresia et al., 1987; Bunner et al., 1985). It may be that the Iraqis discovered some effects of that kind, and that is why they weaponized the toxin.

There has been concern about an increased risk of lung and liver cancer among humans chronically exposed to low-level AFB_1 in grain dust at mixed oral and respiratory intake levels of 0.04 to 2.5 μg per week (Massey, 1996; Autrup et al., 1993; Coulombe, 1993). Mycotoxins have been shown to have mitogenic effects at levels well below clinical toxicity (Griffiths, Rea, et al., 1996). Other than the cancer risks, however, respiratory disease or systemic illness from chronic respiratory exposure has not been found (Coulombe, 1993); Autrup et al., 1993).

There have been some significant studies on animals, although caution must be exercised in generalizing these findings to humans. Sensitivity to aflatoxins varies tenfold among species because of metabolic differences and the balance between activation and detoxification mechanisms (Coulombe et al., 1991), and species vary as to the sites where aflatoxin is activated.

Experimental animals have shown a range of aflatoxin responses from mild inflammation to more striking illness with tracheal epithelial damage, alveolar injury, and pulmonary hemorrhage (Coulombe et al., 1991; Coulombe, 1993; Jakab et al., 1994). Guinea pigs, after a large aerosol exposure, developed hemorrhage and exfoliation of epithelial cells at six hours (Northup et al., 1995). Of particular interest, since the doses are in a range of potential military interest because of high potency, is a report that guinea pigs exposed for four hours to nanogram amounts by aerosol produced hemorrhage and exfoliation of respiratory cells (Northup et al., 1995). Intratracheal aflatoxin in rats appears in the blood in 3 to 12 hours (Coulombe et al., 1991). Minor bronchial mucosal damage occurred in rats that were intratracheally exposed to 300 µg/kg microcrystalline AFB_1, but bronchiolitis occurred with intratracheal dust aflatoxin delivery (Coulombe et al., 1991).

Northup and Kilburn (1978; as cited by Hendry and Cole, 1993) reported tracheal-bronchial cell destruction in hamsters and guinea pigs from acute inhalation of aflatoxin.

Aflatoxin in rats was also retained longer when adsorbed on dust particles than when delivered in its microcrystalline form (Coulombe et al., 1991). Aflatoxins are known for their impairment of resistance to infections, so secondary respiratory and other infections might be expected. For example, macrophage function was impaired for two weeks following exposure to AFB_1 aerosol in rats (16 µg/kg) (Jakab et al., 1994). Pulmonary pathology also occurs experimentally with oral aflatoxicosis, and there was some bronchopneumonia in the Malay outbreak (Fernandez, Ramos, et al., 1995; Fernandez, Verde, et al., 1995; Chao et al., 1991).

Rats given intratracheal aflatoxin B and G for 30 weeks developed carcinomas of the liver, intestine, and kidney (as cited in Hendry and Cole, 1993: Northup and Kilburn, 1978).

Nervous and Musculoskeletal Systems. Aflatoxin is rapidly distributed to gray matter (Larsson and Tjalve, 1996), although no histopathologic descriptions of changes arising from aflatoxin exposure were found in the literature, other than the previously noted cerebral edema and neuronolysis noted in Thai and Malay children and in monkey experiments (Chao et al., 1991; Bourgeois et al., 1971a, 1971b). Animals and humans with high exposures to aflatoxin have seizures. The Malay cases showed widespread edema, with petechial hemorrhages in the white matter; however, these patients were on respirators for prolonged periods, and the brains were necrotic with impression of hypoxic encephalopathy (Chao et al., 1991). The mechanism for neurotoxicity is not clear, although brain cells have high metabolic rates, so disturbances in mitochondria and energy metabolism would be significant. No data have emerged to suggest that peripheral neuropathy is a problem arising from aflatoxin exposure, and there are no reports of musculoskeletal problems.

Studies in mice show that "nontoxic" low-level exposure to AFB_1 reduced brain levels of serotonin and catecholamines (Kimbrough, Llewellyn, and Weekley, 1992). Although the clinical significance of this observation is unknown, it is noteworthy that this type of exposure to AFB_1 affects these important neurotransmitters.

Cardiovascular and Hematologic. No reports of characteristic cardiovascular findings were found. Cardiac hemorrhages have been described in cattle acutely poisoned by aflatoxin (Rajendran et al., 1992). Fatty degeneration of heart muscle (especially atrial and conduction systems) was seen in Thai children efficiently poisoned by AFB (Bourgeois, Olson, et al., 1971).

Hematologic problems, although noted, do not seem prominent. *In vitro* studies have shown dose-related inhibition of myelopoiesis in several marrow culture models (Cukrova et al., 1991; Dugyala et al., 1994). Aflatoxins impair phagocytosis by alveolar macrophages (Richard and Thurston, 1975). The impaired production of prothrombin in the liver in serious intoxications may contribute to the observed bleeding in other tissues.

Other Sites and Systems. Because aflatoxins are soluble in DMSO (McLean and Dutton, 1995), it might be possible to deliver the toxin dissolved in DMSO through the skin. There is no information about acute or chronic cutaneous effects or hazards arising from cutaneous exposure.

Although the conjunctiva binds toxins, there is no information about inflammation or other acute or chronic toxic effects on the eye (Larsson and Tjalve, 1996).

Renal pathology is seen in acute toxicity, but does not appear to be a feature in chronic exposures. Autopsy data show swollen pale cortices with congested medullary regions. Aflatoxins M_1 and M_2 were found more often than B_1 in renal tissue (Chao et al., 1991). Bourgeois, Olson, et al. (1971) noted fatty degeneration of kidneys with proximale tubule damage.

At levels below clinical illness, aflatoxins are immunosuppressive and impair humoral and cell-mediated immunity (Griffiths et al., 1996; Raisuddin et al., 1993; Cysewski et al., 1978; Dimitri and Gabal, 1996). Although acute effects of immunosuppression in animals reversed after two weeks (Jakab et al., 1994), longer exposure has resulted in loss of suppression of toxoplasma cysts (Venturini et al., 1996). It would not be surprising to see reactivation of quiescent infections, such as herpes.

Cross-Systemic and Chronic Effects. Because of human health concerns, efforts are made to keep aflatoxins at low levels in food and milk. Interestingly, mice fed low levels of AFB_1 and AFG_1, within human exposure limits, showed signs of liver and kidney cytotoxicity, although species differences may play a role in this observation (Ankrah et al., 1993). Studies addressing chronic human exposure in occupationally exposed workers to unmeasured AFB in food show increased rates of liver cancer, impaired child health and development, and increased infections from long-term exposure (Groopman et al., 1996). No reports of neuropathy, chronic brain syndromes, skin problems, or arthropathy from chronic oral intake were available. Animal studies have found weight loss, illness, and reproductive problems from respiratory intake (Coulombe, 1993; Aulerich et al., 1993; Bonomi et al., 1995). Teratogenic effects have been observed (Raisuddin et al., 1993).

Combined Interactions

As noted before, there has been discussion of enhanced toxicity from combined exposure to trichothecenes and aflatoxins (U.S. Army, 1990). No reports of combined respiratory exposures were found. Some animal-feeding studies (chickens) found synergism (Huff et al., 1988), and others did not (Harvey et al., 1995), although the latter study showed some synergism in weight loss of a liver enzyme. We have not found a study that looked at synergism in acute respiratory exposures, which would be helpful in understanding the significance of this possible synergism.

What to Look for in the Gulf Context

The intended use of Iraqi aflatoxin weapons is unclear (Zilinskas, 1997). The toxin is stable enough to survive transport through the atmosphere and to persist trapped in dust, creating a secondary inhalation hazard. It is not clear that such transport and contamination occurred, but at low levels it would have been difficult to recognize or detect. The carcinogenic effects of aflatoxins take many years, and the risk from an acute exposure via missile attack does not seem enough to make it a credible objective.

There is insufficient information about respiratory effects in primates. Northup's finding of respiratory injury in animals with nanogram amounts of aflatoxin aerosol raises the possibility that respiratory toxicity is much greater than the better known oral toxicity, which might reflect the intended Iraqi use. Because the entire cardiac output passes the lungs, it might be possible to produce seizures, coma, and liver failure via the respiratory route.

Dramatic illness would have been noticed in the Gulf War if exposure to aflatoxin took place. There are no documented clinical reports of acute symptomatic lower-level human exposures, but extrapolation from animal studies suggests that low doses might produce respiratory irritation, nausea, malaise, and anorexia—symptoms not specifically associated with toxins or other chemical agents, where eye or skin problems would typically be expected. At levels comparable to those grain workers are exposed to, there might be no symptoms, although tissue and immune effects may occur.

Compared to most of the agents under review, it is hard to describe a "typical" aflatoxin case. As a result, it would be difficult to tie individual Gulf War illness cases to aflatoxin poisoning, even if it had occurred.

It is unknown what symptoms a combined low-level trichothecene and aflatoxin exposure would display. Although U.S. Army (1990) mentions synergistic effects, there are some data that prove a synergistic effect (Huff et al., 1988) and some that suggest that such a synergy does not always occur (Harvey et al., 1995). Studies of combined respiratory exposures would be helpful.

Summary, Conclusions, and Recommendations

Why Iraq developed weapon systems for aflatoxin remains speculative; respiratory toxicity at low levels and immunosuppression at low doses may provide hints, although there is little information about primate respiratory toxicity. Oral exposure in Malaysia led to deaths; if exposure at similar levels could be achieved through inhalation, pulmonary and systemic effects would be delayed, and there would have been no detection means (and no effective therapy). The agent, if spread in the vicinity of U.S. troops, would be stable enough to provide recurrent exposures. Although the estimated lethal dose of 2 to 4 mg/kg is not as toxic as some substances, it would be possible to create an aerosol that would deliver the 140 mg of toxin sufficient to kill a 150-pound person (if the Malay experience with children can be generalized). Of course, a full-blown outbreak of this nature would have been noted during the Gulf War. Lower levels of exposure might resemble acute oral exposure in animals, with vomiting, malaise, and nonspecific signs and symptoms.

There is no clear clinical picture that would make recognition of low-level aflatoxin exposure easy. However, there is also no information that aflatoxin was present in the Gulf War, and no descriptions of Gulf War illnesses resemble what might be expected from aflatoxin exposure.

Several steps might still be taken to assess the possibility of aflatoxin exposure in the Gulf. These include following up on a report that aflatoxin antibodies could be detected in exposed persons by measuring antibody levels in Gulf personnel and controls (Autrup et al., 1993). The antibody level in the Danish controls was low compared to that in Kenyans with high dietary intake, so finding antibodies in Gulf war veterans would not be conclusive proof of exposure to military toxin, since food exposure alone could promote antibody formation. Blood and tissue samples proximate to the Gulf deployment would be most useful, but care in study design and use of controls would be necessary. The antibody measurements are not routine but have apparently had substantial use.

Harrison and Garner (1991) detected aflatoxin and adducts in formalin-fixed pathology specimens a long time after the event in Malaysia. AFIP could consider analyzing some of its preserved tissues from Gulf cases for aflatoxins and adducts. Also, an analysis could be made of whether material from other Gulf War veterans shows adducts from aflatoxin. Adducts in Gulf War tissue material higher than those in controls would not prove a particular source of aflatoxin exposure but, if found, would require more research on this toxin.

Aflatoxin is sufficiently stable that it might still be detectable in clothing, equipment, filters, and mask canisters from the Gulf War, if they can be located. It would be useful to ask Malaysian health officials about any long-term effects in the less severe cases from the 1988 outbreak. Such a follow-up period would be about two years longer than the current Gulf War period of observation.

The aflatoxins are potent and poorly understood. They do not seem a likely explanation for the pattern of illnesses in Gulf War veterans, but it does at least appear possible to detect exposure of U.S. personnel to low levels of aflatoxins. Aflatoxins are a poorly understood agent, so further research on their possible military threats should be considered.

The respiratory toxicity of aflatoxins in primates and other species should be evaluated seriously, with some selective evaluation of combined toxicities (e.g., with trichothecenes or infectious agents). A better understanding of the mechanisms of central nervous system toxicity and immune suppression would be helpful (e.g., do aflatoxins alter responses to leishmaniasis, malaria, sand fly fever?).

Aflatoxins are known carcinogens. The induction of cancer has generally been seen in populations with sustained exposures to fairly high dietary levels of the toxin after many years (and in some situations in populations with a high prevalence of chronic hepatitis B infections). A short (few weeks), low-level exposure to aflatoxins should have little risk of increased cancer because the incremental additional amount compared to the background level in Western diets would be small.

Chapter Five

NERVE AGENTS

The military nerve agents are a family of highly toxic phosphoric acid esters, structurally related to the larger family of organophosphate compounds. In fact, development of nerve agents was a by-product of insecticide research and development (OSRD, 1946; Hayes, 1982). Germany developed nerve agents just before and during World War II; subsequently, several countries, including the United States and the Soviet Union, made them the subject of intense research and development and stockpiled them as weapons (SIPRI, 1971; SIPRI, 1973).

Nerve agents have been used in some wars since that period (SIPRI, 1971; UN, 1984; Cordesman and Wagner, 1990, 1991); to suppress internal uprisings in Iraq (Macilwain, 1993); and more recently, in large-scale terrorist attacks (Ohtomi et al., 1996; Morita et al., 1995, Okumura et al., 1996). Nerve agents have also been the subject of much concern during and since the Gulf War. They occasioned considerable defensive efforts and, later, concerns that coalition forces might have been exposed to them during the war (Riegle and D'Amato, 1994; House, 1997; Senate, 1994). The concern was increased by the discovery that U.S. forces had unknowingly destroyed a substantial amount of nerve agents in demolitions at the Iraqi depot at Khamisiyah shortly after the end of the Gulf War, resulting in possible exposure to low concentrations of nerve agents over a large area (OSAGWI, 1997a; CIA, 1997).

There is a great deal of literature on nerve agents and organophosphate pesticides, including several recent books on chemical agents (Somani, 1992; Marrs et al., 1996; Sidell, Takafuji, and Franz, 1997), with one giving a detailed summary of human studies in the UK and United States (Marrs et al., 1996; Smart, 1997; Sidell, 1997; Dunn et al., 1997; Sidell and Hurst, 1997).

This chapter provides an overview of nerve agent effects but looks especially at information about the effects of low, or inapparent, exposures on mood, memory, thinking, strength, and behavior. It also pays particular attention to information that may provide insight on mechanisms for long-term neuropathy.

HISTORY

The first nerve agent of military significance was discovered by Dr. Gerhard Schrader, a chemist conducting insecticide research with organophosphates in 1937. He synthesized ethyl-N-dimethyl-phosphoroamidocyanate, which has had a number of names since then but is most commonly called tabun. The toxicity was personally experienced by the investigators, who found that a small drop of tabun, spilled on a laboratory bench, resulted in pinpoint pupils, dim vision, headache, and difficulty breathing (OSRD, 1946; Harris and Paxman, 1982). Later animal tests showed rapid lethality. Under German law, these findings were reported to the War Ministry, which subsequently developed tabun (in 1939) and a related nerve agent, sarin, later. A third agent, soman, was discovered in 1944 (SIPRI, 1971; SIPRI, 1973). The designation "G" arose from the markings on German chemical weapons found after the war: GA for tabun, GB for sarin, and GD for soman (SIPRI, 1971).

A pilot plant at Munster Lager provided enough tabun for field trials in 1939 (OSRD, 1946). Later, larger production plants were built but encountered considerable delays, with full production of tabun beginning in 1942. Sarin proved more difficult to produce, and only in 1945 were the Germans able to produce several hundred tons of it. Soman was not produced in quantity (SIPRI, 1971; SIPRI, 1973).

Several hundred accidents occurred during the production of nerve agents, and ten workers were killed. Exposure to low levels of tabun was so common that workers were given extra milk and fat rations because it was observed that larger fat consumption had a protective effect (Harris and Paxman, 1982).

The United States and the UK conducted extensive research during World War II on some related compounds, diisopropyl flurorophosphate (DFP) (also designated as agent P-3) being the best known (OSRD, 1946), but these less-toxic variants appeared most suitable as incapacitating agents because of their ocular effects. Achieving lethal concentrations was difficult.

After the war, the United States, the UK, and the former Soviet Union conducted extensive classified research and development. The German plants and technical information were in the part of Germany the Soviets occupied. That appears to have contributed to a very large postwar Soviet chemical effort (Seagrave, 1981; Harris and Paxman 1982; SIPRI, 1971).

The United States began producing sarin on a large scale in the early 1950s; occupational exposures from that period also provided useful data. No worker died, but nearly 1,000 sustained some exposure. Illnesses were generally brief, usually only a few days, sometimes a few weeks (Craig and Freeman, 1953; Gaon and Werne, 1955; Craig et al., 1959; Holmes, 1959; Marrs et al., 1996,

Sidell, 1997). These workers have been subject to only limited follow-up, using small groups and controls (Metcalf and Holmes, 1969).

Defensive research into detection, decontamination, and treatment continues. The perception that soman was a key element in the Soviet arsenal, coupled with recognition of its high toxicity and resistance to therapy, resulted in research emphasis on this agent. The rapidity of action and resistance to oxime therapy lead to the development of pretreatment drugs (carbamate reversible inhibitors), as well as deployment of diazepam drugs with some NATO forces (NATO, 1973; Gall, 1981; Marrs et al., 1996; Sidell, 1997; Dunn et al., 1997).

Problems related to aging chemical munitions in stockpiles and decisions in many countries to eliminate chemical weapons have resulted in research into lower-dose exposures and the longer-term implications of exposure of nonmilitary populations (SIPRI, 1980; Watson et al., 1989; Dacre, 1989).

Meanwhile, development and use of organophosphate-based insecticides has proliferated, and they continue to be widely used in agriculture (Hayes, 1982). Although these insecticides are less toxic than the nerve agents, the illnesses they produce clinically resemble those nerve agents produce (Grob and Harvey, 1953; Hayes, 1982). The toxicity of these insecticides to humans is thus relevant (Haley and Kurt, 1997; Haley, Kurt, and Horn, 1997), and this chapter includes information from pesticide studies where it seems helpful. However, Sidell stresses the clinical differences between the organophosphate insecticides and nerve agents, noting that cholinergic crises from pesticides last much longer than those from military nerve agents (Sidell, 1997; Sidell and Hurst, 1997). On the other hand, reviews of possible long-term effects of nerve agents have regarded organophosphate pesticide experience as being informative (NAS, 1982; Karczmar, 1984; Boskovic and Kusic, 1980; Jamal, 1995b).

It was recognized early that the clinical-pharmacological effects of nerve agents and related organophosphate pesticides resembled the strong actions of the neurotransmitter acetylcholine (ACh). This chemical activates specialized receptors at the nerve synaptic junction, promoting discharge of the nerve on the other side of the synapse and stimulating the action of the nerve. ACh is rapidly destroyed by the enzyme acetylcholinesterase (AChE) (one of a family of serine esterase enzymes), which plays a regulatory role to limit the effects of ACh.

A key mechanism of action of nerve agents is their inhibition of AChE, which results in physiological-pathological overstimulation by excessive ACh (OSRD, 1946; Somani, 1992, Ch. 4). This common mechanism explains the similar effects of many nerve agents and their response to therapy with atropine and oximes.

These agents also inhibit a variety of other enzyme systems (e.g., serine esterases), and their effects impinge on other biological systems via mechanisms that the inhibition of AChE does not fully explain. Increased understanding of neurobiology and neurotransmitters has aided the understanding of these agents (O'Neill, 1981; Prioux-Guyonneau et al., 1982).

WEAPONIZATION

The earliest nerve agents, tabun and sarin, were considerably more toxic than the existing chemical gas weapons, such as phosgene, by a factor of 7 to 40 (Franke, 1967; OSRD, 1946). These agents were hard to detect; even when exposures were insufficient for rapid fatality, they injured and incapacitated soldiers. Liquid contamination of soils, clothing, and material could provide a secondary vapor hazard for variable periods. Artillery shells that detonated the same as ordinary shells could deliver these agents effectively (OSRD, 1946). During World War II, the Germans used aerial bombs and spray tanks for delivery. The vapor density allowed the agent to flow into lower terrain, trenches, bunkers etc., extending the hazard after the attack, which the Germans regarded as desirable.

Subsequently, many agents and potential agents were synthesized and tested. Toxicities turned out to be rather similar (Callaway and Blackburn, 1954). The several G agents varied in the threat they posed via the skin (sarin was not very effective), and efforts were made to mix them with other agents that might enhance skin penetration, such as mustards or lewisite (SIPRI, 1973; Krustanov, 1962). However, a variety of other factors, such as stability, ease of production, and physical properties, may have been more important than toxicity in weaponization decisions (SIPRI, 1971, 1973). Efforts were made to thicken the nerve agents with additives to increase their persistence and penetration (SIPRI, 1973). In the end, several countries adopted sarin, while the former Soviet Union produced soman and thickened soman (SIPRI, 1971, 1973).

The later development of the V agents, such as VX, provided a number of very toxic compounds. Although not very volatile, these could be disseminated in aerosols and provided a very high percutaneous hazard with an environmental persistence far greater than the G agents. Both Western and Soviet forces adopted these agents.

Nerve agents can be delivered by free rockets, guided missiles, and mines, as well as mortar and artillery shells, aerial bombs and submunitions, and spray tanks. Weaponized nerve agents are suitable for a large variety of military operations and for both tactical and strategic use.

Defensively, nerve agents can be used to disorganize forces in assembly areas and reserve formations. The more persistent agents can impede advancing forces, especially by reinforcing other obstacles. During the Gulf War, commanders were reasonably concerned that operations to breach Iraqi defenses might be subject to chemical attack (Clancy and Franks, 1997).

Because of the hazards and difficulties of deploying chemical weapons, the United States (and perhaps other countries) developed so-called binary weapons during the 1970s and 1980s. The ingredients to produce a nerve agent were stored separately in the munitions and then were combined to produce the agent shortly before impact (Rutman, 1976; Eyring, 1976). There are reports that Saddam Hussein claimed Iraq had such weapons,[1] but UNSCOM found none (UNSCOM, 1991, 1992, 1995). The United States found the development of such weapons to be challenging. A variety of ingredients were potentially involved, and some of the reaction by-products were also toxic (Rutman, 1976; McNamara et al., 1979). Sarin and VX are the most commonly discussed binary agents in the U.S. stockpile, but other theoretically highly toxic, although less stable, agents might be produced (Lohs, 1975).

There have been reports of a highly toxic Soviet binary nerve agent, called Novichok, designed to be undetectable by U.S. detectors (Smart, 1997). The information came from a émigré who indicated that Iraq might have acquired agents of this family. Information about these newer Soviet agents (33 and 232) is only to be found in press reports interviews and Internet postings (Englund, 1992a, 1992b; Adams, 1996; Tucker, 1996). No detailed or peer-reviewed scientific data are available.

RELEVANCE TO THE GULF WAR

Nerve agents are relevant to illnesses in Gulf War veterans for two reasons: Iraq had developed a chemical capability and had used nerve agents prior to the Gulf War, and there was some potential for exposure of U.S. troops during the conflict.

Iraq's Capability

Iraq's acts against the Kurds were an early indication of its chemical capability,[2] while the Iran-Iraq War showed considerable and improving Iraqi use of a variety of agents, not all of which were identified (Cordesman and Wagner, 1990). Tabun was definitely used against Iranian forces (UN, 1984). Typical nerve agent casualties were independently confirmed, and tabun was identified in a bomb, mixed with chlorobenzene (a stabilizer) in a percentage quite similar to what the Germans used in World War II (OSRD, 1946). In later fighting, Iraq appears to have used nerve agents with some success in attacks in the southern

---

[1] "Iraqi Threat of Chemical Warfare with Israel" (1990).

[2] "Iraq: How Iraq is Defying the World Concerning the Alleged Use of Chemical Weapons by its Armed Forces Against the Kurdish Population" (1988); Macilwain (1993).

sector (Cordesman and Wagner, 1990). Although sarin and cyclosarin might have been used in these attacks, there was reason to be concerned that Iraq's large chemical program might also have produced soman. More recently, UNSCOM suspected and later documented that Iraq had produced VX. Iraq initially admitted to some research on VX, but admitted to UNSCOM late in 1996 that it had produced 3.9 tons of VX as well as 58.5 tons of precursor chemicals (Miller, 1998).

After the Gulf War, the UN became aware that Iraq had substantial stocks of tabun, sarin, and cyclosarin—with sarin and cyclosarin being present in the 122-mm rockets destroyed at Khamisiyah. A barrage of such rockets can rapidly establish a lethal concentration over a large area, representing great danger to personnel not wearing respirators. Cyclosarin can also be a more persistent threat than sarin and is a greater percutaneous hazard (U.S. Army, 1990).

It seems unlikely that potential use of such agents against coalition forces had been the reason Iraq chose them. Development of weapons takes considerable time, and the coalition formed rapidly. Tabun has some persistence and is the easiest agent to produce. It is also capable of producing incapacity for many military functions at levels well below lethal concentrations (OSRD, 1946). As with other Iraqi nerve agents, tabun is suitable for both offensive and defensive use.

The discovery that Iraq had substantial stocks of cyclosarin was interesting because, although this agent was fairly well known, no major power had adopted it. Iraq may have selected it to provide a more persistent and percutaneously effective agent than sarin, one that also has formidable inhalation toxicity. With a sarin production capability, Iraq may have found it easier to produce cyclosarin than to develop VX. However, Sidell, Takafuji, and Franz (1997) indicates that Iraq may have produced cyclosarin because precursor chemicals for sarin—but not those for cyclosarin (e.g., cyclohexyl alcohol)—had been embargoed.

Coalition forces offered many potential targets to Scud missiles: airfields, ports, assembly areas, and logistic facilities, some proximate to urban areas. The Iraqi Scuds had payloads sufficient to place considerable agent on target, although not with great accuracy. Before the air war began, Iraq had a substantial air force, which had demonstrated some ability to deliver chemical agents (Cordesman, 1990; UN, 1984; Zilinskas, 1997), which threatened both the same targets as missiles did and other tactical targets.

Writings after the war indicated that U.S. commanders were concerned about the threat of chemical agents to their forces, especially during initial efforts to breach Iraqi defenses, when friendly forces would be concentrated in identifiable locations and not be moving rapidly (Clancy and Franks, 1997). Training emphasized protective equipment and, as the attack risk increased, the use of pretreatment medications.

Potential for Exposure

Both before and after the start of the air war, there were many alarms from chemical-agent detection systems. The significance of these alarms remains controversial. They apparently resulted from other environmental contaminants, and confirmatory tests generally did not find proof of an agent, although some allied force reports continue to raise doubts (Riegle and D'Amato, 1994). Some have alleged that a nerve agent was present, perhaps from attacks on Iraqi chemical storage facilities, while the general position of DoD and other analysts has been that sarin would be unlikely to present a hazard after being dispersed over hundreds of kilometers and thus having the opportunity to disperse and to hydrolyze (OSAGWI, 1998b; PAC, 1996b).

In two separate accidental exposures during the 1950s at Dugway Proving Ground, workers developed signs, symptoms, and laboratory evidence of mild nerve agent exposure in a test area three days after a sarin test, when it was thought safe to work without protection. In both incidents, it was noted there was a lot of dust blowing at the time of exposure, but the exact locations with respect to test area were not indicated. At the time, it was suspected that sarin had survived longer than expected because it was trapped on dust particles. No environmental samples were taken. The severity resembled that seen with a vapor exposure CT of 15 mg-min/m^3. This suggests that, in some circumstances, sarin trapped on dust particles may persist for a long time and represent a hazard when stirred into the air (Brody and Gammill, 1954; Craig and Freeman, 1953). Craig and Freeman (1953) described an exposure that took place 24 hours after a test: The safety officer had thought it safe to be in the immediate test area without protection because the weather was warm. Again, exposure seemed to be from dust.

Earlier military research had shown that sarin and the organophosphate pesticide paraoxon trapped on small inert particles were highly toxic to experimental animals (Asset and Finklestein, 1951). Particle delivery is a key means of distributing pesticides. No information was available about the details of the models used to estimate agent dispersion from Iraq to Saudi Arabia, or for the Khamisiyah event, or whether particle trapping is even considered relevant to such models. There are indications that sarin trapped on dust may persist and be dangerous longer than is commonly thought. Declassified reports (Defense Intelligence Agency, 1997) indicate an awareness of Iraqi "dusty mustard," but also noted that other agents might be used in dusty form.

The DoD position has been that Iraq did not use chemical weapons, and there do not appear to have been any readily recognizable casualties from nerve agent attacks. However, as discussed in detail below, there is precedent for misinterpretation of low-level exposures (Gaon and Werne, 1955), and there is some reason to think that the pyridostigmine bromide (PB) pretreatments U.S. troops received could have reduced the intensity of response to low-level challenges (Gall, 1981; Husain, Kumar, et al., 1993; Vijayaraghavan, Husain, et al., 1992).

Controversy thus remains about Iraqi use of chemical weapons,[3] with allegations that there might have been some. Even if the Iraqi higher command had explicitly instructed troops not to use chemicals, they appear to have been present in the operational area.[4] At least some of these lacked distinctive markings, making accidental release feasible. There is no proof that this occurred, however. UNSCOM, as cited in PAC (1997), indicates there were no chemical agents in Kuwait or in Iraq south of Khamisiyah. OSAGWI has also extensively investigated all suspected cases and to date has not been able to confirm chemical weapon exposure except one case for a single individual and in the case of Khamisiyah (OSAGWI, 1997d).

Khamisiyah

It is clear that U.S. forces unknowingly destroyed Iraqi chemical weapons in March 1991 at the Khamisiyah depot, thinking that these were conventional munitions (OSAGWI, 1997a). Rockets containing sarin and cyclosarin were destroyed by explosive charges, releasing some agent into the atmosphere. Several studies have attempted to model exposures from this incident (Babarsky, 1998; CIA, 1997). One study under way (Gray et al., 1998) used the plume analysis to identify troops who had been more and less exposed to the sarin. The case narrative (OSAGWI, 1997a) had indicated that there were no reports of immediate clinical effects on the nearest troops. In an effort to rule out longer-term effects from low-level exposure, the researchers are now comparing the hospitalization experiences of the 61,000 personnel potentially exposed to the plume with a group of 250,000 who had been in the region but not in the plum pattern. Low-level exposure effects are discussed later in this review.

Hypotheses

Unexplained illnesses in personnel returning from the Gulf War generally do not "fit" the pattern of readily recognized disorders associated with nerve agents. Many hypotheses are being tested. Congressional testimony (Riegle

---

[3]"Researcher Claims Iraq Fired Chemical Weapons During Gulf War" (1997).

[4]"Iraq May Have Moved Chemical Weapons into Southern Kuwait" (1990).

and D'Amato, 1994; House, 1997; Senate, 1994) questioned whether a combination of exposures to chemicals might have produced a new delayed-onset disease. The chemicals may have included pesticides, such as the personal repellent diethyl-*m*-toluamide (DEET), the anti–nerve agent prophylactic PB, and perhaps chemical warfare agents.

Veteran Reports

Studies of selected, defined small groups of ill Gulf veterans and controls in the United States (Haley, Kurt, and Horn, 1997; Haley, Horn, et al., 1997; Haley and Kurt, 1997; Hom, Haley, and Kurt, 1997) both found epidemiological indications of unusual exposures (e.g., flea collars, being outside during attacks) and identified three to six clinical syndromes. They found subtle indications of diffuse neurological injury in a smaller group of 23 veterans and suggested a variant of delayed organophosphate neuropathy, with the suggestion, based on animal research, that nerve agents could not be ruled out as being involved (Abou-Donia et al., 1996; Husain, Kumar, et al., 1993; Husain, Vijayaraghavan, et al., 1993). Jamal et al. (1996), studying ill UK Gulf veterans, found indications of subtle neurological injury, with sensory peripheral neuropathy being the most striking, although exposure studies were not reported. Where the Jamal studies correspond to those of Haley and Hom, they do not always agree; for example, Haley and Hom did not detect sensory neuropathy, while Jamal did not find the abnormal evoked responses that Haley and Hom did. There was, however, evidence of some organic neurological disorder in both groups of ill veterans. The significance of these findings is controversial; while the authors considered them statistically significant, others question the statistical techniques.

The RAND report on pesticides (Cecchine et al., 2000) will document the use of anticholinesterase pesticides in the Gulf theater, while self-reported exposure interviews (Haley and Kurt, 1997) document some unauthorized use of commercial "flea-collar" devices that contained chlorpyrifos. Pesticides are discussed here only with respect to possible interactions with nerve agents.

This review cannot determine the causes of illnesses in Gulf War veterans, but it provides a background of information about nerve agent effects to help analyze hypotheses and plan further studies. PB is discussed only in the context of interactions with nerve agents; a separate report has been issued on PB (Golomb, 1999).

CHEMICAL CHARACTERISTICS

The common structural framework for the agents under consideration is shown in Figure 5.1 (key in Table 5.1), with a table showing the particular groups attached in the various agents. The thio-analogs (e.g., thiosarin) substitute

RAND *MR1018_5-5.1*

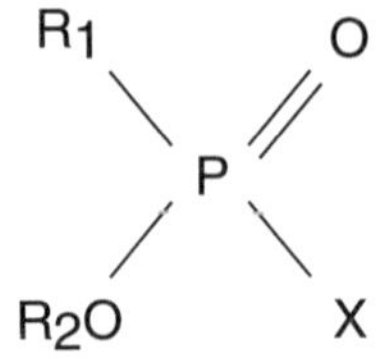

$$ R_1 \diagdown \quad O $$

P

$$ R_2O \quad X $$

SOURCE: AD Little (1986, Ch. 5).
NOTE: See Table 5.1

Figure 5.1—Chemical Structures of Nerve Agents

Table 5.1

Nerve Agent Chemical Structure

Agent	X	R_1	R_2
Tabun (GA)	CN	$N(CH_3)_2$	C_2H_5
Sarin (GB)	F	CH_3	$CH(CH_3)_2$
Soman (GD)	F	CH_3	$CH(CH_3)C(CH_3)_3$
Cyclosarin (GF)	F	CH_3	Cyclohexyl
VX	$SCH_2CH_2N[CH(CH_3)_2]_2$	CH_3	C_2H_5

SOURCE: SIPRI (1973).
NOTE: Keyed to Figure 5.1.

double-bonded S for double-bonded O. The chemical and physical properties are given in Appendix B.

A carbon-phosphorous bond is common to the nerve agents but is rare in the less-toxic organophosphate pesticides (SIPRI, 1973). Thousands of organophosphate compounds have been synthesized. Because of their chemical characteristics, nerve agents slowly degrade in water, with half-lives from 5 to 40 hours, depending on pH.

The military agents are racemic mixtures of stereoisomers. There are (+) and (–) forms of tabun and sarin, while soman has four chiral forms (Benschop, Berends, and de Long, 1981). The different isomers and mixtures thereof have important toxicological and kinetic differences; for example, the (–) isomer of sarin is more toxic than the racemic mixture (SIPRI, 1973; Boter and Dijk, 1969).

RELATED CHEMICALS

Many chemicals are related to the nerve agents. Some are even more toxic (e.g., Tammelin esters, fluorophosphocholines, phosphothiocholates) (SIPRI, 1973; Binenfeld, 1967). Others include such agents as GE, VM, VS, Gd42, Gd83, and

DFP and such pesticides as amidon, parathion, malathion, paraoxon, chlorpyrifos, systox, tetraethyl pyrophosphate. Of note is TOCP, an organophosphate chemical that is a very weak inhibitor of AChE compared to most of the other organophosphates. TOCP, however, produces delayed neuropathy (Hayes, 1982).

DETECTION

Sight and smell are unreliable means of detecting nerve agents (although some have characteristic odors). It has been difficult to develop detectors that are more sensitive than the miotic response of the human eye although that has been the goal.

MILITARY SYSTEMS

A number of measurement systems are not used operationally (Department of the Army, 1996). Field systems include ion mobility spectrometers (the M8A1 alarm and the CAM device), chemical reaction kits (M256A1), enzyme-based detection (the M256A1 and some foreign systems, such as the Czech GSP11), and mass spectrometers (the MM-1 system in Fox vehicles) (DSB, 1994; OSAGWI, 1997f; OSAGWI, 1998b; OSAGWI, 1997c).

The M8A1 alarm system, which U.S. forces use widely, is designed to detect nerve agents as vapors or aerosols. It responds within less than 2 minutes to G agents in the range of 0.1 to 0.2 mg/m^3 and to VX at 0.4 mg/m^3. The bias is toward sensitivity, not specificity, and a large number of interfering chemicals can produce false alarms (smokes, fuels, insecticides, paint fumes, cologne) (OSAGWI, 1997f).

The M256A1 system is used not as an alarm but for confirmatory testing. This is a slower response system than the M8A1 alarm, taking 15 minutes for nerve agent analyses, but it is able to detect nerve agent vapors at 0.005 mg/m^3 of G agents and 0.02 mg/m^3 of V agents. This system is less influenced by the interferants that affect the M8A1 (DSB, 1994).

The UK's CAM also uses ion mobility spectrometry but responds to nerve agents at or below 0.1 mg/m^3 within less than a minute. This device also can detect mustard agent vapors (DSB, 1994).

The Fox nuclear, biological, and chemical reconnaissance vehicle is optimized to detect and mark surface contamination by chemical weapons. The system uses a mass spectrometer that is configured to determine suspected threat chemicals promptly, then determine the spectra of specific agents more definitively. This system is less sensitive than the alarms—requiring levels of about 62 mg/m^3 and 45 seconds to respond to nerve agents. Events during the Gulf War showed that oil fires and oil vapors could interfere with the system and cause some false alarms. The vehicle was also equipped with the M8A1 alarm (OSAGWI, 1997c).

There are also detector papers used to detect droplets, and according to DSB (1994), M8 paper responds to G or V droplets of 0.02 ml with a color change within 20 seconds or less. M9 paper responds with a color change but to smaller 100 μm drops.

Regarding the sensitivity of detectors in comparison with human thresholds for eye effects, the Subcommittee on Toxicity Values for Selected Nerve and Vesicant Agents (NAS, 1997) estimates miosis levels as follows:

- VX—0.09 mg-min/m^3
- cyclosarin—0.2 mg-min/m^3
- soman—0.2 mg-min/m^3
- sarin—0.5 mg-min/m^3 (or somewhat higher)
- tabun—0.5 mg-min/m^3 (or somewhat higher).

This suggests that, for the M8A1 at least, it is quite possible for miosis to occur from VX before detector alarming, with miosis from cyclosarin and soman occurring sooner or at the same time as detection. In the cases of tabun and sarin, the detection is likely to precede miosis.

TISSUES

There has recently been progress in documenting the presence of sarin in body fluids from patients exposed in the Japanese attacks. Frozen serum samples taken from hospitalized cases were found to contain sarin in the range of 0.2 to 4.1 ng/ml. The methodology, too complex to detail here, may be useful for biological monitoring of exposed workers, for confirming exposures, and in patient care (Polhuijs, Langenberg, and Benschop, 1997).

Urinary metabolites of sarin were followed in a patient from the Matsumoto, Japan, incident. Two metabolites—methylphosphonic acid (MPA) and iso-propylmethylphosphonic acid (IMPA)—were identified on the first day after the attack. By day 3, MPA was barely detectable, but IMPA was measured for one week. Total excretion was 2.1 mg for IMPA and 0.45 mg for MPA. Estimated total sarin exposure was 0.05 mg/kg (Nakajima, Sasaki, et al., 1998).

Analysis of urine samples from four Tokyo victims not only documented sarin and sarin metabolites, such as IMPA, but also detected chemicals associated with sarin products, such as ethyl-sarin and its metabolite, ethyl methylphosphonic acid. Other contaminants associated with sarin production were found in substantial amounts: ethyl alcohol, isopropyl alcohol, isopropyl methyl phosphonate, and diethylphosphonate (Minami et al., 1998).

Although congressional testimony (Riegle and D'Amato, 1994) emphasized agent alarms after the start of the air war, there were alarms before then, probably false positives. To conserve battery power, fewer detectors were turned on before the air war and therefore one would expect fewer alarms before the air war (OSAGWI, 1999).

ENVIRONMENTAL EFFECTS AND PERSISTENCE

Compared to other organophosphate compounds, nerve agents are highly to extremely toxic. Nerve agents are highly toxic to vertebrates and invertebrates, and their persistence in soil and water can be quite harmful. Demilitarization research has considered these factors. Table 5.2 describes the persistence of the various agents. The threat that persistent agents pose can affect military operations, e.g., by restricting the use of contaminated facilities.

Table 5.2

Persistence of Nerve Agents

Agent	Persistence
Tabun	Heavily splashed liquid lasts one to two days, depending on weather. Takes 20 times as long as water to evaporate. Persists in water one day at 20°C and six days at 5°C.
Sarin	Little persistence. Evaporates as fast as water or kerosene.
Soman	Heavily splashed liquid lasts one to two days (depending on weather). Takes four times as long as water to evaporate. Thickeners can extend the duration of persistence.
Cyclosarin	Heavily splashed liquid lasts one to two days (depending on weather). Takes 20 times as long as water to evaporate.
Thiosarin	Unknown
VX[a]	Splashed liquid can persist for weeks to months. Calculated to evaporate 1,500 times slower than sarin.

SOURCE: U.S. Army (1990).
[a]Other V agents are similar.

TOXICOLOGY AND TOXICOKINETICS

Nerve agent effects were satisfactorily modeled in the 1940s and 1950s, providing an understanding of the mechanisms of action and the clinical pathological findings and guiding therapy. But this knowledge, based on weapon development and efforts to improve casualty care, focuses on higher-level exposures, rather than the mild to subclinical exposure levels that might be relevant for Gulf War studies. Also, interactions with common pharmaceuticals and other environmental toxins have not been studied, although interactions with heat, cold, and exercise have been.

There are differences in opinion as to how pertinent studies of organophosphate pesticides are to understanding nerve agents. Clinical differences between organophosphate pesticides and nerve agents should be kept in mind, as will be discussed later. Sidell (1997) emphasized the rapid onset of nerve agent effects compared with those of organophosphate pesticides and noted the longer and more-difficult-to treat course of serious organophosphate pesticide poisoning. Likewise, no seriously poisoned nerve agent casualty has been reported to have the intermediate syndrome that Senanayake and Karalliedde (1987) described as arising from pesticide exposure.

Cholinesterase inhibitors have been used therapeutically in the past for glaucoma and are used currently to treat myasthenia gravis (Harrison, 1997). Cholinesterase inhibitors are currently the most established treatment strategy in Alzheimer's disease—several drugs, including tacrine, donazepil, and rivastigmine are in use, and many others are under study (Nordberg and Svensson, 1998).

REASONS FOR CONSIDERING ORGANOPHOSPHATE PESTICIDE EFFECTS

Although organophosphate pesticides are less-potent inhibitors of AChE than nerve agents and have less-steep dose-response curves, the two groups share many features in common: inhibiting AChE and other serine esterases and interacting with receptors similarly. Ignoring the human experience with organophosphate chemicals in looking at lower-dose effects and the possibility of longer-term effects from such exposures and assessing effects from unrecognized exposures would neglect much of the relevant evidence, in the opinion of this author.

At the clinical level, the early signs and symptoms of nerve agents and those of organophosphate pesticides are identical, so there is no ready distinction between them. Early investigators such as Grob and Harvey (1953, 1958) showed equal interest in other organophosphate pesticides and at times included them in studies using nerve agents. Organophosphate pesticides are sometimes used in laboratory models to understand nerve agent effects. Since follow-up information on nerve agents is limited, the somewhat greater human experience with organophosphate pesticides may be instructive in looking for possible effects. Those interested in organophosphate pesticides have also noted common features of longer-term effects (Korsak and Sato, 1977). It is of course impossible to discuss delayed neuropathy without considerable reference to non–nerve agent organophosphates; likewise, experience with organophosphate pesticides illuminates understanding of the common mechanisms of tolerance both classes share. Interactions between environmental exposures to organophosphate pesticides and the effects of nerve agents are also possible.

The model is that these agents inhibit AChE, resulting in excessive ACh effects within the nervous system. The peripheral cholinergic systems are best understood, while the central nervous system picture continues to evolve. Central cholinergic systems are important in protective systems, locomotion, alertness, and memory and in the regulation of a number of cyclic and periodic behaviors (Petras, 1984).

NON-AChE EFFECTS

It became evident over time that inhibition of AChE did not completely explain the effects of nerve agents. Van Meter, Karczamar, and Fiscus (1978) showed that administering sarin or DFP to rabbits, even when the brain AChE was profoundly inhibited by a first dose of these agents with atropine treatment to prevent seizures, that a second dose of agent produced seizures although there was no AChE to inhibit. In their related studies, even when the enzyme was fully protected by physostigmine pretreatment, large doses of the agents were lethal. Therefore, lethality was not closely related to AChE inhibition. They concluded that the agents could act directly on central nervous system sites (see later discussions).

It has also been recognized that nerve agents can also inhibit enzymes outside of the cholinergic system, chiefly serine esterases. O'Neill (1981) reviewed data that indicated a role for anticholinesterase compounds, such as DFP or nerve agents, in altering the metabolism and persistence of important neuropeptides, such as endorphins, enkephalins, and substance P, which are degraded by serine esterases—producing some symptoms of agent exposure that do not respond to atropine. Experimental support of this concept of non-ChE effects on the brain is provided by Clement and Copeman (1984), who found a long-lasting analgesia in mice following exposure to soman and sarin, which was reversed by the opiate antagonist nalaxone. They also infer that inhibition of proteases may increase the effects of endogenous opioids. No information was available on changes in opioid receptors following exposure to anti-cholinesterase drugs.

Before the discovery of nerve agents, it was known that some organophosphorus compounds (e.g., TOCP) could cause a delayed neuropathy occurring weeks after exposure, in people and animals, the effect being quite separate from any AChE effects. This disorder, organophosphate-induced delayed neuropathy (OPIDN), has been the subject of much study (Abou-Donia, 1981; Johnson, 1975; Johnson, 1992). The disorder was complex, with sensitivities varying according to age, species, and chemical. The hen came to be the standard screening model (Johnson, 1975).

An enzyme, neuropathy target esterase (NTE), was recognized as playing a role in the disorder. Naturally, the nerve agents came under scrutiny for their ability to induce neuropathy (see later discussions). Different agents have been found to vary considerably in their ability to inhibit NTE and to produce neuropathy. It was shown (in hens) that repeated subneurotoxic doses of DFP or sarin, in animals protected by atropine and the oxime P2S, could develop delayed neuropathy even at dosing intervals of 16 days (Davies and Holland, 1972).

Prior to the Gulf War, the prevailing view was that some military agents could acutely produce delayed neuropathy only at very high levels, many times the lethal doses of the agents (and requiring "heroic" treatment efforts for the cholinergic problems) (Marrs, Maynard, and Sidell, 1996; Sidell, Takafuji, and Franz, 1997, Ch. 8; Bucci, Parker, and Gosnell, 1992b, 1992c; Gordon et al., 1983). The reviewer did not find discussions of hazards from repeated low-dose exposures, although neuropathy from repeated low doses of other neurotoxic chemicals was known.

But the concern with illnesses after the Gulf War has turned attention toward that possibility. Haley et al. have suggested that an atypical delayed neuropathy might be involved in some Gulf War illnesses (Haley, Horn, et al., 1997; Haley and Kurt, 1997; Haley, Kurt, and Hom, 1997; Hom, Haley, and Kurt, 1997; and Somani, 1997). There is a report that inhaled sarin in mice at daily doses that do not produce cholinergic signs of illness can produce typical delayed neuropathy after 10 days of exposure (the does would be very symptomatic in humans) (Husain, Vijayaraghavan, et al., 1993); see later discussions.

Regardless of the proximate mechanism of action, a complex cascade of effects can follow once the toxic effect of the nerve agent is initiated: seizures and hypoxia, with the excitotoxins the seizures release producing neuronal injury (Lipton and Rosenberg, 1994).

MECHANISM OF ACTION—ACUTE EFFECTS

ACh (Figure 5.2) serves as the neurohumeral transmitter at the endings of post-ganglionic parasympathetic nerve fibers, between somatic motor nerves and skeletal muscle, at preganglionic fibers of both sympathetic and parasympathetic nerves, and at synapses within the central nervous system (Goodman and Gilman, 1990). Normally, as a nerve impulse arrives at a cholinergic synapse, or neuroeffector junction, ACh is liberated in packets from storage vesicles, crosses the synaptic cleft, and stimulates specialized choline receptors of the adjacent neuron, depolarizing the postsynaptic membrane (Figures 5.3 and 5.4). ACh is almost immediately inactivated by the enzyme AChE, producing choline and acetic acid. Transmission of the impulse ceases, and the membrane repolarizes and is ready to respond again.

Nerve agents and organophosphate pesticides bind to the enzyme, first in a reversible way. Many agents then "age" the enzyme, producing a very difficult-to-reverse bond (Figure 5.5). The aging rate varies with the agent and is an important therapeutic consideration. VX ages slowly (many hours), while soman ages rapidly (6 minutes) (SIPRI, 1976; De Jong, 1987). The carbamate inhibitors, such as eserine and PB, also inhibit the enzyme, but reversibly.

As a consequence of nerve agent inhibition of AChE, ACh accumulates at synapses, giving rise to uncoordinated bursts of signals, initially stimulating function and then paralyzing it. This brings about the characteristic signs and symptoms, which are usually grouped as follows (Klaassen, 1996; Goodman and Gilman, 1990; Marrs et al., 1996; Koelle, 1994):

1. **muscarinic**—miosis, increased lachrymation, increased nasal secretions, tightness in chest, wheezing, increased bronchial mucus, increased gastrointestinal tone, cramps, peristalsis, nausea, vomiting, diarrhea, increased sweating, frequent urination, bradycardia, and heart block

2. **nicotinic**—muscle weakness, fasciculations, fibrillation, cramps, difficulty breathing, pallor, elevated blood pressure, and tachycardia

3. **central**—headache, dizziness, impaired memory and alertness, anxiety, tension, irritability, emotional instability, lethargy, ataxia, seizures, insomnia, excessive dreaming, coma, respiratory depression, and paralysis.

The predominant findings in acute intoxication are explained by AChE inhibition as manifested by the above responses and are similar with both nerve agents and organophosphate pesticides. However, the situation in the central nervous system is complex. Receptors activated by ACh can also modulate the release of other neurotransmitters within the brain (Goyal, 1989). Nerve agents may directly affect the release of other transmitters by mechanisms unrelated to cholinergic receptors (Prioux-Guyonneau et al., 1982).

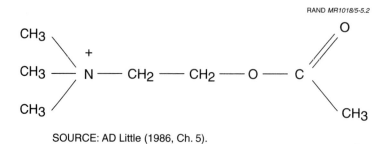

SOURCE: AD Little (1986, Ch. 5).

Figure 5.2—Chemical Structure of ACh

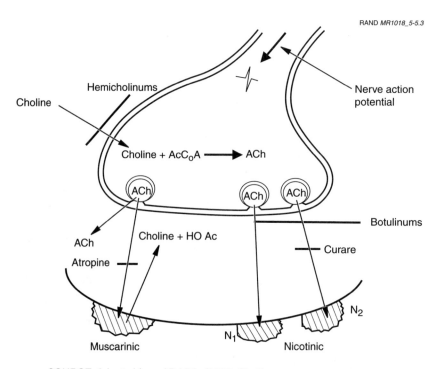

SOURCE: Adapted from AD Little (1986, Ch. 5).

Figure 5.3—Cholinergic Action and Effects of Drugs and Toxins

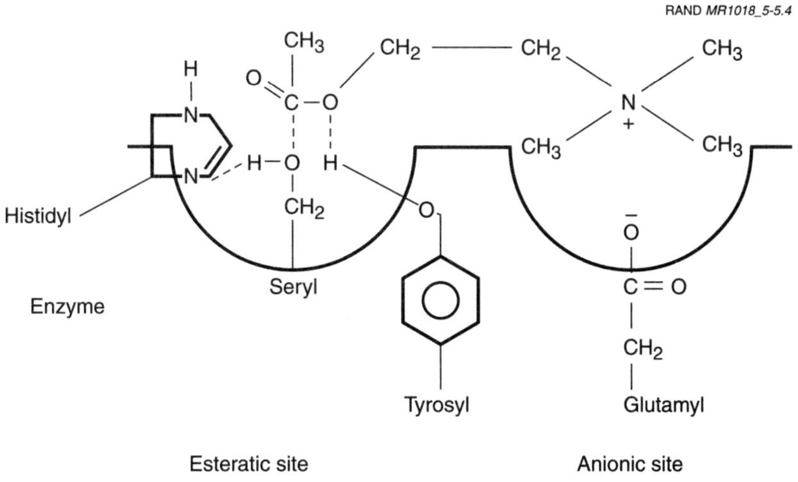

RAND *MR1018_5-5.4*

SOURCE: Adapted from AD Little (1986, Ch. 5).

Figure 5.4—AChE Active Site, with ACh

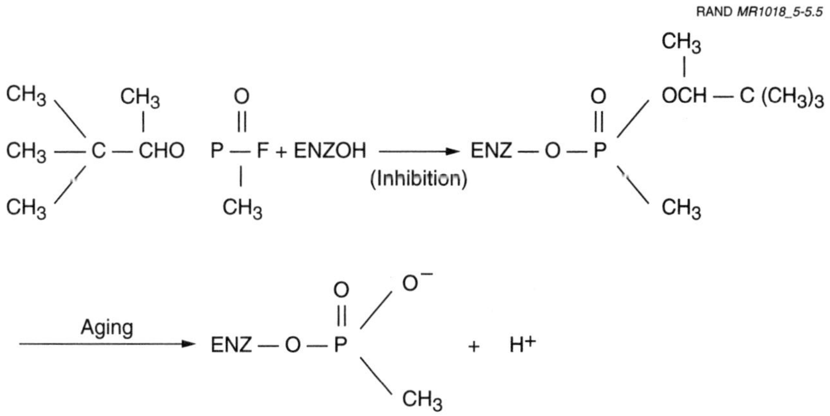

RAND *MR1018_5-5.5*

SOURCE: Adapted from AD Little (1986, Ch. 5)

Figure 5.5—Reaction of Nerve Agents with AChE

AChE INHIBITORS

A common index of the relative potency of various agents is the negative log of the molar concentration required to inhibit 50 percent of the AChE *in vitro* (the pI_{50}). The higher the pI_{50}, the more potent the ability to inhibit cholinesterase and, in general, the greater the toxicity. Because this is a logarithmic measure, a difference of 1 in pI_{50} is a difference of a factor of 10 in actuality. Table 5.3 is more precise in predicting the inhibition of the enzyme than in predicting toxic effects.[5] Animal studies show a correlation between potency and toxicity. Many drugs and chemicals are weak cholinesterase inhibitors, with pI_{50}s of about 2 (e.g., cysteine, glutathione, streptomycin, chloramphenicol, penicillin, quinine, quinidine, antimalarials, antihistamines, and ranitidine) (Root and Hofmann, 1967).

Alkylating agents used in chemotherapy and for immune suppression, such as cyclophosphamide, inhibit AChE and serum cholinesterase, requiring modifications of anesthesia given proximate to their use (PDR, 1998). Sulfur mustard also inhibits cholinesterase (Krustanov, 1962; Dacre and Goldman, 1996).

Toluene, an organic solvent, at levels of 2,000 parts per million, has been shown *in vivo* and *in vitro* to inhibit AChE bound to red blood cell and synaptic membranes (Korpela and Tahti, 1988). Other aromatic and chlorinated hydrocarbons inhibited red cell AChE *in vitro* (Korpela and Tahti, 1986a, 1986b). Another study showed *in vitro* red cell inhibition from a variety of hydrocarbons (including benzene, xylene, and trichloroethylene); ethanol also slightly inhibited the enzyme (Korpela and Tahti, 1986a, 1986b). Lower levels of toluene (300 parts per million) *in vitro* also inhibited red cell AChE.

A comparison of rates of inhibition of eel AChE by oxono (P = O) inhibitors and thiono analogs (P = S) of several agents (paraoxon, fonofos, sarin, and soman) showed that the oxono compounds had substantially higher phosphorylation rate constants than their thiono analogs. This was thought to be due to differ-

Table 5.3

**Anticholinesterase Potency of
Organophosphates**

Agent	pI_{50}
Tabun	8.6
Sarin	8.9
Soman	9.2
Thiosoman	8.9
Cyclosarin	10.1
VX	8.8
DFP	6.5
Parathion	4.9

NOTE: See text for definition of pI_{50}.
SOURCES: (Dacre, 1984; SIPRI, 1973).

---

[5]Other measures of relative potency, such as LD_{50} ratios, have also been explored.

ences in hydrophobicity of the analogs (Maxwell and Brecht, 1992). Aging of the enzyme was not reported.[6] Note that AChE is found in a number of tissues that lack neural connections, such as erythrocytes, lymphocytes, basophils, spermatozoa, and placenta (Sastry and Sadavongvivad, 1979). The functional role of the enzyme in such tissues is not known, and although it is inhibited there by nerve agents, the biological consequences are little understood (Sastry and Sadavongvivad, 1979; Meier et al., 1985).

PRETREATMENTS AND TREATMENTS FOR NERVE AGENT POISONING

This review is not concerned with treatment of nerve agent injury, but the basic pretreatment approach is described below.[7] The term *pretreatment* is used to describe an intervention made before exposure to assist with treatment required after exposure. This is distinct from prophylactic intervention, which may protect to the point that therapy is not required. At one time, there was serious consideration of using atropine (or atropinelike drugs) or oximes (reactivators) as pretreatments (Karakchiev, 1973, SIPRI, 1976).

The main current approach is to use a drug like PB that binds to cholinesterase in a reversible manner, in an amount that leaves many functional sites untouched, avoiding toxicity. When a soldier encounters a nerve agent, such as soman, that binds irreversibly to the enzyme, the sites occupied by the drug are protected from attack. After the dose of nerve agent has reacted elsewhere, the reversible drug PB leaves the enzyme site, restoring function. This approach is needed for agents, such as soman, that "age" and bind rapidly to the enzyme in a way that oxime drug treatment cannot reverse.

Koster (1946) used the carbamate physostigmine to protect cats from DFP. The very rapid aging of the enzyme bound by soman (about 6 minutes) caused great interest in NATO countries in using carbamates to pretreat for this Soviet threat agent. Several countries, including the United States, chose PB (used to treat myasthenia gravis) (Sidell, Takafuji, and Franz, 1997). This drug, the subject of a separate RAND report (Golomb, 1999), ordinarily does not cross the blood-brain barrier because of its polar nature (Goodman and Gilman, 1990).

No discussion was found on the situation of continued PB use after unrecognized exposure to nerve agent. One concludes that an unstated assumption within the research and medical community about PB use was that attacks would be obvious and that PB would not be used after intoxications.

---

[6]This is the only information that emerged from this review on properties of thiosarin. It suggests that thiosarin and thiosoman may be somewhat less toxic than their better-known analogs.

[7]For more information, see the accompanying report on PB (Golomb, 1999).

Adverse Health Effects

Considerable effort went into developing administration regimens for PB that would be safe and effective and that would not impair military performance (Gall, 1981). But the actual use of PB during the war has produced unexpected responses and concern. These issues have been exhaustively investigated in a separate volume of this series (Golomb, 1999).

Treatments

Atropine, the mainstay of treatment agents (Marrs, Maynard, and Sidell, 1998; Grob and Harvey, 1953), antagonizes the effects of ACh on muscarinic receptors. It does not act on nicotinic receptors. Oximes, a second class of treatment drugs, are used to reactivate AChE by displacing the agent from the enzyme, but only before aging has occurred. As noted, the treatment of soman poisoning is difficult, and it was for this agent primarily that pyridostigmine was used as a pretreatment. U.S. forces use injectable forms of atropine, pralidoxime, and diazepam. Diazepam is used for its anticonvulsant effect (U.S. Army Medical Research Institute of Chemical Defense, 1995).

It is known that cyclosarin is somewhat resistant to treatment with some common oximes, including pralidoxime, based on animal and *in vitro* studies (Coleman et al., 1966; Clement, 1992; Worek et al., 1998; Kassa and Bajgar, 1995). However, rhesus monkeys pretreated with pyridostigmine and challenged with intramuscular doses of 5 LD_{50} of cyclosarin, followed by treatment with atropine and 2-PAM (pralidoxime) had 100 percent survival (Koplovitz et al., 1992). This suggests that the treatment means available to U.S. forces during the Gulf War would have been effective against cyclosarin. Oximes have a number of other effects on allosteric sites and receptors and block overstimulated ganglia.

As mentioned above, however, AChE inhibition does not explain all aspects of nerve agent toxicity (Van Meter, Karczmar, and Fiscus, 1978; Kaufer et al., 1998; O'Neil, 1981). Several nerve agents appear to be weak direct agonists of receptors, with VX acting strongly on nicotinic receptor ion channel sites (Albuquerque et al., 1983, 1985; Eldefrawdi et al., 1985). There are also indications of direct agent binding to synaptic membranes (Anderson and Chamberlain, 1988), and soman has also been shown to act directly on the receptor (Hoskins, 1982). Cholinergic stimulation by inhibition of cholinesterase in effect stimulates expression of the proto-oncogene c-fos in the brain. The long-term significance of this is uncertain, as will be discussed later (Kaufer et al., 1998; Friedman et al., 1996).

Nerve agents can also inhibit other serine esterases (e.g., trypsin, chymotrypsin, and thrombin) (Meier et al., 1985; O'Neill, 1981; Walday, Aas, and Fonnum,

1991; Pasternack and Eisen, 1985) and serine proteases involved in regulating neuropeptides (e.g., substance P and met-enkephalin (O'Neill, 1981; Clement and Copeman, 1984). The functional significance of these findings is unclear, although O'Neil (1981) suggests that some signs and symptoms of nerve agent poisoning might be mediated by enkephalins, whose persistence in the brain is prolonged by exposure to DFP, for example.

Delayed Neuropathy and Neuropathy Target Esterase (NTE)

Of particular interest is NTE, which has been implicated in a form of delayed neuropathy known as OPIDN (Abou-Donia, 1981; Johnson, 1975; Johnson, 1992). It has been hypothesized that some of the neurological findings in Gulf War illness patients arise because of combined chemicals including nerve agents that may have produced this type of neuropathy (discussed further under "Clinical Findings," below).

In general it has been very difficult to produce delayed neuropathy in animals using nerve agents. Doses vary in excess of lethal levels, requiring pretreatment and treatment (Gordon et al., 1983). The natural substrate of NTE and the detailed mechanism of toxicity are not known. Toxicity only occurs when a sufficiently large amount of the enzyme is inhibited. There is no known treatment. The enzyme is widely distributed in the nervous system and has also been demonstrated in lymphocytes and platelets, which have been used in screening and toxicity studies (Bertoncin et al., 1985; Lotti, 1991). The hen has become the standard research animal for NTE studies (e.g., Olajos, DeCaprio, and Rosenblum, 1978).

Johnson (1972) noted that only a tiny amount of toxin was required to produce an effect, the rest being dissipated via nonspecific reactions and degradation mechanisms. He raised concern that if another compound overloaded or blocked such pathways, the threshold dose of the neurotoxic compound would decrease.

Phenylmethylsulfonyl fluoride has been used as a pretreatment protective of NTE but increases toxicity if given after a NTE inhibitory agent, such as TOCP or mipafox (Pope and Padilla, 1990). There has been speculation that administration of PB after a toxic exposure might have the same effect (Haley, Kurt, and Horn, 1997; Halley, Horn, et al., 1997; Halley and Kurt, 1997).

The temporal properties of delayed neuropathy are complex. Classically, after an acute exposure to TOCP or DFP at sufficient doses, there is a 10- to 14-day delay before onset of signs and symptoms. In human TOCP cases, there is weakness and then paralysis, chiefly involving the lower extremities. There is degeneration of axons both peripherally and in the spinal cord. Recovery is rare but does occur (Hayes, 1982). Animal studies with organophosphate chemicals have shown that cumulative effects can produce such lesions; in some studies, doses six weeks apart were cumulatively able to produce the neuropathy (Lotti, 1991). Although no reports of the effects of combinations of different chemicals that inhibit NTE emerged, there seems to be some potential for complex interactions.

The classical findings of delayed neurotoxicity have generally been found from the medulla to the periphery (Abou Donia, 1981). Some possibility remains that higher brain centers might be affected. Prendergast, Terry, and Buccafusco (1997, p. 116), point out in the review section of their paper that impairment of AChE does not predict cognitive impairment well in animals and suggest that NTE, which has also been associated with cognitive impairment, might be involved. They did not measure this enzyme in their studies

ENTRY AND FATE

Adsorption

The lipophilic nature of the nerve agents indicates that, as a group, they can readily penetrate the skin, lung, and gastrointestinal tract and, after entering the circulation, can be widely distributed, largely according to regional blood flow. The considerable species variation in sensitivity to these agents appears to reflect differences in the amount and distribution of nonspecific esterases that can bind the agents (Somani, 1992), although there are species differences in AChE affinity for organophosphate agents (Wang and Murphy, 1982).

Dermal

The skin does provide some degree of environmental protection, particularly against vapors. Military agents vary in the threat they pose. Tabun and sarin are rather volatile, and high concentrations (vastly higher than toxic respiratory doses) are required to produce toxicity through the skin by vapor exposure. Humans exposed to CTs of 1,000 to 1,300 mg-min/m^3 of tabun showed only a decline in serum and red cell cholinesterase. Even at a CT of 2,000 mg-min/m^3, subjects had no symptoms (Krakow and Firth, 1949). The NRC's Committee on Toxicology (NRC, 1997) cited 1951 work by McGrath in which humans were exposed to sarin vapor at CTs of 190 to 1,010 mg-min/m^3 without lowering blood enzyme levels. Exposure to levels of 1,225 to 1,850 mg-min/m^3 resulted in declines of ChE from 31 to 90 percent. No illness occurred, but two of nine subjects showed sweating. The committee considered 1,200mg-min/m3 to be a threshold effect ECT_{50} exposure.

Liquid agents applied to the skin are readily absorbed (Blank et al., 1957), but for volatile agents, such as sarin, evaporation reduces the amount of agent available for absorption (Grob et al., 1953). Applying 5 mg/kg of tabun to the skin of volunteers produced no illness but resulted in a 30-percent fall in AChE and notable local sweating (Freeman et al., 1954).

Chlorpyrifos, a pesticide of some Gulf War interest, is very poorly absorbed through the skin (Nolan et al., 1984). Some agents of intermittent volatility (e.g., soman and cyclosarin) present a greater hazard, and VX presents the greatest percutaneous hazard (Sim, 1962).

People show distinct regional differences in skin absorption; for VX, the highest rates are on the head and neck (Sim, 1962). Moisture, heat, and abrasions can increase agent transfer, while the total area exposed is important (Blank et al., 1957). The dermal toxic dose for many agents is considerably higher than for parenteral or respiratory exposure, reflecting not only evaporative and mechanical losses but also the ability of the skin and underlying tissues to bind agents and to inactivate them enzymatically (Fredriksson, 1969). For example, the skin dose of VX required to reduce red-cell AChE by 50 percent in humans is 32 µg/kg, while the intravenous effect is attained with 1 µg/kg. VX, on the other hand, is not hydrolyzed efficiently in the skin.

Ocular

Agents can be readily absorbed from the conjunctival sac and the eye (Grob and Harvey, 1958). Theoretically, dangerous amounts of agent could be absorbed as droplets by this route, but no data suggesting this is likely. The marked local effects of miosis, dim vision, impaired night vision, headache, lethargy, and impaired accommodation are predominant features of eye toxicity.

Respiratory

Vapors and aerosols are well absorbed from the lung. Oberst et al. (1959, 1968) demonstrated that humans exposed at rest to doses of sarin retained 89 percent of the inspired agent, less (79.5 percent) if exercising. The authors noted that CTs were not highly reliable indicators of toxicity. CTs ranging from 7 to 9.7 mg-min/m^3 (exercising men) and 33 to 42.6 mg-min/m^3 of sarin all produced similar absorbed doses. Particles with adsorbed agent can also be dangerous by this route (Asset and Finklestein, 1951).

Gastrointestinal

Gastrointestinal exposure of animals has been extensively studied for organophosphate pesticides, but little has been done with nerve agents. One study suggests that gastrointestinal exposure to a nerve agent produces rapid and serious intoxication (Karakchiev, 1973). Human studies (Sidell and Groff, 1974) with 4 µg/kg of VX taken orally showed a rapid response with fall of red-cell AChE. Maximum inhibition was 70 percent at two to three hours, with mild gastrointestinal disturbances (colic, nausea, vomiting, and diarrhea). Systemic symptoms were rapid at 20 minutes in other studies of sarin (Grob and Harvey, 1953) and VX (Sim et al., 1971).

Metabolism

Intra-arterial administration of sarin (Grob and Harvey, 1953) at 6 µg/kg showed the agent would pass the capillary bed with immediate symptoms and gradual decline of red-cell AChE to 28 percent over one hour. Smaller doses (3 to 4 µg/kg) produced no symptoms and only a minimal decline in red-cell AChE, suggesting that such lower levels may be detoxified.

Animal data show that rapidly acting agents at high dosage levels are not cleared effectively but that there are detoxification systems capable of dealing with lower levels of challenge (Somani, 1992; Fonnum and Sterri, 1981). Guinea pigs metabolize sarin at a rate of 0.013 µg/kg/min and soman at a rate of 0.009 µg/kg/min (Somani, 1992, p. 89). The rates of metabolism probably vary, with the isomers involved as in the case of soman (Benschop et al., 1981, 1984; De Bisschop et al., 1985). Carboxyesterases are important in metabolizing sarin, soman, and tabun (Walday, Aas, and Fonnum, 1991; Maxwell, 1992), but these enzymes are quantitatively much more important in rodents than humans. Nonspecific enzymes in serum and liver (aliesterases) metabolize all agents (Somani, 1992, p. 91).

Female mice are known to have plasma butyrlcholinesterase levels about twice that of matched males, with carboxyesterase levels 1.3 times those of males. The detoxifying or protective effects of these enzymes were not detectable in comparisons of the brain AChE levels in males and females three hours after intraperitoneal injection of 4 mg/kg of DFP or 0.3 mg/kg of sarin (Tuovinen et al., 1997).[8]

Some forms of paroxonase (PON1) in the serum hydrolyze sarin and soman at a high rate, breaking the P-F bond (Davies, 1996). Serum anhydride hydrolase (parathionase) is also active at least against soman (Broomfield, 1992). Variations in the abundance of these enzymes in human populations may produce variations in sensitivity to agents (Mutch et al., 1992).

The serum and some tissues contain an enzyme butyrylcholinesterase (EC 3.1.1.8), whose main biological purpose is unknown. This enzyme can hydrolyze ACh. Nerve agents and carbamates bind to this enzyme. Studies of an Israeli soldier who was hypersensitive to PB showed a variant of this enzyme that had low affinity (1/20th normal) for PB and other cholinesterases

---

[8]These were substantial doses, and they do not exclude a useful role in protection from lower-level exposures.

(Lowenstein-Lichtenstein et al., 1995; Schwarz et al., 1995). This suggests a role for the normal enzyme in decreasing the effects of low doses of anti-cholinesterase agents.

Elimination Excretion

In the case of soman, there appears to be a deposit site, probably in muscle, that does not inactivate the agent but rather stores and later releases it in toxic form. No such phenomenon has been reported for other agents, but the possibility apparently has not been evaluated. The effect lasts hours not days (Van Helden and Wolthuis, 1983; Wolthuis, Benschop, and Berends, 1981; Van Helden, Berends, and Wolthuis, 1984).

In general, the agents disappear rapidly from the blood, with rapid formation of hydrolysis products. The main metabolic product of sarin, IMPA, remains in tissues, although a great deal is eliminated rapidly in the urine, with a half-life of 3.7 hours (Fleisher et al., 1969). Cyclosarin studies show it is hydrolyzed to a similar analog with a half-life of 9.9 hours. Soman metabolism is more complex and biphasic, with half-lives of 3.6 hours and 18 hours, and soman accumulates in the lung (Shih, McMonagle, et al., 1994). Pinacolyl phosphonic acid is a major soman metabolite. IMPA was detected in the urine of Japanese sarin casualties—in one case for a week (Nakajima, Sasaki, et al., 1998; Minami et al., 1998).

Distribution

Sublethal amounts of soman injected intravenously in mice yield only trace amounts in tissues after 1 minute, with most converted to pinacolyl phosphonic acid. Studies show distribution to blood, choroid plexus, and spinal fluid at 2 minutes, with a distinct concentration in hypoglossal and vestibular nuclei, and later in the thalamus and caudate nucleus (Traub et al., 1985).

Blood flow is a key determinant in distribution of all agents (Somani, 1992, p. 79), and the higher percentage of the cardiac output going to the brain increases the risk there. Sites at which the brain is active show increased metabolic activity associated with vasodilation and increased blood flow, raising the possibility that distribution of agent might vary according to brain activity at the time of exposure (Scremin, Shih, and Corcoran, 1991; Scremin and Jenden, 1996).

Regional inhibition of AChE has been used to examine distribution effects, as has alteration of receptor properties. For example, Churchill et al. (1984) report such alteration in the olfactory bulb, hippocampus, and cortex, and such inhibition seems to be long lasting (Shipley et al., 1985). The latter regions are important in memory, while limbic system involvement influences mood and activity. The effects show age differences in the distribution of inhibition (Shih, Penetar, et al., 1990), but the correlation with inhibited AChE and clinical findings is uncertain.

Although the carbamates, such as PB, do not bind to aliesterase (Somani, 1992), there is concern that PB might occupy other binding sites, rendering them unavailable to bind nerve agents and thus increasing the amount of agent available at sites where toxicity is manifested. However, in animal studies with VX and soman, the agent was not increased in the brains with PB pretreatment (Anderson et al., 1992).

EXPOSURE-EFFECT RELATIONSHIPS

Reports of effects vary by study and species. This section does not focus on higher-level exposures, which are less relevant to the Gulf situation. Greater attention is paid to lower-dose studies, some of which examine behavioral consequences of exposure as well as noting factors that might modulate responses to agent.

Acute Exposures, Acute Effects

There is no information on thiosarin, and the information on cyclosarin is sparse. Table 5.4 gives lethality and incapacitation estimates for the others.[9] There has also been a no-effect estimate of a CT of 1.6 mg-min/m^3 for VX (McNamara et al., 1973). However, a study cited by the Committee on Toxicology (NRC, 1997) could not identify an adverse level (no-observed-adverse-effect level) based on VX exposures ranging from 0.7 to 25 mg-min/m^3 (cited report was Bramwell et al., 1963). Lethality and incapacity estimates for cyclosarin are now available based on the extensive review of the Subcommittee on Toxicity Values for Selected Nerve and Vesicant Agents (NAS, 1997), although these are sometimes based on analogies with better-known agents. Some of their findings are included in Table 5.4. Generally, the toxicity of cyclosarin falls between that of soman and sarin (Cresthull et al., 1957), although some authors credit it as being twice as toxic as sarin (Karakchiev, 1973). Appendix B gives effect estimates for other species and modes of exposure. It is of some note that female animals show greater sensitivity to nerve agents (Callaway and Blackburn, 1954, for example), and the rate of recovery of AChE is slower (Woodard et al., 1994). A follow-up study of some Tokyo subway sarin cases

---

[9]See Appendix A for an explanation of CT and other dose measurements.

Table 5.4

Estimates of Nerve Agent Lethality or Incapacitation to Humans

Agent	Skin LD_{50} (mg liquid, 70 kg man)		Respiratory LCT_{50} (mg-min/m^3)			Respiratory ICT_{50}/ Severe Effects (mg-min/m^3)	
	NAS	Somani	NAS	Somani	Other	NAS	Other
Tabun	<1,500	200–1,000	<70	100–200	150–400	<50	100–300
Sarin	<1,700	100–500	<35	50–100	70–100	<25	15–75
Soman	350	50–300	<35	25–50	50–80	<25	5–25
Cyclosarin	350		<35			<25	
VX	<<5	5–15	<15	5–15	30–100	10	5–50

SOURCES: Somani (1992), p. 77; OSRD (1946), U.S. Army (1990), Karakchiev (1973), McNamara et al. (1973), Trask et al. (1959) (NRC, 1997).

found subtle neurological deficiencies in female cases (compared to control) but not in the male cases (Yokoyama, Araki, et al., 1998a).

Also of interest are fairly large-order variations in sensitivity to nerve agents at different times of the circadian cycle, as Elsmore (1981) showed in LD_{50}s of rats given soman at intervals around the clock. Agents also disrupt circadian rhythms (Mougey et al., 1985). This might mean that nerve agents or pesticides might be more toxic to troops at night than in the day, when most human studies have been done.

The U.S. Army Surgeon General has established exposure limits to a number of nerve agents for workers (eight-hour exposures) and the civilian population (MMWR, 1988). Concentration limits were established for exposures (see Table 5.5).

Such exposure limits are selected both to avoid any clinical signs and generally to provide at least an order-of-magnitude safety margin. Estimated remote cumulative doses for the Khamisiyah release appear to be higher: 0.01296 mg-min/m^3 (CIA, 1997).

Behavioral Effects

A study of 29 troops in the mid-1940s (Marrs et al., 1996) found that humans exposed to a CT of 28 mg-min/m^3 of tabun had definite symptoms; all 29 had miosis and vomiting; 26 were depressed; 22 were fatigued; and some night performance was impaired.[10] Recovery took one week, so it seems unlikely a

---

[10]Marrs lists the report as an unpublished Ministry of Defence report, but outside review indicates that this was a 1945 Porton Report by Curwan and Mittner (PRZ2711), which was not available for our review.

Table 5.5

**Nerve Agent Exposure Limits Established by
the U.S. Army Surgeon General**

	General Population (72 hours, mg/m^3)	Workers (8 hours, mg/m^3)
Tabun	3 x 10^{-6}	1 x 10^{-4}
Sarin	3 x 10^{-6}	1 x 10^{-4}
VX	3 x 10^{-6}	1 x 10^{-5}

SOURCE: MMWR (1988).
NOTE: The MMWR summary did not include soman and cyclosarin. The document from the Surgeon General (DAMD17-85R0072, p. 49) on which the MMWR report was based also shows an 8-hour time-weighted average soman of 3x10^{-5} mg-min/m^3. The 8-hour time-weighted average for cyclosarin was the same as for sarin.

similar outbreak in the Gulf would have escaped medical notice. Low inhaled-dose exposure to sarin of 5 µg/kg (calculated from respiratory exposure) did not impair a variety of complex tasks.[11]

An investigation of dermally applied EA1701 (an early designator for VX) using a micrometer syringe, at several levels of exposure, found mood, thinking, and behavioral changes in 93 human volunteers exposed to VX at levels that did not produce gastrointestinal, respiratory, or muscle symptoms, although some experienced nausea. In that study, decreases in red cell AChE correlated with anxiety and decreased mental performance; the exposures were of several levels and some had no fall in AChE (Bowers et al., 1964). These volunteers are presumed to be included in the long-term follow-up study that found no long-term effects (NAS, 1985). The authors did not give the actual doses (perhaps for security reasons) but drew attention to the considerable mental effects without peripheral signs of cholinesterase inhibition.

Another study (Sidell, 1967), using intravenous VX at three levels (three subjects at the lowest, four next, and 18 at the highest), with a placebo control group (four subjects), found no significant blood pressure or heart rate changes. AChE showed 70 percent inhibition. Doses were 1.3 µg/kg, 1.4 µg/kg, and 1.5 µg/kg. There were few peripheral symptoms. Although eight were nauseated and four vomited, these symptoms took an hour to develop. Twelve subjects were dizzy or lightheaded, and nervousness was common. A number facility tests showed a significant decrease only in the 1.5-µg/kg group. Presumably, the volunteers noted above were included in the long-term follow-up study, which did not find long-term effects in volunteers (NAS, 1985), but no short-

---

[11]It was not possible to obtain primary sources from Marrs's references, but the text gives fairly detailed accounts.

term follow-up was included in the reports, so the duration of the effects is uncertain.

Low doses of soman and sarin (1/40th to 1/9 LD_{50}) alter rodent behavioral performance, although the animals appear well. They seemed anxious (i.e., they hesitated on some tasks and were less inquisitive), but only sarin impaired coordination and balance (Sirkka et al., 1990). Behavioral changes were also observed in rats (open field locomotion) given sign-free doses of soman (4 μg/kg) and sarin (20 μg/kg) intraperitoneally lasting over 12 hours (Nieminen et al., 1990).

Marmoset studies (Wolthuis, Groen, et al., 1995) of cholinesterase inhibitors showed little physiological response at low levels, although blood AChE was decreased. However, there was definite disruption in a number of tests (e.g., visual discrimination, eye-hand coordination, and choice-time). There were increases in no-attempt behavior (i.e., failures to respond to rewards). PB had more behavioral effects than had been expected, given that it does not usually pass the blood-brain barrier. The performance decrements took place at levels of agent without overt clinical signs. There have been many studies of animal performance in response to nerve agents, with an emphasis on soman (Hartgraves and Murphy, 1992). At 0.5 LD_{50}, soman and VX were more disruptive of performance than tabun and sarin (Mays, 1985).

Ocular Effects

The eye is sensitive to vapor or aerosols, with clinically and operationally important effects occurring at low levels (OSRD, 1946; NAS, 1997; Sim, 1956). These effects should have appeared if there were significant low-level exposures in the Gulf. Miosis refers to constriction of the pupils but is usually associated with a constellation of other problems: dim vision, pain, impaired night vision, difficulty focusing, and appearance of eye inflammation. CTs for miosis (mg-min/m^3) are 20 for tabun, 2 for sarin, 0.1 for soman, and 0.09 for VX (OSRD, 1946; Karakchiev, 1973; McNamara et al., 1973; Sim, 1956; Johns 1952). Human night vision is impaired via a retinal effect at 5 CT of sarin (Rubin and Goldberg, 1957b). The no-effect level for VX is 0.02 mg-min/m^3 (McNamara et al., 1973). The recent report of the Subcommittee on Toxicity Values for Selected Nerve and Vesicant Agents (NAS, 1997), which used multiple sources that may have been different from the above citations, determined the CT for miosis of sarin to be 0.5 mg-min/$m^{3,}$ a much lower figure than that noted above, although they noted that there were also reports of no effects at this level of exposure.

Dermal Effects

Dermal exposures generally require higher doses to generate the effects seen through other routes (see Appendix B). They are associated with slower onset of symptoms, fewer eye and respiratory symptoms, more cardiovascular symptoms, and nervous system symptoms. Reducing blood AChE by 50 percent required total doses of 400 mg of sarin, 65 mg of soman, and 30 mg of cyclosarin (Marrs et al., 1996; note the difference in dermal effect between sarin and cyclosarin). Parenteral (e.g., intravenous) and gastrointestinal routes of exposure were reviewed but do not seem relevant to Gulf War situations. Sweating is the common marker of dermal exposure and can be rather persistent.

Combined Effects

Tabun and mustard show a marked increase in toxicity and lethality when animals are exposed to both, and serum cholinesterase recovers more slowly than when the agents are used singly (Krustanov, 1962). The recognition of possible mixed use of sarin and cyclosarin prompted study of their combined toxicity; animals did not show unique toxicity, and therapy with standard measures was satisfactory (Clement, 1994). (See the earlier discussion on treatment mentioning the resistance of cyclosarin to oxime.)

Stress and Steroid Effects

How stress influences the effects of agents has not been studied extensively. Adrenalectomy did not alter the toxicity of sarin and soman in Wistar rats. Pretreatment with ACTH, adrenal cortical extract, cortisone, prednisolone, or corticosterone did not decrease soman toxicity. Soman toxicity was significantly decreased by pretreatment with prednisolone or cortisone plus atropine, compared to atropine alone (Stabile, 1967).

Modulation by Pretreatment

Humans exposed to a CT of 5 mg-min/m^3 (30 min) of sarin after PB pretreatment had an altered miosis course with less conjunctival irritation and a shorter course of symptoms (i.e., two to three days versus seven to ten days) (Gall, 1981). This demonstrates that the clinical response of pretreated persons to low doses of agents may be modified by the pretreatment, possibly decreasing or preventing some of the signs and symptoms.

There has been concern, however, that pretreatment medications might enhance the toxicity of some agents. Physostigmine after DFP did not protect but rather enhanced toxicity (Koster, 1946).

There are limited indications that PB, not followed by treatment (e.g., with atropine or oxime), may decrease the duration and severity of symptoms and perhaps their occurrence in humans and animals exposed to low doses of an agent (e.g., sarin). Husain, Vijayaraghavan, et al. (1993) showed that sign-free PB and physostigmine pretreatments, also not followed by any treatment, provided a definite, favorable modification of the pulmonary function decreases in rats exposed to a CT of 51 mg-min/m^3 of sarin. Rats are less sensitive to sarin than humans; the LCT_{50} for the rat is about 220 (Callaway and Blackburn, 1954), and the estimated LCT_{50} for humans is about 75 mg-min/m^3 (NAS, 1997). Related studies by the same group (Vijayaraghavan et al., 1992) showed that, in rats exposed to sarin at a CT of 51 mg/m^3 aerosol, pretreatment with carbamates, PB (0.075 mg/kg intramuscular), or a "symptom free" dose of physostigmine 20 minutes before sarin exposure protected lung AChE and increased survival. Physostigmine afforded better results. No treatment was given.

Longer Exposures and Tolerance

There is less information about chronic exposures, especially with measured doses. There are no reported exposure levels in the accidental occupational exposures reviewed, some of which may have reflected low-level exposure. Hartgraves and Murphy (1992) provide a substantial review of the behavioral effects of low-dose exposures to agents, some of which were subchronic or chronic. Chronic low doses of soman impaired primate responses, but the responses were not exacerbated by physostigmine pretreatment (Blick et al., 1993).

Animals and humans exposed repeatedly to sublethal levels of anticholinesterase compounds (inhibitors, such as nerve agents, organophosphate pesticides, drugs, carbamates, and carbamate pesticides) over time (days to a week) develop a condition known as tolerance, in which further administration of the inhibitor does not produce further signs and symptoms of exposure. Animal models have also shown behavioral tolerance to sustained sublethal exposures to DFP (Costa et al., 1982; Modrow and McDonough, 1986; Russell et al., 1975; Wolthuis, Philippens, and Vanwersch, 1991; Chippendale et al., 1972). Behavioral tolerance to soman in rats was seen, although performance decrements were noted on days of soman administration (Russell, et al., 1986). Doses of 35 µg/kg were given subcutaneously three times a week for four weeks (Modrow and McDonough, 1986). Dogs exposed to 25 µg/kg/day of sarin vapor for five days were symptomatic but showed signs of developing tolerance (Cresthull et al., 1960). A large, long-term study designed to simulate occupational exposures used beagles, exposing them daily to 10 mg-min/m^3 of sarin for six months (Jacobson et al., 1959), which resulted in some illness, no direct mortality, signs of tolerance, and full recovery after the end of study.

Russell et al. (1986), showed that prolonged administration of soman (11 doses over 22 days, 35 µg/kg—0.3 log of the LD_{50}) produced few signs of toxicity, although body temperature fell initially and then showed tolerance. Hypoalgesia continued, but tolerance was shown after initial decrements for a variety of temporal and performance activities. Brain AChE levels stabilized during the study despite continued administration of soman, implying some compensating regulatory activity (Russell, et al., 1986).

In contrast a single sublethal dose of soman in rats (100 to 150 µg/kg, intramuscular) did not produce seizures immediately but greatly altered spontaneous motor activity and test performance lasting for over 21 days. Some animals were very excitable and developed seizures when handled (Haggerty et al., 1986).

Nonspecificity

Tolerant organisms show decreased response not only to the inducing chemical but also to other anticholinesterases and cholinergic compounds such as carbachol and oxytremorine. They also show increased sensitivity to the effects of antagonists, such as atropine (Costa et al., 1982; Modrow and McDonough, 1986).

It has been shown that tolerance to the organophosphate pesticide disulfoton and the agent DFP can be induced by administering small doses that do not produce any overt signs of toxicity (Schwab and Murphy, 1981). A similar finding has been observed in humans taking the inhibitor echothiophate for glaucoma (DeRoetth et al., 1965). Tolerance has been seen in pesticide workers (Hayes, 1982) and is the probable explanation for the production and laboratory workers in the U.S. nerve agent program who had very low levels of cholinesterase but who reported no symptoms (Freeman et al., 1956; Holmes, 1959).

Extensive research has excluded increased metabolic clearance of the inhibitors as an explanation of tolerance. The uptake of choline and synthesis of ACh in the presynaptic tissues is not impaired (Costa et al., 1982).

Receptors

There are two main classes of receptors for ACh: muscarinic (with three subgroups of differing affinities) and nicotinic. Peripheral tissues, such as the gastrointestinal and pulmonary systems, are muscarinic, while skeletal muscles are nicotinic. The central nervous system contains both types of receptors, but their role is less well understood than in peripheral tissues and the autonomic nervous system. The receptors are primarily found on postsynaptic membranes, although there are some presynaptic muscarinic receptors (Costa et al., 1982).

Decreases in the abundance of both muscarinic and nicotinic receptors in response to sustained exposure to anticholinesterases has been demonstrated and seems to be the paramount mechanism of tolerance (Costa et al., 1982; Schwab et al., 1983; Bartholomew et al., 1985). Receptor decrease has been seen in tissue cultures, as well as *in vivo*. There may be additional mechanisms distal to the synapse involved in tolerance (Schwab et al., 1983).

Muscarinic receptors have been the most studied. Their abundance is decreased by chronic exposure to anticholinesterases or direct-acting cholinergic compounds (downregulation), while the binding affinity of the receptors is not altered (Costa et al., 1982). Indications are that receptors are internalized within the cell much as ligand-bound insulin receptors are. *De novo* synthesis of new receptors is required for recovery of normal abundance of receptors. In addition to decreases in receptor abundance, the function of the remaining receptors is altered, with decreased binding of agonists and antagonists in animals tolerant of organophosphate pesticides (Schwab et al., 1983; Costa et al., 1982; Schwab et al., 1981).

Nicotinic receptors appear to be more stable, although desensitization of nicotinic cholinergic motor end plates is fairly rapid. Other nicotinic receptors are slower to decrease than muscarinic receptors, although downregulation does occur. (Buccafusco et al., 1997).

The extent of downregulation in different parts of the central nervous system varies considerably—e.g., the brain stem showed much less downregulation in muscarinic receptors of rodents than did the striatum and cortex (Bartholomew et al., 1985). A single sublethal dose of soman in rats produced a reversible decline in muscarinic receptors of the telencephalon but an irreversible decline in the pyriform cortex (Pazdernik et al., 1986). Downregulation from low levels of anticholinesterases has also been demonstrated *in vitro* (isolated synaptic membranes of the bovine caudate nuclei) (Volpe, Biagioni, and Marquis, 1985).

Carbamates also induce tolerance, although their binding to AChE is reversible. Short-acting carbamates, such as physostigmine, require sustained infusions to induce tolerance. Tolerance to neostigmine has been shown in people and animals. The mechanisms of tolerance with carbamates may be more complex than with organophosphate agents, but downregulation of muscarinic receptors has been shown with them.

Duration

For indirectly acting cholinergics (anticholinesterases), the duration of cholinesterase inhibition is the critical factor, since anticholinesterase level appears to be the ultimate regulator of sensitivity to these chemicals. Prolonged exposure to anticholinesterases produces a decline in receptor abundance (Schwab et al., 1983).

The separate RAND report on PB (Golomb, 1999) also considers receptor effects. Most studies of this compound as a pretreatment have been fairly short, many of three to five days of exposure (Gall, 1981). Prolonged use of this drug, which is fairly long acting (the oral half-life is about four hours), might induce tolerance, at least in peripheral tissues, thus decreasing the effects of nerve agents by a mechanism additional to its reversible binding to AChE.

As noted previously, there is now reason to suspect that, under severe stress conditions, PB can pass the blood brain barrier and can act centrally as well as peripherally in downregulating receptors (Friedman et al., 1996).

Tolerance May Not Be Beneficial

The decrease of muscarinic and nicotinic receptors in the brains of animals tolerant to organophosphates raises the possibility that the balance of neuronal connections might be modified, with effects on higher brain functions. Such effects, rather than being protective, might represent a pathological process (Taylor et al., 1979). Animal studies have shown correlations of reduced memory and decreased abundance of brain nicotinic receptors (Gattu and Buccafusco, 1997).

Research inspired by illnesses in Gulf War veterans (Buccafusco et al., 1997; Wickelgren, 1997) has demonstrated decreased (over 50 percent) abundance of nicotinic receptors in cortical striatal and hippocampal neurons of rats exposed to sign-free doses of DFP (0.25 mg/kg/day for 14 days). Three weeks after withdrawal of DFP, treated animals showed impaired learning of a water maze, although previously trained animals retained their maze memories. There was no recovery of hippocampal nicotinic receptors three weeks after stopping DFP. A report in *Science* (Wickelgren, 1997, p. 1404) indicates that DFP-treated rats given nicotine before the water maze test learned adequately. Related studies in nonhuman primates given DFP 0.01 mg/kg/day for 25 days did not show altered performance in a delayed-matching-to-sample task, although red-cell AChE fell to 76 percent of control. Similar results occurred with 0.015 mg/kg/day for 15 days. Impaired performance was encountered at levels of 0.02 mg/kg/day, but these animals showed mild overt toxicity (Prendergast, 1998).

Induction of C-fos

The emerging picture of how cholinesterase inhibitors rapidly induce the expression of the transcription factor for c-fos points the way for possible long-term effects and added mechanisms of tolerance. It also appears that severe stress-induced release of ACh in animal models can also induce c-fos expression. The changes in gene expression initially enhance and later inhibit neuronal excitability mediated by muscarinic receptors. C-fos, an early immediate transcription factor, mediates selective regulatory effects on long-lasting activities of genes involved in ACh metabolism. This appears to create a situation in which the effects of cholinesterase inhibitors might persist long after the agents are no longer present (Kaufer et al., 1998). The role of c-fos and other intermediate early genes (IEGs), such as c-Jun, that seem to play an important role in translating stimuli into longer-term adaptive responses of cells is vast and complex and eventually may explain the longer-term effects of brief chemical exposures. A brief summary of recent information on IEGs and c-fos can be found in Appendix C.

The finding that cholinergic stimulation or stress can induce the expression of immediate early genes, such as c-fos, is not surprising in view of the variety of stimuli that activate this transforming factor. The possibility of this proto-oncogene playing a role in producing long-term effects from exposure to agents that produce cholinergic activity seems great, but the details remain to be demonstrated. This might be the mechanism by which short-term exposures produce long-term effects without killing large numbers of cells.

Although stress of various kinds increases c-fos, the regions involved vary with the stress model employed. It remains to be demonstrated which, if any, cholinergic stimuli produce effects convergent with stress responses.

Delayed Effects

The clinical manifestations of typical OPIDN begin about two weeks after exposure, with a progressive peripheral neuropathy, which can also involve the central nervous system, with axon degeneration and later demyelination. Sustained lower doses are as toxic as single exposures to larger doses, provided some threshold is crossed, with chronic dermal exposure being suspect (Cherniack et al., 1986; Hayes, 1982). Additive effects with long intervals between exposures (up to six weeks) have been demonstrated (Hayes, 1982; Davies and Holland, 1972; Abou-Donia, 1981).[12] No human case of typical delayed neurotoxicity arising from nerve agents has been reported. Sarin in repeated sublethal exposures did produce a typical neuropathy in mice (Husain, Vijayaraghavan, et al., 1993).

Sarin can produce delayed neurotoxicity in animals. However, very high levels of acute exposure (30 to 60 times LD_{50}) are required to produce the effect in hens protected from cholinesterase toxicity by treatments (PB, oximes, atropine) (Gordon et al., 1983). It was recognized that some humans with

---

[12]Note that a toxicity threshold would make the importance of negative studies less clear.

analogously high acute doses might survive as battle casualty treatment improved, possibly resulting in delayed neurotoxicity. But after examining sustained exposure of rodents to sarin aerosol, Husain (Husain, Vijayaraghavan, et al., 1993; Husain and Pant, 1994) questioned the impression that it took very high levels of repeated challenge with sarin to produce delayed toxicity. Husain et al. did not produce delayed neuropathy in Wistar albino rats with daily 20-minute sarin exposures for ten days (250 mg-min/m^3 exposures). However, white albino mice given 5 mg/m^3 of sarin for 20 minutes (i.e., 100 CT) daily for ten days developed classic delayed neurotoxicity (weakness, ataxia, and twitching) beginning at day 14 and confirmed by tissue pathology. The mice were not initially ill from sarin exposure and manifested no symptoms of anti-cholinesterase intoxication. The doses would be lethal in the range for humans (NRC, 1997). Since the hen has become the standard animal for OPIDN studies, there is less information about the effects in mice.

AChE levels in the brain were reduced by only 19 percent. Platelets and the spinal cord showed marked decreases in NTE levels, although less than in mipafox controls. This report has not been replicated. Rodents have generally been considered resistant to delayed neuropathy and have been used in research on the subject. The authors did not discuss why the species differed. The hen has become the standard animal for OPIDN toxicity studies with less information from mice.

Studies of the effects of the isomers of soman and sarin hinted at the possibility of nerve agents producing NTE effects at lower levels of exposure. A trend of increased inhibition of lymphocyte NTE in hens exposed to Sarin II (an isomer of sarin) suggested that longer exposures at lower levels might cause cumulative toxicity (Crowell et al., 1989). The P+ isomer of soman is a potent inhibitor of NTE, suggesting that this isomer alone could produce neuropathy at unprotected LD_{50} levels (Johnson, Read, and Benschop, 1985).

There has been considerable comment that this "low-level" exposure raises the possibility that sustained exposures in humans might result in neuropathy. The exposures in the study are at the upper range of LCT_{50} for rodents. Rodents, however, are more resistant to nerve agents than humans, and the mice in question did not require any treatment. However, the results are not congruent with earlier studies with sarin in hens or with the experience in dogs (which are not a standard animal for NTE research). Dogs do develop delayed neuropathy from DFP (Johnson, 1975). However, chronically exposing dogs to sarin vapor did not produce any neuropathy (Jacobson et al., 1959). The main weight of information makes it difficult to attribute delayed neuropathy to sarin or cyclosarin, given the very low levels calculated for the Khamisiyah release.

The studies of Gordon et al. (1983) demonstrated that soman and tabun did not produce delayed neuropathy at doses 38 times the LD_{50} of soman and 82 times the LD_{50} of tabun. In these studies, animals were provided the appropriate chemical therapy to enhance survivability following supra doses of agent. The same studies looked at the molar concentrations of agents required to inhibit *in vitro* 50 percent of the two enzymes, NTE and AChE, and calculated the ratios of the two (Table 5.6). The presumption was that the larger the number, the greater the likelihood of encountering delayed neurotoxicity from the agent in question. The results of other studies are summarized in Table 5.7.

A measure of the complexity and difficulty of this field is demonstrated by the Lenz et al. (1996) finding that sustained infusion of high daily doses (57 µg/kg/day) of VX in rats not provided chemical therapy reduced brain NTE by 90 percent at 14 days. No study of pathology or clinical response was reported. VX was not previously thought to be capable of significant NTE affects.

Severity-Sequelae Relationships

It is uncertain whether sequelae always correlate with severity at onset, although it seems intuitively obvious. Holmes (1959) reviewed the experiences of a group of workers exposed to sarin at various levels (although none so severely as to suffer seizures). He found that the more seriously exposed were ill longer. However, Stephens et al. (1996), in a study of groups exposed to organophosphate pesticides, found no correlation between acute exposure effects and the severity of performance shortfalls in later neuropsychological testing. In the reports of accidental cases, there are instances of patients with mild initial symptoms who had rather protracted later symptoms (Gaon and Werne, 1955; Brody and Gammill, 1954; Craig and Freeman, 1953).

Table 5.6

Molar Concentration of Agent Required to Inhibit Half of Enzyme Activity

	NTE	AChE	AChE/NTE
DFP	9.3×10^{-7}	1.05×10^{-6}	1.1300
Sarin	3.38×10^{-7}	1.9×10^{-9}	0.0056
Soman	3.77×10^{-7}	4.6×10^{-10}	0.0012
Tabun	6.65×10^{-6}	3.5×10^{-9}	0.0005
VX	2.5×10^{-4}	3.6×10^{-10}	10^{-6}

SOURCE: Reprinted by permission from *Archives of Taxicology*, Gordon et al. (1983), pp. 71–82. ©1983 Springer-Verlag, Berlin, Germany.

NOTE: Cyclosarin was not studied.

Table 5.7

Results of Other Delayed-Neuropathy Studies

Tabun (GA)	A 90-day study in hens at maximum tolerated dose (plus atropine) did not demonstrate delayed neuropathy (Willems et al. 1984).
Soman (GD)	To date, only repeated doses on the order of 150 times the LD_{50} have produced delayed neuropathy (Gordon et al., 1983; Willems, Nicaise, and De Bisschop, 1984). In a 90-day subchronic study at daily doses of GD insufficient to produce clinical signs, no delayed clinical or histological neuropathy resulted (Hayward et al., 1990).
Cyclosarin (GF)	GF has not been studied as extensively as the other agents. Vranken, De Bisschop, and Willems (1982) demonstrated that GF *in vitro* is a very potent inhibitor of NTE, but at doses where some lethality was encountered, no neuropathy occurred (Willems, et al., 1983).
VX	Most *in vitro* and *in vivo* studies fail to suggest that VX has any delayed neuropathic potential (Gordon et al., 1983; Vranken, De Bisschop, and Willems, 1982; Willems, Nicaise, and De Bisschop, 1983). However, Lenz, Maxwell, and Austin, (1996) raises some doubts about this conclusion.
Thiosarin	There is no information about this agent.

CLINICAL FINDINGS

A diligent effort to locate data about human clinical experience from exposures to nerve agents, while examining organophosphate pesticide experience for comparison, produced the following reports providing descriptions and consequences of exposures:

1. **Books and manuals:** NATO (1973), Grob (1956), OSRD (1946), Marrs et al. (1996), SIPRI (1971), SIPRI (1973), Lohs (1975), Karakchiev (1973), SIPRI (1976); Boskovic and Kusic (1980); Marrs et al., 1996); Sidell, Takafuji, and Franz (1997); Somani (1992)

2. **Organophosphate pesticide data:** Hayes (1982)

3. **Reviews:** IOM (1997), Jamal (1995b), Karczmar (1984), AFEB (1994), Grasso (1984), Clark (1971), Lotti (1995), Grob and Harvey (1953)

4. **Reports of intentional poisonings, Iran and Japan:** UN (1984); Perrorta 1996); Nozaki and Aikawa (1995); Nozaki et al. (1995); Okumura et al. (1996); Yokoyama, Ogura, et al. (1995); Yokoyama, Yamada, et al. (1996); Yokoyama, Araki, et al. (1998a, 1998b); Masuda et al. (1995); Hatta et al. (1996); Suzuki et al. (1995); Yasuda et al. (1996); Kato and Hamanaka (1996); Nohara and Segawa (1996); Inoue (1995); Morita et al. (1995); Ohtomi et al. (1996); Nakajima, Sato, et al (1997); Nakajima, Ohta, et al. (1998); Suzuki (1995); Murata et al. (1997)

5. **Reports of accidental and occupational exposures to nerve agents and pesticides:** Kaplan et al. (1993), Savage et al. (1988), Gershon and Shaw (1961), Whorton and Obrinsky (1983), Korsak and Sato (1977), Sim et al. (1971), Metcalf and Holmes (1969), Stephens et al. (1996), Tabershaw and Cooper (1966), Dille and Smith (1964), Seed (1952), Callaway (1950), Duffy and Burchfiel (1980), Cullen (1987), Sparks et al. (1994), Bell et al. (1992), Burchfiel and Duffy (1982), Holmes (1959), Callaway and Blackburn (1954), Sidell (1973), Senanayake and Karalliedde (1987), Sidell (1974), Brody and Gammill (1954), Freeman et al. (1956), LaBlanc et al. (1986), Craig et al. (1959), Finesinger et al. (1950), Vale and Scott (1974), Namba et al. (1971), Coombs and Freeman (1954), Richter et al. (1986), Kundiev et al. (1986), Rengstorff (1994), Cadigan and Chipman (1979), Craig and Freeman (1953), Gaon and Werne (1955)

6. **Experimental studies of human exposures:** Marrs et al. (1996); Sim (1956); Sim (1962); Sidell (1967); Rubin, Krop, and Goldberg (1957); Freeman et al. (1954); Oberst et al. (1959); Oberst et al. (1968); Grob and Harvey (1953); Cresthull et al. (1963); Sim et al. (1964); Bowers et al. (1964); Krachow (1947); Neitlich (1965); Rubin and Goldberg (1957a, 1957b); Grob and Johns (1958); Grob and Harvey (1958); Grob et al. (1947); Sidell and Groff (1974); Craig et al. (1959); Wilson (1954); Burchfiel (1976); Oken and Chiappa (1986); Freeman et al. (1952).

The reports of sarin and tabun accidents from the U.S. test and production efforts in the 1950s were especially helpful for this review, because many provided case descriptions and included at least short-term follow-up (Holmes, 1959; Craig and Freeman, 1953; Brody and Gammill, 1954; Gaon and Werne, 1955; Finesinger et al., 1950). Longer-term follow-up of sarin workers and pesticide workers has been difficult to locate, but some reports are available. Research subjects also had short periods of follow-up but were the subject of long-term review by the NAS in 1985. Experimentation on human subjects stopped at Edgewood Arsenal in 1975, with 1,300 having been exposed to anticholinesterase chemicals. Most studies with nerve agents had begun after 1954, with few after the mid-1960s (NAS, 1982). So, follow-up was in the 20- to 30-year range (NAS, 1985). The recent experience in Japan, where sarin was released in urban areas, provided information from well-equipped, well-staffed hospitals, with follow-up information for at least three months, with limited longer (six- to eight-month) reports.

This section concentrates on ocular, dermal, and respiratory exposure routes, emphasizing lower levels of exposure and clinical severity and information about long-term consequences and any patterns of illness similar to illnesses in Gulf War veterans. Earlier case reports suggest that clinicians did not expect long-term symptoms to arise from very mild exposures and sometimes considered alternate explanations for such patients when encountered (e.g., chronic anxiety). There is not much information about repeated or sustained exposures.

The amount of information about specific agents is uneven. There is much information about human exposures to sarin, but much less for tabun, soman, and VX. The only information available on human experience with cyclosarin is from secondary sources. The 1982 NAS review indicated that 27 volunteers were exposed to cyclosarin and that there were apparently both some sensory and oxime treatment studies. No information about thiosarin is available.

For nerve agents and pesticides, it is not always easy for the clinician to determine if an exposure has occurred, and AChE levels correlate poorly with the clinical findings. Holmes (1959) stated, with respect to a sarin production facility, that

> The examiner frequently asks himself the question "Is this a true exposure?" If so how serious is it? Except possibly for miosis, there seems to be no single symptom which occurs in every exposure. Only in the more severe exposures was miosis present in every instance. It is apparent that in milder exposures a single symptom related to a system occurs. When this happens it raises a question as to whether a particular symptom is a result of exposure or represents a symptom related to some other medical problem, such as a cold etc. When several symptoms related to a system occur, there is little doubt in the examiners mind both that this is a true exposure and in all probability a fairly severe exposure. When there is a scattering of symptoms related to different systems then the question arises if an exposure has occurred. Correlation with acetylcholinesterase is unreliable—in many instances a person is judged to have a mild exposure when the red cell acetylcholinesterase shows a greater drop than expected.

Acute Effects

Table 5.8 summarizes signs and symptoms arising from nerve agent exposure by several routes. No clinical differences are expected between various nerve agents. The clinical signs and symptoms from other organophosphate pesticide exposure are also quite similar (Hayes 1982; Namba et al., 1971). Table 5.9 classifies the severity of poisoning and is the basis of classifications used through this report. The emergency department of a Japanese hospital in Tokyo (Okumura et al., 1996) has summarized its experience with 640 victims of the subway attack. The department treated and released 82 percent (528) of the cases. The detailed findings in this group have not been reported, but these cases were considered to have been full recoveries. Of the 111 patients (17.3 percent of those in emergency department) admitted, 107 were considered moderate cases (16.7 percent) and four were considered severe. One of these

Table 5.8

Signs and Symptoms Following Short-Term Nerve Agent Exposure

Site of Action	Signs and Symptoms
Ciliary body	Frontal headache, eye pain on focusing, blurred vision
Conjunctivae	Hyperemia
Nasal mucous membranes	Rhinorrhea, hyperemia, but this may also be present after systemic absorption
	Following systemic absorption of liquid and prolonged vapor exposure
Bronchial tree	Tightness in chest sometimes with prolonged wheezing, expiration suggestive of bronchoconstriction or increased secretion, dyspnea, slight pain in chest, increased bronchial secretion, cough, pulmonary edema, cyanosis
Gastrointestinal	Anorexia, nausea, vomiting, abdominal cramps, epigastric and substernal tightness (cardiospasm) with "heartburn" and eructation, diarrhea, tenesmus, involuntary defecation
Sweat glands	Increased sweating
Salivary glands	Increased salivation
Lachrymal glands	Increased lachrymation
Heart	Bradycardia
Pupils	Slight miosis, sometimes unequal, later maximal miosis (pinpoint pupils); sometimes mydriasis is observed
Bladder	Frequent, involuntary microurination
Striated muscle	Easy fatigue, mild weakness, muscular twitching, fasciculation cramps, generalized weakness including muscles of respiration with dyspnea and cyanosis
Sympathetic ganglia	Pallor, occasional elevation of blood pressure
Central nervous system	Ataxia, generalized weakness, coma with absence of reflexes, Cheyne-Stokes respiration, convulsions, depression of respiratory and circulatory centers resulting in dyspnea and fall in blood pressure; emotional effects very often occur

SOURCE: NATO (1973).

died. Table 5.10 summarizes the clinical findings in the moderate and severe cases. There were two deaths, one in the emergency department and one later and 638 patients were considered to have made a full recovery. The moderate cases were hospitalized for 2.4 days (mean).

Table 5.11 summarizes the mild cases encountered in the workers accidentally exposed to "G" agents (tabun and sarin) studied by Craig and Freeman (1953). These cases show a lesser prevalence of eye, gastrointestinal, and nervous system findings but more rhinorrhea than in the Japanese cases, but the Japanese cases were a single event, while Craig and Freeman summarized multiple events. Their table is somewhat misleading in that, as in the Japanese cases, miosis was the most consistent finding (48 of their 53 cases). Most of their cases recovered rapidly, 78 percent within two days, most of the remaining ten cases within one week, with one case still symptomatic at 20 days.

Table 5.9

Severity Classifications for Organophosphate Pesticide Poisoning

Term	Description
Latent	No clinical manifestations
	Serum cholinesterase activity is 50 to 90 percent of normal
Mild	Fatigue, headache, dizziness, nausea and vomiting, increased salivation and sweating, chest tightness, abdominal cramps or diarrhea, can still walk, numbness of extremities
	Serum cholinesterase activity is 20 to 50 percent of normal
Moderate	Unable to walk, generalized weakness, difficulty talking and fasciculations, in addition to the symptoms but more miosis associated with mild poisoning
	Serum cholinesterase activity is 10 to 20 percent of normal
Severe	Unconsciousness, loss of pupillary light reflex, fasciculations, flaccid paralysis, moist rales in lungs, seizures, respiratory difficulties and cyanosis, secretion from mouth and nose
	Serum cholinesterase activity is less than 10 percent of normal

SOURCE: Modified from Namba et al. (1971); AD Little (1986), Ch. 5.

NOTE: Namba's classification, developed from experience with parathion and methyl parathion poisoning, has been adopted for classification of nerve agent exposures.

Commonly, cases are stratified clinically according to severity, as follows:

1. **latent:** exposed but asymptomatic so far

2. **mild:** distinct symptoms but ambulatory

3. **moderate:** unable to walk, distinct symptoms but conscious, able to sit

4. **severe:** seizures, coma, prostration.

The following subsections discuss these in reverse order (omitting the latent stage). A discussion of delayed effects follows.

Severe Intoxications. Several severe intoxications will be described, from accidents and the incidents in Japan to give a clinical picture of the problems that confronted military planners in the Gulf and to describe some of the sequelae of severe intoxications. Sidell (1973, 1974) reported two severe intoxications requiring hospitalization. The first was a 33-year-old man who sustained an accidental combined respiratory, cutaneous, and mucosal exposure to soman (less than 1 ml). He immediately decontaminated himself, was asymptomatic on arrival at the emergency room about five minutes later, but then collapsed. He was cyanotic with labored breathing, had a blood pressure of 180/80 mm Hg, and had a heart rate of 150/min. His conjunctivae were very inflamed; hehad marked oral and nasal secretions and widespread fasciculations. He was given intravenous atropine and 2-pyridine aldoxime methiodide (2-PAM). Cyanosis worsened, but he became conscious about 30 minutes later. Fascicu-

Table 5.10

**Signs and Symptoms in Patients with Moderate
to Severe Sarin Exposure**

	Sign or Symptom	Patients	
		Number	% (n=111)
Eye	Miosis	110	99.0
	Eye pain	50	45.0
	Blurred vision	44	39.6
	Dim vision	42	37.8
	Conjunctival injection	30	27.0
	Tearing	10	9.0
Chest	Dyspnea	70	63.1
	Cough	38	34.2
	Chest oppression	29	26.1
	Wheezing	7	6.3
	Tachypnea	28	31.8[a]
Gastrointestinal tract	Nausea	67	60.4
	Vomiting	41	36.9
	Diarrhea	6	5.4
Neurologic	Headache	83	74.8
	Weakness	41	36.9
	Fasciculations	26	23.4
	Numbness of extremities	21	18.9
	Decrease of consciousness level	19	17.1
	Vertigo and dizziness	9	8.1
	Convulsion	3	2.7
Ear, nose and throat	Running nose	28	25.2
	Sneezing	5	9.0
Psychological	Agitation	37	33.3

SOURCE: Okumura et al. (1996). ©1996 American College of Emergency Physicians (ACEP). Reprinted by permission.
[a]n=88.

lations continued, and he was restless, with nausea and vomiting, and electrocardiogram changes showed sinus tachycardia and then atrial fibrillation for 20 hours. His physical condition improved more rapidly than his psychiatric condition. He was observed to be depressed and withdrawn and had bad dreams that improved with scopolamine treatment. He had difficulty calculating. AChE remained low, but other laboratory tests were normal. By six weeks, he was back to his premorbid level and was doing well at six months.

The second was a 52-year-old man whose mask malfunctioned in a sarin-filled room. He noted respiratory difficulty; on arrival at the emergency room 5 to 10 minutes later, he was cyanotic and having seizures. He was given intravenous atropine and oxime and required respiratory assistance for apnea. Fasciculations were prominent, and he had marked wheezing, developed an S4 gallop, and later had electrocardiogram changes typical of ischemia. He resumed

Table 5.11

**Incidence of Symptoms in Workers Accidentally
Exposed to Tabun and Sarin (mild cases)**

Symptoms	Number of Workers	% Exposed Workers
Respiratory symptoms	41	77
Pressure sensation	35	
Localization not recorded	17	
Throat	2	
High sternum	3	
mid sternum	9	
low sternum	3	
not localized	1	
Cough	20	
Unproductive	15	
Productive	5	
Wheezing	9	
Inability to obtain a satisfactorily full inspiration	8	
Increased exertional dyspnea	7	
Dyspnea at rest	1	
Rhinorrhea	31	58
Eye Symptoms	29	55
Dim vision	24	
Impaired accommodation	13	
Pain on accommodation	6	
Central Nervous System Symptoms	27	51
Headache	17	
Headache as only CNS symptom	7	
Disturbed sleep	13	
Mood change	12	
Easily fatigued	10	
Increased perspiration	3	
Dizziness	2	
Gastrointestinal symptoms	14	26
Anorexia and/or nausea	9	
Increased GI activity	6	
Diarrheal stool	6	
Vomiting	2	
Miscellaneous		
Unpleasant taste to tobacco	10	
Poor driving	6	

SOURCE: Craig and Freeman (1953).

breathing one hour later. This patient was more alert at three hours and was able to ambulate at nine hours. He was rehospitalized four months later because of fatigue and dyspnea on exertion and was diagnosed with depression at six months. He died of myocardial infarction 18 months after exposure (Sidell, 1973, 1974).

There were two major sarin events in Japan, the first at Matsumoto in June 1994 (seven deaths and about 600 persons poisoned). The second was in Tokyo in March 1995 when sarin was released into the subway (11 died and 5,000 were poisoned) (Morita et al., 1995; Okumura et al., 1996). A third event was a man sprayed with VX (Nozaki and Aikawa, 1995).

The Japanese cases were well-documented. Some patients were comatose on admission, with miosis, seizures, fasciculations, flushing, tachycardia, hypotension, and respiratory distress; hypoxia was common. Many required intubation. Creatine kinase and glucose levels were elevated; many patients were acidotic at pH 6.8. Reports on secretions varied (Suzuki et al., 1995; Nozaki and Aikawa, 1995). Many recovered well, but some reported dysesthesias. One person had retrograde amnesia for 70 days (Hatta et al., 1996), and another was delirious and had hallucinations for over one week (Inoue, 1995). There were few deaths following hospitalization, but one man remained in a vegetative state in Matsumoto six months later.

The VX patient initially presented with blurred vision; seizures, fasciculation, and sweating followed. There was no miosis. The patient became cyanotic and was on a respirator for several days. He required atropine drip and intravenous diazepam. He was released after 15 days with brachial plexus neuropathy and antegrade and retrograde amnesia. Unlike the sarin cases, bradycardia had been prominent (Nozaki and Aikawa, 1995).

Moderate Exposures. At the hospital receiving the largest number of patients from the Japanese subway attack, 111 were categorized as severely or moderately injured (4 severe and 107 moderate) on admission (see Table 5.10). In these patients, miosis (99 percent) and headache (75 percent) were the most frequent symptoms, followed by dyspnea (63 percent) and nausea (60 percent); bradycardia was uncommon. Even at discharge, headache and eye pain were common. All but one made full recoveries (one severe case died), although 37 (33 percent of the 111) had acute stress disorders and four were diagnosed with PTSD at three months (Okumura et al., 1996). Of 213 patients seen initially at another Tokyo hospital, none had complaints at three-month follow-up (Yokoyama et al., 1996), similar to other Japanese reports.

In a three-week follow-up of some 117 mild and moderate cases in Matsumoto (Morita et al., 1995), the initial symptoms included rhinorrhea (78), headache (53), dark vision (52), sneezing (24), fatigability (18), dizziness (17), and nausea (14). Others reported diplopia, dysesthesia, vomiting, dysphagia, increased tearing, or gait disturbances. Most of these symptoms cleared by three weeks. At six months, five people visited hospitals regularly, with diverse complaints. One man with no history of lung disease was mildly hypoxic, and another had low-grade fevers.

Grob et al. (1953) reported a moderately severe reaction to percutaneous sarin in a volunteer. Illness was delayed several hours after exposure, lacked immediate eye or respiratory findings, and ran a protracted course with waves of recurring symptoms over four to five days. The dose was about 0.18 mg/kg through abraded skin. After 2-3/4 hours, there was local sweating; at 5-3/4 hours, the patient experienced general sweating, giddiness, and abdominal cramps. Blood pressure rose, and he was given atropine. One hour later, nausea, sweating, generalized weakness, and fatigability existed. He was short of breath with abdominal cramps but no wheezing. Maximum symptoms occurred at 10 to 11 hours, with dilated pupils and decreased vital capacity. He had mild symptoms with atropine at 13 hours, was fatigued and weak at 21 hours, and had insomnia and nightmares at 40 hours, finally recovering over the ensuing days.

Mild Exposures. *Respiratory.* Review of the inhalation exposures of sarin, tabun and some V-agent accidents supports the description in Wilson (1954) of mild intoxication, of symptoms that develop rapidly and then evolve over time:

> The chief effects consist of a feeling of constriction in the throat and chest, a tendency to cough, and eyes that quickly become red and painful with contracted pupils such that the subject finds it painful to focus on near objects. A severe and persistent frontal headache usually follows, and he becomes dejected and not inclined to bother to do anything unless he must. At night he is restless and has difficulty getting to sleep, and when he does has vivid dreams and nightmares; these symptoms may last 3–5 days. With larger doses, there is anorexia, nausea, vomiting, abdominal pain, salivation and diarrhea. There is sweating and generalized muscle weakness and fasciculations. Psychological changes include restlessness, irritability and insomnia. The appearance of the symptoms bears no relation to the plasma cholinesterase activity.

The occupational experience related to sarin production and testing was extensive. Holmes (1959) analyzed 991 cases in two groups, stratified by four levels of red-cell cholinesterase levels, with initial and follow-up examinations. All but a few cases were mild, and there was little treatment. These cases did not have long-term follow-up of the whole group, but cases were followed enough to determine that 10 percent had symptoms lasting two or more weeks. Appendix B includes information from this extensive report.

Several other reports also shed light on this issue: Brody and Gammill (1954), 75 cases; Gaon and Werne (1955), 244 persons; Craig and Freeman (1953), 53 cases; and Finesinger et al. (1950), 40 cases. Sarin was the primary agent to which people were exposed, but Freeman also reported four tabun exposures and two combined tabun-and-sarin exposures. The reports arose from medical examinations of exposed persons and later follow-up exams. The symptoms are those shown in Table 5.11 (Brody and Gammill, 1954; Craig and Freeman, 1953, had similar findings). Data from Holmes (1959) suggest a tendency for persons with higher percentages of cholinesterase inhibition to have more symptoms and longer periods of illness. Gaon and Werne (1955) could not make such an assertion; their cases, which lasted over three weeks, showed 47 percent with no significant reduction in enzyme level. In a series of 182 cases, they reported that 106 (58.2 percent) had recovered in three days, 34 (18.6 percent) in one week, 19 (10.4 percent) in two weeks, but 23 (12.6 percent) took three weeks or more. They did not describe their follow-up process but documented two cases with persisting symptoms 10 to 11 months after exposure (recurring headaches, dizzy spells, fatigue, syncope, and weakness for one; memory problems, inattention, and fatigue in the second).

Table 5.11 gives an idea of the prevalence of symptoms, with eye problems being acutely the most prevalent, as was noted previously. Note the considerable percentages of symptoms related to the central nervous system, including mood changes, thinking problems, and fatigue.

Although most cases resolved within three days, some 12 percent of Gaon's cases persisted for three weeks or more (Gaon and Werne, 1955). Many exposed patients did not attribute their symptoms to exposure but rather to colds.[13] Some patients who had asymptomatic miosis and/or depressed AChE levels experienced no symptoms, while some obviously exposed and symptomatic individuals had little decrease in AChE levels.[14]

In an effort to understand factors related to accidental exposures, it was noted that accidents seemed more common in colder weather; the authors attributed this to workers seeking shelter from the cold in heated shacks, where agents trapped on clothing could evaporate in a closed space, causing some sustained exposures (Brody and Gammill, 1954). The specific symptoms in patients with prolonged symptoms were not reported, which was also the circumstance with Holmes (1959). He did not report beyond "two weeks or more." His smaller group of 156 cases noted 10.9 percent lasting two weeks or more, while in his larger group of 635 cases, 20 percent were symptomatic for three weeks or more.

Those recovering were prone to motor vehicle and other accidents. It became the practice to forbid driving or night work for several weeks. Speaking clearly, thinking, and remembering were significant problems for some, lasting for weeks. Some individuals experienced an initial euphoria or giddiness; emo-

---

[13]These patients came to attention because their supervisors referred them; because other findings had been noted for them, such as miosis and abnormal blood tests; or because they came from settings in which exposures were suspected, e.g., coworkers were obviously sick.

[14]The authors of these early papers did not mention the possibility of tolerance arising from repeated exposures, altering the clinical response to further exposures. One would expect tolerant persons to have depressed AChE levels.

tional problems and irritability with family members and supervisors were documented frequently (Gaon and Werne, 1955). Some individuals became less careful and reliable and were thought to be "acting silly," which was out of character. Protracted fatigue and weakness were common, lasting two months in some cases. It was common for workers to report that the taste of cigarettes was lost or unpleasant. One soldier thought smoking worsened his weakness (Gaon and Werne, 1955).

Brody and Gammill (1954) frequently noted a distaste for cigarettes in their 75 cases. They also provide individual case descriptions, such as that of a 23-year-old man who was wearing protective equipment, but not a hood, who collected samples after an aircraft spraying flight of sarin on November 10, 1953. He was able to detect the odor of sarin and tightened his mask, but he developed a frontal headache and rhinorrhea. Four hours later, he had pinpoint pupils, photophobia, headache, and eye pain. Mild substernal pressure and dyspnea on exertion were noted. He was mildly ataxic and reported that his joints felt stiff. He took oral atropine and was continued in work status.

That night, he was restless; the headache continued, and he awoke from several nightmares. On arising, he was disoriented and had numb legs. His nausea quickly improved. His night vision was poor. He continued to work despite continued headache.

On November 12, he had headache, small pupils, and trouble reading and focusing. That night, he woke every two to three hours. He reported that 0.4 mg of oral atropine helped with the symptoms. He remained somewhat unsteady. He worsened at work during the day: The rhinorrhea increased; he vomited after lunch and then started diarrhea with 12 loose stools. He developed a cough productive of thick mucous.

That evening, he had vertigo and nearly fell. He took atropine, but sleep was frequently interrupted. He felt confused and numb all over. The next day, his "memory was no good," at times blank—he said things he did not remember saying. His joints were stiff, and he developed heartburn and belching. He vomited a few times. He felt very depressed—"nothing mattered any more." He gradually improved and recovered after several days. His ChE level was initially about 30 percent of normal.[15]

Gaon and Werne (1955) use one patient to illustrate late development of symptoms. The patient had two sarin exposures; symptoms of the first cleared in one day, and symptoms of the second cleared in three days. Eight months later, the patient complained of absentmindedness, an example being a near

---

[15]This case, although technically "mild," appears fairly incapacitating for many types of work.

accident when he failed to look both ways while driving across railroad tracks. He complained of difficulty with arithmetic and forgot lighted cigarettes around the house. He felt "lazy" and "draggy." He stated that his potency was impaired and his legs were weak. In several other cases, physicians tended to be skeptical of the relation to sarin exposure. Used to exposures in which most symptoms were over in a few days, they had difficulty accepting the possibility of long-term effects arising from mild exposures.

Two experimental studies of respiratory exposure of humans to measured low-level amounts of sarin appear relevant to understanding low-level effects (Oberst et al., 1959; Freeman et al., 1952). In these, the absorbed doses were in the range of decimals to a few micrograms per kilogram. Since the minute volume of respiration is proportional to the degree of physical activity, the amount of absorbed nerve agent (at a given concentration) is also proportional to the minute volume.

In a large study (141 subjects), Oberst et al. (1959) studied inhalation exposures of sarin vapor at varying levels for 2 minutes, in men at rest or exercising. The amount of sarin absorbed and the inhibition of red-cell AChE were measured. The amounts of sarin retained ranged from 0.1 to 4.9 µg/kg. At rest, 87 percent of the sarin inhaled was retained; minute volumes averaged 7.9 l/min. During exercise, 79.5 percent of the sarin was retained; minute volumes averaged 42.9 l/min. The degree of inhibition of erythrocyte AChE was proportional to the retained dose, with 3.8 to 4.2 µg/kg required to inhibit 50 percent of the enzyme activity. Absorbed doses of 0.1, 0.2, and 0.3 µg/kg showed enzyme inhibitions of 3, 2, and 4 percent, respectively. Absorbed doses of 0.5 µg/kg showed inhibitions ranging from 0 to 25 percent, with the line of least square regression showing 8 percent inhibition. Absorbed doses of 1 µg/kg produced inhibition of 0 to 54 percent, with a mean of 14 percent. CT exposures ranged from 2.4 to 46.2 mg-min/m^3. The authors note the unreliability of CTs, since CTs of 33 to 46 in resting men and 7 to 9.7 in exercising men produced similar absorbed doses. Comparing animal enzyme and lethality data, they estimated human LD$_{50}$ to be in the range of 11.9 to 26.2 µg/kg. Unfortunately, they did not describe any of the clinical responses of the subjects to these measured levels of absorbed sarin. The reviewer notes that, although the group data were consistent, there was considerable individual variation in the degree of inhibition from a given dose of sarin. How much of the variation reflects differences within the lungs (mucous trapping, tissue absorption) and how much reflects differences in detoxifying metabolism are not known. Given the paucity of data about clinical effects from measured, documented human exposures, it might be worthwhile to see whether the medical records of this large number of subjects, which we believe to still be on file at Edgewood Arsenal, contain clinical observations about their response to defined dosages of sarin.

Fortunately, the second study (Freeman et al., 1952), although smaller, obtained data on signs and symptoms, neuromuscular function, EKGs, pulmonary function, and red-cell and serum AChE levels arising in controls (six), men at rest (eight), and men exercising (nine). The latter two groups breathed sarin vapor for 2 minutes via a tube in the mouth and without eye exposure. The amount of sarin retained was measured. The total absorbed dose in the resting group ranged from 0.08 to 0.16 µg/kg (average 0.12 µg/kg). The exercise group ranged from 0.22 to 0.99 µg/kg (average 0.56 µg/kg). There were no significant differences before and after in the three groups in ChE levels, hand grip and fatigue, vital capacities, maximum breathing capacity, and EKGs. (Two exposed subjects showed declines in ChE levels of about 10 percent.) The control group had no signs, but one subject experienced cough and a sense of incomplete inspiration, which was not present 24 hours later. Of the exposed resting group, two developed signs (transient rhonchi and inspiratory wheezing on examination of the chest), while six (including the two above) noted cough, chest pressure, and incomplete inspiration (doses ranged from 0.08 to 0.16 µg/kg). All these symptoms had cleared 24 hours later, but one subject (0.13 dose) reported disturbed sleep. Of the exercise group, three developed signs (inspiratory wheezing, scattered rales, and rhonchi) at 0.22 to 0.71 µg/kg, while five developed cough, chest pressure, and incomplete inspiration (0.22 to 0.99 µg/kg). At 24 hours, two had continued chest pressure, and one of these had developed headache. The authors did not report CTs, which the reviewer estimates to represent levels of 0.5 to 0.6 mg-min/m^3. Individual variation is again noted, with some exposed persons reporting no symptoms. The levels of exposure are slightly above those known to produce miosis and are at levels that could be measured by standard detectors.

Dermal. Low-level dermal exposures to G and V agents are documented. Some exposed persons are asymptomatic but have depressed AChE levels (Freeman et al., 1956). In general, dermal exposure produces symptoms more slowly, with eye and respiratory symptoms occurring later. Results from the literature are given in Table 5.12. Note that the cyclosarin result suggests it represents a serious cutaneous hazard (Marrs et al., 1996).

In 33 of 40 subjects exposed dermally to VX, AChE fell to 50 percent from doses of 5 to 20 µg/kg (Sim, 1962). Signs and symptoms appeared in 28 subjects, and eight required treatment. Local signs were sweating, erythema, and itching; systemic signs were weakness, fasciculations, dizziness, headache, abdominal cramps, vomiting, and diarrhea. One patient had orthostatic hypotension.

In a V-agent accident (Freeman et al., 1956), a chemist had bilateral forearm exposure. She developed a headache that night, and had unusual sweating of forearms the next day. Later that day, she developed chest pressure, which

Table 5.12

Signs and Symptoms of Dermal Exposures to Nerve Agents

Tabun vapor, 2,000 CT	No symptoms and fall in AChE in masked subjects (Krakow and Fuhr, 1949)
Tabun (5 mg/kg) liquid, 400 mg (total dose)	Produced local sweating and a fall in AChE by 30 percent, with sweating lasting 8 to 14 days for most subjects, but one had sweating for 95 days (Freeman et al., 1954)
Sarin liquid, nonpersistent application 6 mg (total dose)	No symptoms, no fall in AChE (Grob and Harvey, 1953)
Sarin liquid, sustained exposure, 20 mg (total dose)	No symptoms, fall in AChE by 23 percent (Grob and Harvey, 1953)
Soman liquid, 35–75 µg/kg	Study I—There was some vapor exposure with chest tightness and miosis—cleared in 3 hours Symptoms began at 35 µg/kg. Testing, which lasted 3 minutes, stopped at 75 µg/kg (Neitlich, 1965)
	Study II—2–8 mg/man produced local sweating, slight fall in AChE (Neitlich, 1965)
Soman liquid, 65 mg (total dose)	Sweating, fall in blood AChE by 50 percent (Mumford, 1950, in Marrs, Maynard, and Sidell, 1996)
Cyclosarin liquid, 30 mg (total dose)	Sweating, fall in blood AChE by 50 percent (Mumford, 1950, in Marrs, Maynard, and Sidell, 1996)
VX vapor, exposure of arms, 28–681 CT	No symptoms, AChE maximum inhibition 43 percent (Marrs, Maynard, and Sidell, 1996)

lasted three days. She became extremely fatigued but continued to work; the sweating lasted 36 hours. She had previously been exposed to sarin, which had made her "slap happy"; her experience with the V agent produced an emotional tenseness that she found unpleasant.

Ocular. Most respiratory exposures involve the eye, and vice versa. The clinical effects of the various agents are similar, although their potencies differ. V agents produce miosis, headache, dim vision, impaired accommodation and conjunctivitis (Freeman et al., 1956) quite similar to tabun (OSRD, 1946) or sarin. Grob and Harvey (1958) instilled 0.3 µg of sarin into the eye producing miosis lasting 60 hours. There were local symptoms of pressure.

Miosis was very common in Japanese victims, with dim vision, eye pain and conjunctival injections (inflamed appearance) in 40 to 80 percent (Kato and Hamanaka, 1996; Nohara and Segawa, 1996). Discomfort with accommodation, due to ciliary spasm, occurred in 15 percent. Rengstorff (1994) studied two sarin accident exposures, and found little effect on vision, despite miosis. Japanese clinicians have reported a variety of abnormalities ranging from blurred discs to field defects. Rubin and Goldberg (1957a, 1957b) showed that night vision is impaired by sarin by a central mechanism, corresponding to the experience with U.S. accident cases. Narrowed field of vision and photophobia were found in dose-effect studies of sarin in producing miosis (Sim, 1956).

Intermediate Syndrome. An acute neurotoxic syndrome can follow the cholinergic period of organophosphate pesticide poisoning. The syndrome includes paralysis of limb and respiratory muscles and cranial nerves and occasional peripheral neuropathy, which seems different from classic delayed polyneuropathy. This intermediate syndrome has only been reported after substantial organophosphate pesticide exposures (Senanayake and Karalliedde, 1987) and has not been recognized with human or experimental nerve agent exposure, not even in the large Japanese experience (Ohtomi et al., 1996).

Long-Term Effects

It was to be expected that there would be interest in possible long-term effects from such highly toxic chemicals as nerve agents. The view of early experts in the field of nerve agent and organophosphate pesticide toxicity was that "recovery from moderate intoxications from nerve gas has always been complete" (Grob and Harvey, 1953). Long-term effects were only expected after severe intoxications, especially in cases experiencing severe hypoxia that was known to have damaged the brain. Soviet authors also considered that prolonged sequelae, such as vegetative-asthenic and extrapyramidal syndromes or toxic encephalopathy, were only expected after severe exposures (Karakchiev, 1973).

In occupationally exposed sarin workers, the duration of short-term symptoms, measured in days and weeks, showed some rough correlation with severity of initial symptoms and degree of cholinesterase inhibition, but exceptions were common (Holmes, 1959).

Other investigators, such as Gaon and Werne (1955) and Craig and Freeman (1953) were diligent in documenting the duration of signs and symptoms after exposures, with most follow-up reports ending at three weeks.

This diligence is part of the reason that Sidell and Hurst (1997) discounted the idea that long-term effects would be overlooked, citing alertness of supervisors in referring workers to medical care who did not seem "right."

Volunteer Follow-Up. NAS-NRC undertook a follow-up study of volunteers exposed to many different chemicals in studies at Edgewood Arsenal. NRC (1982) reviewed the known effects of "anticholinesterase compounds," including nerve agents (and some organophosphate pesticides) and then reviewed in detail the clinical records of 15 percent (219 cases) of the volunteers exposed to these agents. Of the 1,406 volunteers, 246 were exposed to sarin, 740 to VX, 26 to tabun, 21 to cyclosarin, 83 to soman, 11 to DFP, 32 to EA3148, 27 to PB, and 10 to malathion. Some volunteers received treatments, others not.

The 1982 panel concluded that, in the doses used, there was no evidence of long-term effects from the compounds surveyed, but noted that the survey under way might add further information. They suggested it would be possible to conduct studies of electroencephalograms (EEGs) in volunteers and controls to look for the changes reported by Duffy and Burchfiel (1980).

The final report (NAS, 1985) contacted volunteers about their health status, reviewed morbidity data from hospitalizations (including hospitalizations for mental illness), and reviewed overall mortality, including cause of death. Results were also analyzed in a stratified manner by class of agent and by specific agents. No unusual pattern of mortality or morbidity was identified and there were no indications of adverse long-term effects in the volunteers exposed to anticholinesterase agents.

Iranian clinicians have documented later consequences of mustard exposures in Iranian casualties of the war with Iraq, but apparently have not published reports of long-term health problems in their casualties from nerve agents.[16]

Limitations of Follow-Up Studies. While the above information supports the conventional view that long-term effects are not to be expected from nerve agent exposures except in the most severe intoxications and that there is little reason to be concerned about long-term health effects from lesser exposures, the situation is, regrettably, not so clear cut. Other medical and scientific personnel have expressed concern about possible long-term health effects of nerve agent exposure while also drawing on the larger human experience with organophosphate pesticides (Lohs, 1975; Boskovic and Kusic, 1980; Cadigan and Chipman, 1979).

Lohs (1975) noted there was little information about the effects of nerve agents, but considered that the chemical and toxicological effects of organophosphate pesticides made comparisons valid. He drew attention to the problem of evaluating long-term effects in trying to determine whether the patient had a history of acute poisoning or whether a subacute course of poisoning had been brought on by imperceptible doses.

The U.S. occupational and accidental exposure reports did not discuss the possibility of long-term health effects arising from subacute exposures. Although it was common to encounter workers with depressed levels of cholinesterase who did not seem ill, no follow-up studies of such workers has appeared.[17]

---

[16]Although patients take pyridostigmine for prolonged periods for myasthenia gravis and although anticholinesterase drugs are used in the treatment of Alzheimer's disease, we did not look at follow-up studies on these conditions, believing that the effort would be beyond the scope of this review.

[17]Longer-term studies were confined to workers with symptomatic exposures (Metcalf and Holmes, 1969).

Lohs (1975) cites and quotes Spiegelberg's studies of German World War II workers involved in nerve agent production. Lohs indicates that there were long-term effects in these workers, although the nature of their exposures or other exposures to organophosphate pesticides is not discussed (see the later discussion on longer-term psychological effects). One group had indications of autonomic dysfunction and decreased libido intolerance to alcohol, nicotine, and medications. A second clinical group had depression, syncope, and indications of neurological dysfunction. According to Lohs, Spiegelberg noted that some persons exposed to nerve agents recovered completely.[18]

Japanese Follow-Up Reports. Several Japanese reports claim patients are free from sequelae at three months (Ohtomi et al., 1996; Yokoyama, Araki, et al., 1998a), but Morita et al. (1995) identified a small number with problems at six months. Reports are now emerging of specialized follow-up studies in small groups of Japanese exposed to sarin. Yokoyama et al. (1998a) reported computerized static posturography studies in 18 exposed persons from the 1995 subway attack (nine men and nine women) and 53 matched controls. The exposed had reduced serum cholinesterase levels on the day of exposure, and their clinical findings (mild to moderate) were documented. They had recovered rapidly and, at the time of study (six to eight months later) were asymptomatic. Women subjects showed significant differences in eye open anterior sway and area of sway, which was interpreted as indicating delayed vestibular-cerebellar effects (Murata et al., 1997). These findings corresponded to similar findings in organophosphate pesticide workers (Sack et al., 1993).

The authors also referred to other work they had done in clinically recovered cases six to eight months later (Yokoyama, Araki et al., 1998b) who showed significant declines in neurobehavioral testing. The study compared 18 currently asymptomatic individuals, who had been exposed to sarin six months previously in the subway attack, with controls matched for age and gender. PTSD checklist scores were high for the sarin group, but the scores did not correlate with the neurological test findings. Brain stem auditory evoked potentials and visual evoked potentials showed prolonged latency in the sarin group. Electocardiographic R-R interval variability was different in the sarin group and correlated with AChE levels determined immediately after the attack. The authors concluded the neurotoxic effects of sarin, not PTSD, accounted for the differences (Yokoyama et al., 1998b).

Two further Japanese studies have looked for longer-term effects in patients and workers exposed in the Matsumoto event, where it is now estimated 12

---

[18]Because the primary documents are currently unavailable, this information should be viewed with caution. Note that the exposures are vague in Lohs (1975), and there is no mention of control subjects.

liters of sarin were released from a point source in a housing area at night (Nakajima et al., 1997; Nakajima, Ohta, et al., 1998). Nakajima and colleagues conducted a survey of all the inhabitants in an area 1 km downwind from the release site and 850 m wide. They contacted 2,052 people, of whom 1,743 responded to the survey. Those with symptoms were followed at four months and one year; 471 sarin victims were identified. Muscarinic symptoms were common to all victims, but nicotinic signs were confined to the most severely injured. Three weeks after the intoxication, 129 patients still had symptoms, such as dysesthesia of extremities. Some victims were experiencing asthenopia. The prevalence of that symptom had increased at four months. Although victims generally felt that the symptoms had decreased over the year, some were still troubled by eye complaints.[19]

A second study was smaller and followed the effects on rescue workers who had been involved in the event at different times after the release. Of 52 workers, 18 experienced some symptoms of sarin exposure. These were generally the earliest-arriving workers. The only worker who required hospitalization was one of the first who had been very active. The symptoms encountered were typical: eye pain, dimmed vision, narrowed visual field, nausea, vomiting, headache, sore throat, fatigue and dyspnea. On examination three weeks later, no worker had abnormal physical or neurological findings. In one-year follow-up, no rescuer had symptoms, unlike the residents: Seven residents were killed; 76 percent of the residents had symptoms; 28 percent were admitted to the hospital; and 21 percent consulted physicians (Nakajima, Sato et al., 1997).

There are examples of acute cerebellar signs in sarin exposure (Brody and Gammill, 1954; Gaon and Werne, 1955). Some animal data indicate that females are more sensitive to nerve agents (Callaway and Blackburn, 1954; Woodard et al., 1994) and recover more slowly.[20]

In summary, the Japanese studies, which primarily follow up moderately severe cases from the Tokyo attack, show victims who appear to be well but have subtle neurological changes detectable by special tests. PTSD has also appeared in victims of the attack and complicates evaluation of nerve agent effects. Long-term follow-up of mild cases has not been reported. Some were apparently included in the survey of cases after the Matsumoto attack, but it is unclear how many of the mild group were among those with illness at six months and one year. Overall, the vast majority of Japanese cases have made clinical recoveries, according to reports available.

---

[19]Asthenopia is a set of eye symptoms: blurred vision, eye fatigue, discomfort, lachrymation, and headache. Similar prolonged symptoms have been reported after organophosphate pesticide poisoning (Tabershaw and Cooper, 1966).

[20]It should be remembered that the cerebellum has important cortical projections and has functions beyond balance and coordination.

Focused Occupational Studies. Metcalf and Holmes (1969) reported follow-ups of two different groups of workers exposed previously to sarin and compared them with controls who were not exposed to chemicals. The authors did not describe how they selected their cases. In their 1952 study of 52 workers and 22 controls, the workers reported a high prevalence of aches and pain, fatigue, and drowsiness. Again in 1969 using a control group, workers who had not been exposed to sarin in the preceding year showed disturbed memory and soft neurological findings, suggesting incoordination. Their EEGs differed from the controls, although they were not clearly pathological.

A somewhat controversial study of 77 workers exposed to sarin more than a year previously and 16 controls found differences in the automated EEG interpretations of the two groups without readily diagnosed pathology (Duffy and Burchfiel, 1980).

Effects of Assumptions on Observations. Some accident reports document cases with substantial health effects—especially on memory and thinking, with fatigue prominent at 10 to 11 months after mild exposures (Gaon and Werne, 1955). In other reports (Brody and Gammill, 1954), it was clear that investigators had difficulty accepting the idea that mental problems four months after exposure could be related to the exposure. Gaon's use of a "possible" late effect also reflects this doubt. It seems possible that some long-term effects of nerve agent exposure may have gone unrecognized because clinicians' preconception that they did not occur.

The review indicates there is some possibility and evidence of long-term health effects arising from mild symptomatic exposures to nerve agents. The relationship to exposure levels or repeated exposures is unknown. The long-term effects, if any, of cumulative subacute clinically inapparent exposures have not been studied with respect to nerve agents. Single low-dose exposures of volunteers have not resulted in long-term problems. It has been shown that longer-term (months) decrements in performance on tests of mental function can occur from clinically inapparent organophosphate pesticide exposure (Stephens et al., 1996).

Delayed Neuropathy. The organophosphate compounds indirectly referred to are TOCP and leptophos, which are inhibitory to esterases, including AChE. These chemicals were associated with massive outbreaks of delayed neuropathy.[21] The organophosphate TOCP was recognized as causing delayed neuropathy ("ginger jake paralysis") by classic research of Smith et al. (1930),

---

[21]Recent review comments note that Smith et al. (1930, U.S. Public Health Service 45, pp. 2,509–2,529) preferred the classic research, which identified the basis for large outbreaks of neuropathy. We have been unable to obtain this paper.

who were concerned with the etiology of a peculiar form of paralysis afflicting large numbers of the population. During the 1970s, the highly publicized problem with OPIDN had focused on the insecticide leptophos, which brought to the forefront the health risks concerning insecticide manufacture in use. It was also appreciated that DFP, an anticholinesterase developed in World War II (OSRD, 1946), could produce a delayed neuropathy. There was understandable concern that other agents might have neurotoxic effects, although no delayed neuropathy was recognized in the approximately 900 occupational exposures to sarin (Holmes, 1959). There was no indication of delayed neuropathy in the NAS follow-up studies of volunteers exposed to agents (NAS, 1985).

Later experience with pesticides showed that some organophosphate pesticides, such as mipafox and leptophos, could also produce a delayed neuropathy. The leptophos experience is interesting in that the typical delayed neuropathy was not immediately evident; the pattern was a peripheral one, involving legs more than arms and sparing higher brain functions. In the case of leptophos, workers were diagnosed as having multiple sclerosis, encephalitis, or psychiatric disorders (Abou-Donia, 1981). Hayes (1982) reviewed this disorder in the case of TOCP and found in long-term follow-up that some of those exposed had dementia, although other factors could not be excluded (Hayes, 1982; Johnson, 1975; Abou-Donia, 1981). Kaplan et al. (1993) also found delayed-onset neuropathy among eight persons who had minimal or no acute symptoms after household exposure to the pesticide chlorpyrifos, generally considered to have low potential for neuropathy.

There is no established therapy for delayed neuropathy (Hayes, 1982). Oximes do not help (Johnson, 1975). Phenylnicotinamide may compete for binding sites and has shown some promise in TOCP-poisoned hens (Lotti, 1991).

Longer-Term Psychological Effects. One study (Coombs and Freeman, 1954) evaluated workers soon after accidental exposure to sarin and then three to six months later, when recovery was assumed to be complete. The researchers used a battery of intellectual performance tests (Wechsler Bellevue, nonverbal, and block design) to evaluate high-exposure and low-exposure groups. The mildly intoxicated "higher" group showed consistent declines in subtest scores for comparison and similarities on Wechsler tests, but the lower level group was normal. Both groups were normal on later testing (Coombs and Freeman, 1954). The long-term NAS follow-up study (after 20 or more years) of U.S. volunteers exposed to nerve agents did not find evidence of long-term health effects (NAS, 1985).

The SIPRI paper (Lohs, 1975) on long-term effects of nerve agents referred to Spiegelberg's studies of German nerve agent production workers many years after exposure. Spiegelberg's studies reported psychiatric syndromes consisting of lowered vitality and drive; defective autonomic regulation (headaches, gastrointestinal symptoms, and cardiovascular symptoms); intolerance to medicines, nicotine, and alcohol; premature aging; depressive symptoms; syncopal attacks; slight to moderate amnesia and dementia; and extrapyramidal neurological changes. No control group was described.

Beginning in 1952 and continuing into the late 1960s, Metcalf and Holmes (1969) of the University of Colorado Medical Center were involved in long-term evaluations of workers exposed to sarin. The sarin production facility did not use modern practices of occupational health surveillance. It does not seem to have occurred to anyone to include in the long-term studies persons from that workplace who did not report acute symptoms. These workers had symptomatic accidental acute exposures previously recorded. Initially, these were shorter term studies during recovery, but later, longer-term (months to years) studies concentrated on psychiatric and neurological effects, performance on behavioral tests, and EEGs. In 1952 (summarized in the 1969 report), 52 exposed workers and 22 controls had psychiatric interviews and evaluations. Muscle aches and pains, drowsiness, and fatigability were significant problems in the exposed group. The 1969 study evaluated men previously exposed to sarin. They had psychiatric interviews, neurological examinations, psychological tests and EEGs. The exposed group showed disturbed memory and difficulty in maintaining alertness and attention. Neurological findings were soft, with an impression of minor coordination deficits. Interviews showed higher numbers of the exposed patients were nervous or irritable or had changes in memory, decreases in libido, changes in sleep habits, or increased fatigue. The nature, time, and amount of exposure, along with the initial symptoms, were not reported. The authors had a control group but did not study workers from the sarin production facility who had not reported symptoms. However, none had exposure within the year. Post-hyperventilation EEGs differed from those of controls, and night EEGs showed many with a narcoleptic pattern. The authors concluded that the collective deficits indicated the deep midbrain effects of organophosphate pesticides.

In a study of 77 workers previously exposed to sarin (none in the year preceding the study) (Duffy and Burchfiel, 1980; Burchfiel and Duffy, 1982), 41 had three or more exposure episodes in the previous six years. There were 38 controls. Inspection of EEGs by blinded interpreters could not distinguish the groups. Spectral analysis by computer, however, showed significantly higher beta activity, lower alpha, and more rapid-eye-motion (REM) sleep in the exposed group.

In another study (Sim et al., 1971; Burchfiel, 1976), rhesus monkeys were injected with enough sarin for serious intoxication or for asymptomatic levels.

EEGs taken a year later were different from those at the time of injection for both groups, although more so with the higher-dose group.[22] The clinical significance of these two studies is uncertain, but it seems clear that doses of sarin that did not produce overt illness in the animals over several days of exposure (1 μg/kg for ten days) can produce long-term changes in EEGs.[23]

Karczmar (1984) reviewed acute and long-term consequences of organophosphate toxicity, summarizing the short- and long-term mental effects of nerve and organophosphate pesticide agents, and reviewed the follow-up studies conducted on sarin workers. The key long-term effects were affect (i.e., mood) and memory deficits, exacerbation of preexisting psychiatric problems, sleep disorders, insomnia, hallucinations and delusions, and psychotic and paranoid reactions. Most of the studies Karczmar reviewed pertained to pesticide experience.

Organophosphate Pesticide Experience. Other studies of organophosphate pesticides provide further insight into neurological, psychiatric, and psychological long-term effects of this class of chemical, including nerve agents. Workers with sustained organophosphate exposure but without toxic symptoms showed definite impairment in trail-making tests and visual gestalt tests, indicating left-frontal-lobe dysfunction. Abnormal EEG changes were also observed (Korsak and Sato, 1977).

Twenty-two farm workers became ill when exposed at mild to moderate severity to two organophosphate pesticides in combination. Nineteen were followed for over four months. Blurred vision lasted over two months, and anxiety that began at three weeks continued. Weakness cleared by two months, but it took two to three months for most to improve (Whorton and Obrinsky, 1983).

Savage et al. (1982, 1988), working from cases of documented organophosphate exposures in a registry, performed hearing, eye, clinical, laboratory, EEG, neurological, and psychological tests on exposed persons and controls. Exposed persons showed larger decreases in memory and abstraction and had more mood changes than controls. On psychological testing, the exposed group had Halstead-Reitan scores in the range seen with cerebral injury.

---

[22]There has been some critique of the primate model, which used implanted electrodes, but the control animals were similarly treated. The method of EEG analysis has also been criticized and rebutted (Oken and Chiappa, 1986). In a 1988 Federal Registry notice, the Centers for Disease Control found the changes to be not clinically significant. The findings need not indicate illness, but long-term rearrangements of brain electrical activity after low-dose exposure to nerve agent indicate of an effect that requires further attention.)

[23]Having an abnormal EEG does not constitute a disease process. However, the fact that a rather modest exposure to a nerve agent can produce what seems to be permanent rearrangement of rhythmic activity in the brain is a substantial effect. It suggests that other long-term neurological and behavioral complaints attributed to low agent exposure must be taken seriously.

Other investigators have identified similar changes in neurologic status or mental health of those exposed to organophosphate pesticides. Among the more interesting:

- several cases each of gastrointestinal problems, headaches, chest pain, and nervousness, plus three motor vehicle deaths among 235 persons exposed to organophosphate pesticides within the previous three years (Tabershaw and Cooper, 1966)

- a distinct decrement in performance on syntactic-reasoning and symbol-digit substitution tests among sheep dippers exposed to organophosphate pesticides; there was no correlation between test performance and prior symptoms of exposure (Stephens et al., 1996).

Jamal (1995b) has reviewed and summarized studies of organophosphate (including sarin) exposure (see Tables 5.13 and 5.14). Most of the clinical experience with nerve agents arises from exposures whose actual levels were unknown and not measured, arising from accidental exposures, from occupational exposures and from human volunteer studies. (Jamal did not review any actual attack experience.)

CLINICAL ASPECTS OF EXPOSURE

Asymptomatic Exposures

It is possible to have exposures that do not produce symptoms but that can lower serum and blood cholinesterase levels greatly (Holmes, 1959; Gaon and Werne, 1955; Freeman et al., 1956). No longer-term follow-ups on such persons are available, although papers reporting the measures of return of enzyme levels mention no problems. The general experience with the occupational exposures was that cholinesterase levels did not correlate well with clinical findings (Craig and Freeman 1953; Gaon and Werne, 1955).

Acute Effects

The effects of acute exposure are sometimes incorrectly interpreted as being due to other common health problems, such as respiratory infection, allergy, asthma, flu, or gastroenteritis, as was the case for workers who knew they were around nerve agents (Gaon and Werne, 1955; Craig and Freeman, 1953).

Acute effects vary by route of exposure. Vapor and aerosols produce eye and upper and lower respiratory symptoms, followed by other symptoms of mental confusion, gastrointestinal distress, and neuromuscular findings with weakness. At lower levels of exposure, it may take one hour from exposure for symp-

Table 5.13

Summary of Published Work on Chronic Effects of Long-Term Exposure to Small or Subclinical Organophosphate Quantities

Exposed Groups	Result[a]	Controls	Agent	Source
Workers Scientists	Psychiatric +ve Anecdote[b]	None	Organophosphate insecticide	Gershon and Shaw (1961)
Workers	Major psychiatric +ve Anecdote[b]	None	Organophosphate insecticide	Dille and Smith (1964)
Workers	EEG +ve Psychology test +ve	High/low	Organophosphate insecticide	Metcalf and Holmes (1969)
Sprayers	Behavior −ve	Nonexposed	Organophosphate insecticide	Rodnitzky (1975)
Farmers	Behavior −ve	Matched (small number)	Organophosphate insecticide	
Primates	EEG +ve	Control animal and preexposure EEG	Sarin	Burchfiel (1976)
Sprayers	Anxiety +ve	Nonexposed	Organophosphate insecticide	Levin et al. (1976)
Farmers	Anxiety +ve	Nonexposed		
Workers	EEG +ve Psychology +ve	None	Organophosphate insecticide	Korsak and Sato (1977)
Workers	EEG +ve Multivariate analysis	Nonexposed	Sarin	Burchfiel and Duffy (1982)
Rhesus monkeys	EEG +ve	Nonexposed		Duffy and Burchfiel (1980)
Workers	Psychometric tests −ve	Nonexposed	Diazinon	Maizlish et al. (1987)
Mice	End plate potential Jitter +ve		Mipafox	Kelly et al. (1994)

SOURCE: Reprinted with permission from Jamal (1995b)

[a]+ve and −ve are standard expressions used in toxicology to mean positive and negative, respectively.

[b]Reports from scientists working with organophosphate pesticides; not examined in detail.

Table 5.14

Summary of Published Work on Delayed Effects of Acute or Symptomatic Organophosphate Intoxications

Exposed Groups	Result[a]	Controls	Agent	Reference
Workers	EEG +ve Anecdote	None	Organophosphate insecticide, sarin, DFP	Holmes and Gaon (1956)
Workers	Psychiatric +ve Visual +ve etc.	None	Organophosphate insecticide	Tabershaw and Cooper (1966)
Rhesus monkeys	EEG +ve	Controls matched	Sarin	Burchfiel (1976)
Workers	EEG +ve Behavior +ve	Low-dose above	Organophosphate insecticide	Korsak and Sato (1977)
Workers	EEG +ve Psychiatric +ve	None	Organophosphate insecticide	Hirshberg and Herman (1984)
Workers	EEG –ve Psychometric test +ve	Controls matched cohort	Organophosphate insecticide	Savage et al. (1988)
Rats	Neuronal necrosis	Untreated	Fenthion	Veronesi et al. (1990)[b]
Workers	Psychometric test +ve	Controls matched	Organophosphate insecticide	Rosenstock et al. (1991)
Mixed	Neurobehavioral +ve Neurological +ve Neurophysiological +ve	Controls	Organophosphate insecticide	Steenland et al. (1994)

SOURCE: Reprinted with permission from Jamal (1995b), p. 89.

[a]NOTE: +ve, positive result; –ve, negative result.

[b]Repeated dosing for 2 or 10 months.

toms to develop (Craig and Freeman, 1953). Dermal exposures are slow in onset and only show eye and respiratory effects late in their course, with mental, gastrointestinal, neuromuscular, and circulatory effects preceding them (Bowers et al., 1964; Sim, 1962).

Eye effects of miosis (difficult and painful accommodation, blurred vision, dim vision, impaired night vision, and dilation of blood vessels in the conjunctivae with an associated headache) are the most consistently observed effects of vapor or aerosol exposures to nerve agents and, at very low levels of exposure, may be the only finding (Craig and Freeman, 1953; Holmes, 1959; Okumura, 1996).[24] In a combat environment, it would be surprising if impaired vision and night vision would go unnoticed and unreported, even if some of the other findings might be misdiagnosed. How much PB might modify the response of the eye to nerve agent is not known. In one study, standard pretreatment with PB for three days in volunteers did not prevent miosis from a CT of 5 mg-min/m^3 sarin but did decrease the severity and duration of the effect (Gall, 1981).

Respiratory effects—upper effects of rhinorrhea and lower effects of chest tightness, coughing, and wheezing—are very common but less specific to nerve agents than are the eye effects. There are no human data on how PB might alter respiratory clinical responses to nerve agents, although some animal data suggest some decrease in effect after PB pretreatment (Husain, Kumar, et al., 1993).

Gastrointestinal effects—nausea, vomiting, abdominal cramps, and diarrhea—occur later than respiratory effects. Excessive salivation is uncommon, except in higher exposures. A common report following exposures was a loss of taste or distaste for cigarette smoking (Holmes, 1959; Gaon and Werne, 1955).

Central nervous system effects of confusion, dizziness, difficulty thinking, and incoordination followed by muscle fasciculations and weakness are common and evolve over time but are present early. Less common are indications of peripheral nerve involvement with numbness and tingling of the hands and feet (Holmes, 1959; Morita et al., 1995). Since PB does not normally reach the brain, no protective effect on central effects of agents is expected from pretreatment.

Mental effects, with impaired thinking and memory, anxiety, and nervousness, have been documented in cases of dermal exposure in which the volunteers experienced no other systemic symptoms or signs (Bowers et al., 1964). Mental effects observed in exposed workers included altered behavior, impaired work performance, irritability, sleep disorders with vivid dreams, and frequent acci-

---

[24]Actual measures of low exposures have been uncommon; miosis without other complaints was often noted in production workers.

dents at work and driving (Gaon and Werne, 1955; Craig and Freeman, 1953; Brody and Gammill, 1954). As Craig and Freeman (1953) noted "inhalation of sarin may effect psychological disturbances of serious consequences for both the individual and those dependent on their judgment."[25]

With dermal exposures, there are skin signs, with excessive sweating, which may be prolonged for many days. Itching and erythema can occur (Sim, 1962; Freeman et al., 1954).

Recovery

The general experience has been that recovery from mild exposures is rapid, although in some studies some 20 percent had continued symptoms at or beyond two weeks, and 10 percent had them at or beyond three weeks (Holmes, 1959; Gaon and Werne, 1955). As will be discussed in longer-term effects, there were examples of much longer periods of symptoms (Gaon and Werne, 1955). Rapid resolution of moderately severe exposures was also the experience in Japan (Okumura et al., 1996). The milder cases in Japan do not seem to have been included in follow-up studies.[26] The muscle weakness encountered in some of Gaon and Werne's cases (1955) may be related to the disorder of myoneural junctions seen with anticholinesterase poisoning in animals (Gupta et al., 1987a, 1987b), but as with the animals is associated with recovery after exposure stops.

SUMMARY OF ACUTE EFFECTS

The conventional view that recovery from mild acute exposures is to be expected is further supported by the NRC follow-up studies (NAS, 1982; NAS, 1985), which found no adverse health effects in volunteers exposed to nerve agents.

Neuropathy Target Esterase Effects (Delayed Neuropathy)

No typical syndrome of delayed neurotoxicity of the type related to NTE has been described as occurring after nerve agent exposure, involving at least 7,000 persons. Animal studies have required very high acute exposures or repeated exposures to produce any neuropathy and could not produce the effect with some agents, such as VX (Gordon et al., 1983). The function of NTE is not known, and it is found in both neural (brain, spinal column, and sciatic nerve)

---

[25]There is also a considerable literature on mental and neurological effects of organophosphate pesticides, e.g., Gershon and Shaw (1961), Tabershaw and Cooper (1966), Stephens et al. (1996), and Korsak and Sato (1977).

[26]Also note other comments about the Japanese experience later, in "Longer-Term Effects."

and nonneural (lymphocytes, platelets) tissue. Higher brain functions are not affected in typical organophosphate delayed neuropathy. Other organophosphate chemicals have produced some atypical syndromes, however. Workers whose toxicity was from leptophos had a variety of diagnoses—mental illness, multiple sclerosis, encephalopathy—made before the nature of their toxicity was recognized (Abou-Donia, 1981). A family that developed neuropathy after exposure to chlorpyrifos (normally not though highly likely to produce neuropathy) also had a variety of mental symptoms (Kaplan et al., 1993). Follow-up of TOCP cases (Hayes, 1982) showed some with dementia and other mental changes, raising questions about the possibility of atypical syndromes.

Epidemiology

In analyzing epidemiological data for indications of low-level nerve agent exposure, the conditions that were commonly mistaken for the agent effects, such as respiratory infections, allergies, and gastroenteritis, should be kept in mind. Two organophosphate pesticide experiences are instructive. There were significant increases in outpatient clinic visits on an Israeli collective farm for eye, respiratory, and headache complaints on days when organophosphate pesticides were sprayed nearby (Richter et al., 1986). A generally higher morbidity for many different complaints has been reported for organophosphate pesticide-exposed greenhouse workers than for controls (Kundiev, Krasnyuk, and Viter, 1986).

Accidents

Changes in management and operational assignments evolved after the early observations that sarin workers with mild intoxications after release to duty were prone to industrial and vehicular accidents (Gaon and Werne, 1955; Brody and Gammill, 1954), although no statistical studies were done on the prevalence and duration of the problem. It became the practice to take exposed workers off night work and driving for several weeks. No studies were available that correlate farm-worker accidents with organophosphate pesticide exposure. However, in their 1966 follow-up study, Tabershaw and Cooper noted without comment that three cases were lost to follow-up by reason of death from motor vehicle accident, and clinical notes show that several others were injured in motor vehicle accidents. No data were available with which to compare this experience.

Many factors no doubt contributed to accidents during the Persian Gulf War and to the motor vehicle accidents that accounted for increased mortality in returned veterans (Kang and Bullman, 1996). Other studies of the motor vehicle accidents are under way, and the findings noted above might be kept in mind as another factor for analysis.

Tolerance

Tolerance to anticholinesterases occurs in humans but has not been the subject of follow-up studies (Hayes, 1982). Some of the nerve agent workers with very low cholinesterase levels who reported no symptoms were perhaps tolerant (Freeman et al., 1956). Tolerant persons do not show typical signs and symptoms when exposed to agents at lower levels, which would otherwise be symptomatic. Tolerance is not specific for particular agents but rather a tolerance for anticholinesterases in general, so that persons made tolerant to organophosphate pesticides would be expected to be tolerant of low doses of nerve agents as well. There is no information on whether there were "tolerant" personnel in the Persian Gulf theater. Individuals potentially could have become tolerant from unauthorized use of "flea collars" containing chlorpyrifos. Other than reduced response to further exposure to anticholinesterases, tolerant persons are expected to show increased sensitivity to atropinelike anticholinergic drugs.

LONGER-TERM EFFECTS (FOUR MONTHS OR MORE)

The possibility of long-term effects from severe exposures is well accepted, although not inevitable (Sidell, 1974; Morita et al., 1995). It seems impossible that severe cases would have gone unreported during the Gulf War.

Six-month follow-up studies of one-moderate-exposure and many-mild-exposure rescue workers in Japan did not reveal any ill health (Nakajima, Sato, et al., 1997). Surveys of exposed residents of Matsumoto, Japan, did note some ill health in those who had mild and moderate exposures at six months, with fewer cases ill at one year (Nakajima, Ohta, et al., 1998).

At six months, a small group of Tokyo victims that had moderately severe intoxications seemed well but had subtle changes on special tests, woman showing more effects than men (Yokoyama, Araki, et al., 1998a).

There are at least three reports of workers with mild exposures (or two in one case) who had problems with memory fatigue, concentration, and irritability four to ten months after their exposures (Gaon and Werne, 1955; Brody and Gammill, 1954). Because at the time it was commonly assumed that recovery from nerve agents was rapid, there was a possibility of underdiagnosis of long-term problems after exposure, since such effects were not thought possible. Some clinical notes of that period reflect doubt that nerve agents were related to the mental symptoms reported.

Metcalf and Holmes (1969) reported on two different groups of sarin workers compared to controls. In the second group, no worker had been exposed to sarin within the year, although some workers had multiple exposures in the past. Compared to controls, this group reported poorer health more mental and emotional problems and had neurological findings suggesting poor coordination. There were nonspecific EEG changes that were greater than in controls. Burchfiel and Duffy (1980) studied workers who had not been exposed to sarin in the previous year, comparing them to controls. They found more abnormal but nonspecific EEG changes in the exposed group.

Lohs (1975) reports studies by Spiegelberg on German World War II nerve agent production workers in follow-up after the war. Exposures are not defined, but this group was said to be in poor health with several clusters of disorder suggesting autonomic dysfunction, depression with intolerance to nicotine alcohol and medicines. The primary report is unavailable, and there may have been many confounding variables.

Organophosphate pesticide follow-up studies of several years' duration to several different chemicals at undefined levels have found health and mental function changes in formerly intoxicated patients (Tabershaw and Cooper, 1966; Savage et al., 1988).

It remains unknown whether unrecognized exposures can cause long-term effects, since no long-term follow-up of asymptomatic persons with low cholinesterase levels from agent exposure has been done. Likewise, no survey or study of production workers who did not report symptomatic exposures has been done. It is unwise to assume that there can be no long-term effects from unrecognized exposures. The organophosphate pesticide study of Stephens et al. (1996) documented exposures in sheep farmers, but mental performance decrements in formal tests conducted several months later showed equal degradations in farm workers who reported no signs and symptoms as in those who did.

"UNRECOGNIZED" EXPOSURES

There are several different categories of unrecognized exposures, with differing prospects for having long-term effects:

- **Acute exposure at a very low level in the "no effect" range, at which detoxification mechanisms eliminate agents, and little inhibition of cholinesterase occurs**—This may have been the situation with the very low levels of agent exposure projected from the Khamisiyah release—with no expectation of long-term effects. Subacute exposures are levels that do not produce overt symptoms but that over time produce substantial decrements in cholinesterase levels, more from repeated small exposures than a single exposure. Such exposures might result in the condition of tolerance.

- **Individuals with low cholinesterase levels but without symptoms**—It is not known whether such persons have long-term consequences, since the matter has not been studied. The report of sheep farm workers exposed to organophosphate pesticides (Stephens et al., 1996) indicates that it is possible to have substantial mental performance decrements after exposures that were not clinically apparent, some months after exposure. It may be possible to have long-term effects from this "unrecognized" category of exposures. It is believed that this group, which may arise from more sustained low-level exposures, could not have existed in the Gulf War, since exposures were all thought to be acute. However, agents trapped on dust or clothing, brought into shelters or vehicles, and released in closed spaces might provide some longer exposure opportunities (Gaon and Werne, 1955; Holmes, 1959; Freeman et al., 1956).

- **Individuals whose clinical response to an otherwise notable exposure to a nerve agent is modified by tolerance developed from sustained exposures to another anticholinesterase chemical (e.g., chlorpyrifos from flea collars)**—There have been no follow-up studies of tolerant persons. The possibility of long-term effects remains an open issue.

- **Individuals whose clinical response to nerve agents is modified by pretreatment with PB**—It is known that the severity and duration of mild exposures of the eye are diminished by pretreatment (Gall, 1981), but it is not known how much benefit may arise in decreasing other signs and symptoms. The matter has not been reported in low-level studies of animals, and human trials are unlikely.

- **Individuals exposed to amounts of nerve agent that produce symptoms and signs that are misidentified as arising from common illnesses, as has been noted in occupational settings**—It may be unlikely that there are long-term effects from mild or unrecognized exposures, but there is reason to think that such effects are possible, with some evidence that long-term effects have occurred (Gaon and Werne, 1955; Holmes, 1959).

PATHOLOGY AND PATHOPHYSIOLOGY

This section provides a picture of the spectrum of effects on various physiological systems following nerve agent exposure. More detailed studies from experimental animals are available, although they primarily deal with higher level exposures (McLeod, 1985; Baze, 1983; Koplovitz et al., 1992; Johanson, Anzueto, et al., 1985); however, subchronic studies have been reported, which were largely negative (Bucci et al., 1992a, 1992b, 1992c, 1992d). Myopathy and myoneural junction degeneration have been studied extensively (Gupta, 1987a, 1987b; Dettbarn, 1984; Ariens et al., 1969).

Recognition has been growing that nerve agents initiate processes with "cascade" effects that continue after direct agent effects have stopped. For example, agents induce seizures, which in turn release excitotoxic neurotransmitters that induce calcium influx into the cells, resulting in lipid peroxidation with ongoing oxidative and free radical damage to cells (Pazdernik et al.,

1996), possibly inducing apoptosis. Nerve agents can also induce massive, cardiotoxic, adrenergic outpouring (Filbert et al., 1993). However, no massive intoxications were encountered in the Gulf War, and animals with lower-level exposures or without seizures have not shown these dramatic changes (Petras, 1984).

Nervous System

This is the main site where the effects are seen. Both peripheral and central dysfunction occur at low levels of exposure (Sim, 1962; Bowers, Goodman, and Sim, 1964). Most animal studies (except for the negative subchronic studies, Bucci et al., 1992a, 1992b, 1992c, 1992d) have focused on the histopathology of higher-level intoxications. For many years, hypoxia was considered the precipitating factor in seizures and in brain injury. However, hypoxia preceding seizures has been ruled out by well-monitored primate studies (Johnson, 1985; Johnson et al., 1988; Johnson, Anzueto, et al., 1988). More-recent information gives a central role to seizures (directly caused by nerve agents) as the inciting stimulus for brain injury (Olney, 1990; Lipton and Rosenberg, 1994). When seizures are prevented, lesions are prevented or reduced (Baze, 1993; McDonough et al., 1995). However, sublethal doses of soman and sarin induced tissue changes without producing seizures, although such changes were not seen with DFP or metrazol (Kadar et al., 1992). Lesions show neuronal degeneration and necrosis with edema. Lesions in primates are concentrated in the frontal cortex, entorhinal cortex, amygdaloid complex, caudate nucleus, thalamus, and hippocampus, a distribution resembling anoxic damage (McLeod, 1985; Petras, 1984; Baze, 1993).

There is evidence of progression of injuries with encephalopathy, mineralization, encephalomalacia, and hydrocephalus in animals surviving substantial intoxications (McLeod, 1985; Wall, 1985). Animals surviving a single LD_{50} dose of sarin showed progressive neurological damage, initially in the hippocampus, pyriform cortex, and thalamus, but extending to other regions over three months (Kadar et al., 1992, 1995). Soman was more likely to produce frontal cortex damage.

The effects of nerve agents and other organophosphate compounds on sensory systems have been studied less than other systemic effects. Cutaneous peripheral receptors, but not mechanoreceptors, showed a reduction following subcutaneous soman administration 2.5 µg/kg/day for ten days in cats, or 5 µg/kg/day for five days. The studies involved the tibial nerve (Goldstein, 1985). In cats, low doses of soman in the range of 3 to 15 µg/kg intravenously were studied with respect to visual sensory performance. There was an abrupt decrease in visual evoked potential with doses above 5 µg, as well as decreases in contrast sensitivity and system gain (De Bruyn, 1991).

Nerve agents cause vascular dilation and increase cerebral blood flow in a manner that might influence their distribution (Scremin, Shih, and Corcoran, 1991). Soman, for example, causes some local constriction in cerebral flow (Sellstrom 1985). The mechanism seems independent of seizure activity (Drewes, 1985). Because of the effects on cerebral blood vessels, there has been suspicion that agents might alter the blood-brain barrier. In severe intoxications, the barrier can become more permeable, but this effect only occurs with seizures (Petrali et al., 1984; Drewes, 1985). Anticholinesterases alter the eye-blood barrier, an analogous situation, independent of seizures (Pshenichnova, 1985). Sublethal injection of soman (0.1 to 0.7 LD_{50}) permits the penetration of Sindibis virus, which usually cannot cross the blood-brain barrier (Grauer et al., 1996), indicating that soman at least might alter the blood-brain barrier without seizures. Increased permeability may make possible the entry of other toxicants, but also the entry of therapeutic agents.

A 51-year-old man was severely poisoned by sarin in the Tokyo attack and was in a vegetative state until he died some 13 months later. Neuropathological examination revealed marked nerve fiber decreases in the sural nerve and moderate decreases in the sciatic nerve. The dorsal root ganglia, dorsal roots, and posterior columns of the spinal cord were normal. It was considered that the dying back distal peripheral axonopathy was a late result of sarin intoxication (Murayama 1997; Himuro et al., 1998).[27]

Studies to identify sarin metabolites were conducted on the stored, formalin-fixed cerebellums of four fatal sarin cases from the Tokyo attack. Sarin-bound AChE was solubilized from the cerebellums, purified, and digested, and a search for sarin hydrolysis products was conducted by gas chromatography. MPA was identified, but IMPA was not and was presumed to have undergone hydrolysis during storage. This appears to be the first report of identifying nerve agent metabolites in formalin-fixed tissues (Matsuda et al., 1998).

Respiratory System

The main cause of death from nerve agents is respiratory failure, primarily failure of central driving mechanisms (Rickett, 1981; Johnson, 1985); Johnson, Anzueto, et al., 1988), but influenced by weakening of respiratory muscles and airway obstruction from bronchospasm and secretions. Mild respiratory symptoms—bronchospasm, rhinorrhea, and increased secretions—are an early sign of exposure. Even at a CT of 5 mg-min/m^3 of sarin can produce symptoms (Marrs et al., 1996), although effects at this level clear rapidly.

---

[27]These findings are not typical of NTE-delayed neurotoxicity pathological findings, which also involve the cord.

Rats exposed to fairly high doses of sarin showed increased cellular proliferation in the lungs with interstitial thickening by day 4; by day 16, there was sign of bronchiolar damage, loss of alveolar spaces, and consolidation. Vigorous standard therapy prevented these changes (Pant et al., 1993).

Johnson, Anzueto, et al. (1988) compared respiratory and cardiopulmonary responses of anesthetized baboons to agent vapors delivered through a respiratory support apparatus in the upper airway using doses of soman or sarin in amounts in the range of estimated LD_{50}, from 0.5 to 2.0—all very severe exposures. The animals were followed for 28 days. Pulmonary artery pressure rose; hypoxia only arose after apnea occurred but continued after respirations resumed. Cardiac output fell, and arrhythmias were noted. Seizures preceded hypoxia. There was evidence of direct pulmonary damage from sarin and more from soman, with persisting neutrophil increase and decrease in alveolar macrophages extending four days beyond exposure (Anzueto et al., 1990). It was suggested that such effects might predispose to pulmonary infection. Soman has been shown to have a direct effect on bronchial smooth muscles, promoting constriction (Fonnum et al., 1984).

Cardiovascular and Circulatory System

Nerve agents and organophosphate pesticides induce myocardial injury, with subendocardial hemorrhage and myonecrosis (McLeod, 1985, Saidkarimov et al., 1985; Singer, Jaax, and McLeod, 1987). Unlike skeletal muscle injury, which is reversible, cardiac injury progresses to fibrosis (McLeod, 1985). This effect is only obvious in serious intoxications (Koplovitz et al., 1992) and resembles the cardiac injury sometimes seen from massive sympathetic outflow in central nervous system catastrophes. Prevention of seizures in animals can prevent the cardiac lesions in some situations (McDonough et al., 1989) but is not always effective (McDonough et al., 1995; Filbert et al., 1993).

Dangerous cardiac arrhythmias (e.g., ventricular arrhythmias (Johnson, Anzueto, et al., 1988)) are a frequent complication of nerve agent and pesticide poisoning. Hypotension and tachycardia with decreased cardiac output are common following large exposures (Johnson, 1985; Johnson, Anzueto, et al., 1988). The tachycardia probably reflects adrenergic effects (Marrs et al., 1996).

Some serious accident patients showed signs of ischemia but may have had premorbid atherosclerosis. Soman, in animal studies, induces coronary vasospasm with decreased coronary blood flow (McKenzie and Ballamy, 1993).

Musculoskeletal System

There is clinical and pathological evidence that nerve agents and other cholinesterase inhibitors can produce myopathy. Muscle pain and weakness were common in occupational cases and serum creatine kinase levels were elevated (indicative of muscle injury) in many Japanese patients. Rhabdomyolysis with myoglobinuric renal failure has not been a feature of this apparently reversible injury. Early responses to substantial agent exposures are extensive twitching followed by flaccid paralysis (Marrs et al., 1996).

A subject of great attention has been the myopathy associated with motor end-plate degeneration, seen with nerve agents, organophosphate pesticides, and carbamate anticholinesterases. These effects are produced well below lethal levels. Two hours after agent administration, there is eosinophilia and swelling of sarcoplasm with loss of muscle striation. Later (within one day), there is leukocyte and histiocyte infiltration (Ariens et al., 1969). Activity and stimulation of motor end plates appears to initiate and exacerbate the problem. Oxime treatments that restore cholinesterase function are protective. The predominant evidence is that this myopathy is reversible. After tabun administration, recovery was seen in seven days (Gupta et al., 1987a).

Other Effects

Skin. The skin shows little reaction to the passage of agents. Increased sweating is seen, and V agents have produced erythema and itching (Sim, 1962). The stratum corneum may trap the agent and later serve as a reservoir for release.

Eye. The eye is extremely sensitive to nerve agents and can suffer effects at doses lower than other organs or systems. Agents coming into contact with the eye produce miosis, and induce vasodilation of conjunctival, scleral, and ciliary blood vessels, with ciliary muscle spasm producing pain. In some cases, intraocular pressure is lowered. There can be retinal effects with lowering of voltage in electroretinograms and decrease in dark adaptation with impairment of night vision, although the latter effect appears to be a central phenomenon (Rubin and Goldberg, 1957a; Rubin and Goldberg, 1957b; Rubin, Krop, and Goldberg, 1957). Eye changes from dermal exposures occur late in the intoxication, and in the case of this exposure route, pupillary dilatation is more likely than miosis. Japanese clinicians have reported a variety of other changes, including blurred disc margins and altered visual fields (Kato and Hamanaka, 1996; Nohara and Segawa, 1996).

Gastrointestinal Tract. Agents are rapidly absorbed from the gastrointestinal tract and produce early local symptoms (Karakchiev, 1973; Grob and Harvey, 1958; Sim et al., 1964), but gastrointestinal effects arise from all exposure routes, with cramping, increased peristalsis, vomiting, and diarrhea, even from low-level exposures. There is not an abundant literature about pathological changes in the bowel, and chronic diarrhea was not a long-term effect reported in occupational studies. Liver injury is reported from some organophosphate pesticide poisonings (parathion) but has not been a clinical or pathological factor in nerve agent toxicity (Hayes, 1982).

Hematological. Hematological effects resulting from agent exposures have been identified, but they do not seem to be clinically important. It is not surprising that some hypocoagulation abnormalities have been seen (Kaulla et al., 1961), since thrombin is a serine-esterase. *In vitro* inhibition of thrombin by sarin has been demonstrated (Thompson, 1969).

Johnson (1985) mentions bone marrow depression in severely poisoned baboons but did not provide details. Sastry and Sadavongvivad (1979) mentioned ACh receptors on stem cells. Nerve agents and organophosphate pesticides may impair immune function, but they may also increase resistance to infection (Mierzejewski, 1970a, 1970b). Clement (1985) found indications of high-dose soman-induced immune suppression in mice, although soman-induced hypothermia could not be excluded as a factor.

Mutagenesis. There is little evidence that sarin, soman, and VX are mutagens (there is no information on cyclosarin), and they do not injure DNA (Goldman et al., 1987). Tabun at high doses is a weak mutagen (Wilson, Nicaise, and De Bisschop, 1994). The presence of a number of sarin production by-products (diethylmethylphosphonate [DEMP], diisopropylmethylphosphonate [DIMP], and ethylisopropylmethylphosphonate [EIMP]) and metabolites (such as ethylmethylphosphoic acid [EMPA)) in the urine of Tokyo sarin victims lead to the conduct of sister chromatid exchange studies using peripheral lymphocytes in nine exposed persons and in controls with positive findings in the victims.

German scientists have stressed the alkylating properties of organophosphate agents (Lohs, 1975), but apart from some pesticides, that does not appear to be a feature of military agents. With the exception of tabun's weak effect at large doses, such agents do not appear to be mutagenic (Goldman and Dacre, 1989; Wilson, Nicaise, and De Bisschop, 1994). A decrease in DNA repair systems *in vitro* has been seen with sarin but not soman (Klein et al., 1987).

Genitourinary. Although there is often increased urinary frequency from bladder-stimulation effects, renal disorders are not a clinical problem encountered with nerve agent exposure (Sidell, Takafuji, and Franz, 1997; Marrs et al., 1996). The kidneys receive considerable blood flow and eliminate agent metabolites, but renal problems related to agents have not come to light (Sidell, Takafuji, and Franz, 1997; Marrs et al., 1996). There are examples of renal failure associated with organophosphate pesticide intoxication (Abend et al., 1994).

Development. There is no evidence of developmental toxicity from sarin (Laborde, 1996). Resumption of weight gain in subacutely exposed young rats given sarin or tabun is an indication of tolerance (Dulaney et al., 1985).

Endocrine. Endocrine systems normally demonstrate considerable periodic activity—circadian variations in corticosteroids and growth hormone, or monthly menstrual cycles. DFP-treated animals did not show altered circadian patterns, although prolactin levels were elevated (Kant et al., 1991). Clement (1985) conducted extensive studies in rodents using several levels of soman subcutaneously. There were increased levels of corticosterone, thyroxine, and T3, which returned to normal in 22 hours. ACTH and testosterone levels were decreased, but only with high-level exposures. Repeated low exposures to soman in rats at 30 µg/kg/day did not produce signs of intoxication or changes in hormone levels. Higher doses (40 µg/kg) produced toxicity and increased levels of glucose and corticosteroids (Peoples et al., 1988). Severe soman intoxication impaired ACTH and prolactin responses (Kant et al., 1991). No detailed endocrinologic studies of humans exposed to low doses of nerve agents are available. It is known that some carbamate anticholinesterases can affect growth hormones (Cappa et al., 1993).

SHORT-TERM EXPOSURES AND LONGER-TERM EFFECTS

This section reviews the literature related to longer-term effects from short-term exposure. The reader should keep in mind that what is possible is described, but whether exposure took place in the Gulf or not is beyond the scope of this report.

Assumptions

Severe and moderately severe poisonings from nerve agents, which clearly can produce long-term effects, would have been recognized during the Gulf War. Nerve agent exposures, if they occurred, were therefore at lower levels capable of producing only mild intoxications, or none.[28] No assumptions were made that only single acute exposures could occur or that repeated or sustained lower level exposures did not, since such matters seemed still to be under investigation.

Information

As is often the case, there is an abundance of data on nerve agents, but studies that directly address the specific issues of concern here are not to be found. Most human data on the effects of nerve agents come from events for which the actual levels of exposure are unknown (accidents and attacks). Most information is short term (weeks at best). Studies of persons who may have been exposed but were not sick are rare. There is more follow-up information about

---

[28]This level of effects has been the main focus of the review.

patients who were hospitalized than patients who were not. The expectation that recovery from all but the most serious poisonings was always to be expected may have introduced a bias to decrease recognition of long-term effects. The situation with respect to animal studies is similar, with more interest in higher-dose exposures and limited follow-up. There is often more interest in demonstrating an effect, such as receptor downregulation, than there is in following the resolution of the effect—i.e., when do receptor levels return to normal? In thinking about longer-term effects, it should be kept in mind that, for rodents whose lives are short, an effect lasting several weeks could be considered a long-term effect in terms of life span.

Questions

Some specific questions about the effects of nerve agents seem relevant to the analyses of the Gulf War:

- Is it possible to have nerve agent effects from lower-level exposures to nerve agent without obvious typical signs and symptoms?

- Is it possible to have long-term effects from mild exposures?

- Is it possible to have delayed effects from unrecognized exposures?

The prevailing view of many experts (Sidell and Hurst, 1997; Marrs et al., 1996; Elson, 1996) and review panels (DSB, 1994; IOM 1996; PAC, 1996a, 1996b) is that long-term effects from exposure to lower levels of nerve agent are not to be expected, especially when no signs and symptoms are recognized. There is substantial evidence to support these views, ranging from the negative findings of long-term effects in volunteers exposed to nerve and other anticholinesterase agents (NAS, 1982; NAS, 1985), through largely negative findings in follow-ups of Japanese casualties (Nakajima and Sato, 1997). There is no evidence that nerve agents are carcinogens, and only tabun has been shown to be a weak mutagen in some assays. Likewise, there has been no expectation of long-term problems from exposures to organophosphate pesticides without overt toxicity (Sidell and Hurst, 1997; Hayes, 1982).

The lack of reports of overt toxicity resembling nerve agent exposure has caused many to dismiss a role for nerve agents in the varied illnesses of veterans of the Gulf War. Sidell (1997) is of the view that long-term effects in sarin workers would not have escaped attention because of the alertness of supervisors and plant physicians to workers whose behavior was unusual.

This review has found information that—from cases of unrecognized exposures, long-term effects from mild exposures, and perhaps delayed effects—makes the above reasonable points of view less certain. The variability of response to nerve agent by gender, time of day, and interactions with drugs and chemicals has already been discussed. The clinical material above discussed a variety of circumstance where exposure might not be recognized at differing levels of exposure. With that in mind, the following subsections discuss the specific questions raised here.

Is It Possible to Have Nerve Agent Effects from Exposures That Are Unrecognized? Based on the published literature, the possibility cannot be ruled out, for the following reasons:

It is well documented that occupationally exposed persons were found who reported no acute signs and symptoms and who had very low cholinesterase levels (Gaon and Werne, 1955; Holmes, 1959; Freeman et al., 1956). Such persons were not subject to any special follow-up but in some cases were observed to be asymptomatic during the period when their cholinesterase levels were returning to normal.

Some of these individuals could have become tolerant of the agent as a result of their exposures. Similar situations are documented in organophosphate pesticide workers, in whom tolerance without preceding symptoms was found (Hayes, 1982). It is not certain that tolerance is without ill effects, but the situation is little studied. A clinical effect in tolerant persons and animals is an increased sensitivity to atropinelike anticholinergic drugs.

Although tolerance has been demonstrated in humans, the receptor downregulation of cholinergic receptors has only been demonstrated in experimental animals (Costa et al., 1982). However, there seems no reason to doubt that such downregulation occurs in humans. Tolerance induced by other non–nerve agent anticholinesterases (e.g., chlorpyrifos flea collars) would be expected to produce diminished clinical responses to low-level nerve agents.

Substantial mental changes (impaired thinking, memory, and calculating ability and anxiety) were documented in volunteers exposed to VX at levels that were asymptomatic for most (Bowers et al., 1964). No study of their recovery period was found; they were included in the negative findings of the NRC follow-up study (NAS, 1985).

There are several animal studies in which animals given doses of sarin, soman, or DFP were "sign free"—lacking overt signs of cholinesterase effects—showed definite behavioral and performance test decrements (Sirkka, 1990, intraperitoneal; Wolthuis, Groen, et al., 1995, intramuscular, acute; Buccafusco, 1997, repeated small doses). Only Buccafusco studied the process of recovery, documenting learning impairments and decreases in brain nicotinic receptors several weeks after exposure (a long-term effect for a rat).

There is comparable mental-effect information from a prospective study of organophosphate pesticide exposure in sheep farmers, which found that farmers exposed to pesticides who reported no clinical symptoms showed decrements in performance on psychological tests some months later comparable to that of farmers who reported symptoms (Stephens et al., 1996). Korsak and Sato (1977) also reported deficits in varied neurobehavioral tests in organophosphate pesticide workers who had never reported having overt symptoms. The latter investigators noted the similarity to nerve agent effects.

Misinterpretation of nerve agent signs and symptoms of exposure as being due to other common illnesses is well documented in occupational settings (Gaon and Werne, 1955; Craig and Freeman, 1953; Holmes, 1959).

Nonhuman primates given doses of sarin that produced no signs or symptoms (1 µg/kg/day for ten days) showed EEG changes not present in controls a year after exposure (Sim, 1971; Burchfiel, 1976) This study has been controversial. The effect may not be clinically important but shows a long-term alteration of brain function.

A surprising report is that of Husain, Vijayaraghavan, et al., 1993, in which mice exposed daily for ten days to inhaled sarin (5 mg/m^3 for 20 minutes) developed typical delayed NTE type neuropathy by day 14. The notable matter is they showed no anti-AChE symptoms at any time.

In summary, there is evidence of asymptomatic or unrecognized nerve agent (and organophosphate pesticide) exposure producing effects of various durations in humans and animals. Alterations of mental function are the best-documented effect.

Is It Possible to Have Longer-Term (Months to Years) Effects from Mild, Lower-Level Exposures? The answer is yes. It does not seem to be common for a single mild exposure to produce long-term effects. The possibility of observer bias causing some cases to be overlooked was discussed earlier.

There are documented case reports of workers with mild exposures (one or two exposures) who had problems of fatigue, poor memory and concentration, and irritability 4 to 10 months after exposure (Gaon and Werne, 1955; Brody and Gammill, 1954).

Workers who had not been exposed to sarin within the previous year, (compared to nonexposed controls) with reported single or multiple mild exposures were found to report poorer health, to have poorer performance on psychological tests, and to have "soft" neurological findings of poor coordination. EEGs were nonspecific but differed from controls. Some of these workers may also have worked with organophosphate pesticides (Metcalf and Holmes, 1969).

In another study of workers a year after their last exposure to sarin, compared to nonexposed controls, Duffy and Burchfiel (1980) found nonspecific EEG changes in the workers that differed from controls.

The single exposures in Japan have shown little in terms of long-term effects. Some moderately severe cases have shown subtle changes on special tests of neurological function six months after exposure. A survey of Matsumoto residents, some of whom were moderately poisoned and others mildly so, showed some nonspecific "asthenia" and poor health at six months, with fewer such symptoms reported at one year (Nakajima, Ohta, et al., 1998). The many mild cases of exposure in Japan have not been reported in the available follow-up studies.

In summary, there is some evidence that mild exposures can have long-term effects. The evidence that a single mild exposure can produce long-term effects is slight, and there is more evidence that repeated mild exposures can result in effects a year or more after exposure.

Is It Possible to Have Delayed Effects from Low Doses of Nerve Agents? There is no compelling evidence that documents latent effects of nerve agents appearing long after unrecognized exposure or resolution of initial signs and symptoms. The subjects of previously noted follow-up studies were not observed during the year before study, and there is no indication that the findings noted had developed just at the time of study. See Table 5.14.

No human cases reported from nerve agent exposures clearly resemble NTE-delayed neurotoxicity, and the main weight of evidence is that nerve agents have little potential for producing delayed toxicity, which typically appears two to three weeks following an acute exposure. At very high doses, soman and sarin can produce the disorder in animals from acute exposures (Gordon et al., 1983), while sarin has produced delayed neurotoxicity in mice from repeated exposures to sarin that did not produce signs of inhibited AChE effects (Husain, Vijayaraghavan, et al., 1993). The whole matter of NTE-delayed neurotoxicity is difficult, since the natural function of the inhibited enzyme and the mechanism by which inhibition causes injury are not known. The effect can be produced in animals with repeated doses of other organophosphate chemicals at intervals of six weeks (Lotti, 1991), and there is a potential for complex interactions of multiple chemicals. Typical delayed neurotoxicity would be readily recognized. Reports of atypical presentations with more central nervous system manifestations in organophosphate poisoning with leptophos (Abou-Donia, 1981), or chlorpyrifos (Steenland et al., 1994), or late dementia in TOCP cases (Hayes, 1982) make it uncertain that the full clinical spectrum of NTE-based toxicity is understood.

Likewise, the mechanisms of long-term effects of nerve agents are not well studied. No studies emerged of animals exposed to low doses of nerve agents with later neurophysiological and biochemical studies. Mechanisms other than inhibition of AChE are required. The long-term effects of nerve agents on receptor abundance and function have not been studied.

The detailed mechanism by which IEGs affect adaptations in the brain merits attention. An interesting concept is that of Kaufer et al. (1998), as demonstrated in animals, that a variety of cholinergic stimuli (stress, PB, organophosphate pesticides, or nerve agents) are all capable of inducing the expression of an IEG c-fos, a regulatory gene that directs the expression of the regulatory protein FOS, known to influence the expression of genes involved in cholinergic brain mechanisms. The duration and end-effects of such induction are not known. The concept does provide an interesting hypothesis of how several environmental factors of interest might converge on a common biochemical pathway in the brain capable of producing longer-term changes in the brain.

In summary, there is no evidence of nerve agents producing delayed effects similar to those associated with NTE, but there is reason not to ignore the possibility totally, given the incomplete understanding of NTE delayed neuropathy and indications that there may be atypical syndromes from this mechanism.

WHAT TO LOOK FOR IN THE GULF CONTEXT

The eyes are highly sensitive to the effects of nerve agents (NAS, 1997). Clinical and epidemiological reviews of the Gulf War should note that vasodilation of conjunctival vessels from nerve agents can resemble conjunctivitis, but pain on focusing, dim vision, impaired night vision, and miosis all point strongly to anticholinesterase effects. Impaired night vision would likely have been reported by affected persons in a combat environment.

Upper and lower respiratory symptoms of rhinorrhea, tight chest, cough, or wheezing are not very specific and have historically been confused with other causes of these symptoms. The same is the case for gastrointestinal symptoms of nausea, abdominal cramps, and diarrhea. Reports of a distaste for cigarettes is common in low-dose nerve agent exposure and, if reported, suggest exposure. Mental changes, disturbed sleep, irritability anxiety, and muscle weakness are commonly found in mild nerve agent exposures but also might be overlooked or misdiagnosed.

However, if several of the different physiological symptoms noted above are present, suspicion should be high that they were produced by nerve agents (Holmes, 1959).

Cholinesterase levels are not a very effective biomarker, other than indicating that an exposure has occurred. Early experience with nerve agents showed poor correlation between enzyme levels and clinical findings, some cases showing no inhibition for a day or more (Craig and Freeman, 1953). Serum levels rise within days after the end of exposure; red-cell levels stay depressed until the affected cells are replaced (about 90 days). Even if frozen serum or red cells from the Gulf War period were available, lowered levels of enzyme would not distinguish between nerve agents and other AChE inhibitors (e.g., chlorpyrifos or PB).

Should Gulf War material thought to have been exposed to nerve agents, such as mask filters or protective clothing, become available, there are now sensitive chemical techniques that might detect degradation products of the agents if they existed (Department of the Army, 1996).

The Armed Forces Institute of Pathology (AFIP) might be consulted on the possibility of obtaining evidence of nerve agent exposures from tissue material in their holdings from the Gulf War and the period immediately after.

Normal autopsy studies are directed at finding a cause of death. It might be useful to explore with AFIP whether material might be examined for indications of anticholinesterase activity, such as examining myoneural junctions for typical pathology.[29] Coronary blood flow is decreased in animals exposed to nerve agents (McKenzie and Ballamy, 1993). Review of material from heart attacks during the Gulf War might also be considered, looking for atypical findings.

AFIP's views could also be sought on the practicality of detecting degradation products of nerve agents in tissues, likely to be found from lower-dose exposures. There is some existing methodology for such measures (Sidell, Takafuji, and Franz, 1997, p. 296), but the applicability to formalin-fixed tissues is unknown to the reviewer. Japanese pathologists using large volumes of formalin-fixed tissues (the cerebellum) from fatal sarin cases have demonstrated sarin degradation products in formalin-fixed tissues (Matsuda et al., 1998), but such methods may or may not be applicable to lower levels of exposure. This is not a study suitable for random screening but might be considered, say, if there were material from a fatal accident after proximate exposure to the plume from a known release.

Any reviews of accidents during and immediately after the Gulf War should be aware of the historical information of high accident prevalence in workers following mild exposures to nerve agents (Gaon and Werne, 1955).

Epidemiologic studies of illnesses in veterans of the Gulf War might keep in mind the unproven possibility that the effects of several cholinergic stimuli (stress, organophosphate pesticides, PB, and nerve agents) might converge to produce longer-term changes in brain chemistry, resulting in a greater effect than any one of the factors alone. Looking at aggregate exposures of individuals and units over time might show correlations with later clinical problems that might not be evident in single-factor analysis. An example would be the previ-

---

[29]This would not, however, distinguish between nerve agents and other anticholinesterase effects.

ously mentioned increased clinic visits to a collective farm clinic on days when organophosphate pesticides were sprayed in the region (Richter, 1986).

There is a possibility that some persons in the theater may have become tolerant to anticholinesterases, including nerve agents. Such persons might come to attention because of adverse reactions to anticholinergic medications with atropine-like effects.

Although c-fos and FOS using PCR and immune methods could probably be detected in AFIP material, their clinical significance is not understood well enough to make such studies worthwhile at this time.

SUMMARY, ANALYSIS, AND COMMENT

Nerve agents inspire respect and fear. They are highly toxic and have steep dose-response curves, tabun being the least toxic and VX the most. They produce lethality in doses measured in micrograms per kilogram.

Their main effects are produced by irreversible inhibition of the enzyme AChE, producing signs and symptoms primarily resulting from excess ACh, overstimulating parts of the nervous system.

They also inhibit a variety of other enzymes in the body, but the biological consequences of this are poorly understood. The same situation applies to their direct interactions with neural receptors and cell membranes.

The nerve agents tabun and sarin are quite volatile, representing a considerable respiratory threat but with low persistence. Their volatility makes them less of a threat from dermal exposure. Soman and cyclosarin are somewhat less volatile and more persistent, and both pose significant dermal and respiratory threats. VX is not very volatile and is very persistent. It represents a serious dermal threat but has dangerous respiratory toxicity delivered as an aerosol in very fine droplets. All are subject to hydrolysis and degradation in the environment, lasting hours to a few days.

Severe intoxications with these agents produce signs and symptoms of seizures, respiratory distress, unconsciousness, and circulatory collapse (impossible to overlook during the Gulf War), which can produce brain and cardiac injuries that are sometimes long lasting. Moderately severe cases from Japan have usually recovered, but at six months, some cases showed subtle neurological changes on special tests despite generally seeming normal.

Delayed neuropathy from inhibition of NTE by nerve agents has never been reported in humans. Only sarin and soman have produced this neuropathy in animals, but exposure to extraordinarily high levels or prolonged exposure is required to produce the effect.

The effects of lower-level exposures to nerve agents have been less extensively studied in animals than those of higher doses. Most human cases of nerve agent exposures have been in the domain of mild or no symptoms. Since the most exposures arose from accidents or attacks, the exact exposure levels of these cases are unknown.

The eye is consistently the organ most sensitive to the effects of nerve agents applied by vapor or aerosol—with constriction of pupils (miosis), pain and difficulty focusing, dim vision, and dilated conjunctival vessels. NAS (1997) estimates these levels causing these effects to be as shown in Table 5.15.

Respiratory symptoms, headache, confusion, anxiety, dizziness, incoordination, nausea, gastrointestinal distress, and weakness all can arise in milder cases, at somewhat higher levels. The upper boundary of exposure that produces mild symptoms (patient can walk and talk but is definitely symptomatic) is not rigorously defined but is probably close to the ICT_{50}, as estimated in NAS (1997); see Table 5.16.

The onset of mild symptoms from lower-level respiratory exposures can be delayed for up to one hour, while it may take longer before symptoms from dermal exposures arise. The historical experience of mild recognized exposures is that symptoms last for hours to a few days before recovery, with 10 to 20 percent reporting effects to two to three weeks or beyond. Long-term effects are not expected.

The precise nature and amount of exposures, if any, of U.S. personnel to nerve agents during and after the Gulf War remains uncertain, as does the role of such exposures in producing illnesses in Gulf War veterans. The conventional view is that, historically, most low-level nerve agent exposures that were recognized produced interesting symptoms, which were cleared in a matter of days or weeks. Effects on memory, thinking, attention, and emotions were known but were considered to fade rapidly. For the majority of exposures, the number and duration of symptoms corresponded to the severity of the initial event. Neither the U.S. production experience nor the experiences in Japan (over 6,000 cases) produced a sustained set of complaints resembling the illnesses in the veterans of the Gulf War.

The low persistence of sarin makes it less likely that there have been effects from prolonged low-level exposures and from long-distance transportation from remote locations. Sarin absorbed in dust particles might persist longer or travel further. Cyclosarin might be more persistent, and less is known about this agent, although it has not been found to produce delayed neuropathy. There seem to be no reports of the dim vision or impaired night vision that would have been expected from low-level exposures, and these would have cre-

Table 5.15

Estimates of Threshold Levels
for Eye Effects of Selected
Nerve Agents

Nerve Agent	mg-min/m^3
Tabun	0.5[a]
Sarin	0.5[a]
Soman	0.2
Cyclosarin	0.2
VX	0.09

SOURCE: NAS (1997).
[a]Possibly higher.

Table 5.16

Estimates of Incapacitat-
ing Levels of Selected
Nerve Agents

Nerve Agent	mg-min/m^3
Tabun	≤50
Sarin	≤25
Soman	≤25
Cyclosarin	≤25
VX	10

SOURCE: NAS (1997).

ated concern during a war. The exposure to nerve agents of U.S. experimental subjects does not seem to have produced notable long-term effects.

Humans retain about 85 percent of inhaled sarin, but some is trapped in the mucous of the respiratory tract and, when absorbed, encounters a number of nonspecific binding chemicals and enzymes in blood and tissue capable of hydrolyzing and degrading it. For very low-level exposures remote from Khamisiyah, these protective systems may have provided a "no effect" level of exposure. For example, the 0.01296 mg-min/m^3 exposure to sarin at Khamisiyah found in the CIA model can also be expressed as 0.01296 μg. During a 1-minute exposure for a human breathing 10 l of air per minute, 89 percent (0.115 μg) of the total inhaled sarin (0.12986 μg) would be absorbed. As a point of comparison, Somani (1992) estimates that a guinea pig can metabolize (degrade and detoxify) sarin at a rate of 0.013 μg/kg/min. Although the rate at which humans metabolize sarin has not been determined, if it is similar to the rate in guinea pigs, a 70 kg human should be able to metabolize 0.91 μg of sarin per minute. This calculated degradation rate is much higher than the calculated exposure from Khamisiyah. Studies of low-dose inhalation exposures with absorbed doses of 0.08 to 9 µg/kg (Oberst et al., 1959; Freeman et al., 1952) indicate considerable individual variation in response and suggest that humans are less able to detoxify sarin than guinea pigs. Intraarterial administration of 3 to 4 µg/kg to humans produced no symptoms (Grob and Harvey, 1953).

The very low estimates of exposure arising from the Khamisiyah release make sarin-cyclosarin–induced delayed neurotoxicity essentially impossible. The amount of sarin required to produce this effect may be less than originally thought by researchers, but rather substantial amounts are required nonetheless.

On the other hand, it is not possible to eliminate nerve agents categorically from playing a role in some cases of illnesses of Gulf War veterans because of other information about the effects of nerve agents and related organophosphate pesticides.[30] The reasons include the following:

1. From occupational experience, it is known that persons have been discovered who had quite low cholinesterase levels, indicating exposure, who had not experienced any acute signs and symptoms, even many years later. Such persons were not studied after their cholinesterase levels returned to normal.[31]

2. Although there is no clear evidence of long-term effects arising from a single acute exposure producing mild effects, there are several reports of sarin workers with one or two mild exposures experiencing problems of fatigue, impaired memory and concentration, and irritability four to ten months after exposure.[32]

3. The population of workers who were in the plants where sarin was made but who did not report symptoms was never included in any long-term follow-up study. Any health problems they may have encountered could have been unrecognized as related to agent exposure. (Follow-up studies of field workers involved with organophosphate pesticides who had not reported clinical symptoms showed a variety of deficits on psychological testing long after exposure was possible; Korsak and Sato, 1977).

4. Follow-up studies of workers with mild responses to sarin exposure (some multiple) a year after the last sarin exposure, showed more health complaints, deficits on psychological testing, neurological findings of poor

---

[30]This falls in the category of agents that "could" do certain things; whether they "did" is quite another matter.

[31]There is also a lack of information about persons with similar findings from organophosphate pesticides.

[32]There may have been problems recognizing long-term effects, since the prevailing view at the time was that they did not occur.

coordination, and nonspecific EEG changes than the controls. Another study with controls found nonspecific EEG changes in workers who had not been exposed to sarin in the previous year.

5.   It is possible to have substantial mental effects from acute nerve agent exposure (VX) (impaired thinking, memory, calculating ability, and anxiety) at levels where other clinical signs and symptoms were absent (Bowers et al., 1964).

6.   Similar data from animal studies with sarin (acute), soman (acute), and DFP (repeated doses) showed impaired test performances and altered behavior at levels not associated with other signs of toxicity. Recovery times for acute exposures were not reported, but the DFP study found impaired learning several weeks after stopping the agent.

7.   The above studies make the point that some mild exposures with effects may be unrecognized and that, at least for some repeated low-level exposures, there can be long-term effects. Comparable data from organophosphate exposures of sheep farmers found decrements in the performance on psychological tests in asymptomatic individuals who were exposed that was comparable to that of those with symptoms, weeks to months after exposure (Stephens et al., 1996).

8.   The controversial study that showed EEG changes lasting a year in non-human primates given 1 µg/kg of sarin for ten days, which did not produce any evident illness, may not be "clinically" important but does show a long-term change in brain function from doses that were without clinical signs (Duffy and Burchfiel, 1980).

9.   The experience with occupational exposures is that it is possible for signs and symptoms of mild exposures to be misinterpreted as being due to other common health problems, such as upper respiratory infections or allergies, because of the nonspecific nature of the symptoms. The possibility that such misinterpretation could have occurred during the Gulf War should not be dismissed.

10. Based on self-reported exposures (Haley, Horn, et al., 1997), there is a possibility that some persons with sustained use of unauthorized flea collars containing chlorpyrifos (or other anticholinesterase exposures) might have developed tolerance to anticholinesterases and would not be expected to show typical signs and symptoms when exposed to nerve agents—providing yet another opportunity for unrecognized exposures.

11. Recovery from the tolerant state has been little studied, and the long-term effects (if any) are unknown. In animals with repeated exposures to DFP, there are suggestions of decreased abundance of nicotinic receptors being

associated with impaired performance on memory tests, for some weeks after stopping the agent (Buccafusco et al., 1997).

12. The effects of PB in modifying the clinical effects of low-level exposures have not been much studied. There is a report that humans pretreated with pyridostigmine and then exposed to 5 CT (mg-min/m^3) of sarin had less-severe miosis and a shorter period of visual symptoms (Gall, 1981). There are reports that pretreatment with PB (and other carbamates) lessens the effects of respiratory exposures to sarin at doses of about 50 CT in experimental animals (without other treatment) (Vijayaraghavan et al., 1992). This raises the possibility that PB pretreatment might modify some low-level exposures to a point where they would not be recognized. Since PB does not normally penetrate the blood-brain barrier, it would not be expected to protect the central nervous system from the effects of milder exposures. There is an animal study at somewhat higher levels using labeled sarin in pretreated and control animals that did not find increased label in the brains of the pretreated animals.

13. There are indications that there can be atypical syndromes, with more indication of central nervous system effects in NTE neurotoxicity (although not from nerve agents). The mechanism of toxicity is not well understood. Nerve agents alone seem unlikely to produce NTE effects, but nothing is known about their effects when combined with other organophosphate chemicals. Some organophosphate chemicals have shown development of toxicity when administered at six-week intervals. Cyclosarin has not been shown to produce delayed neurotoxicity in acute animal models, but it is a potent inhibitor of NTE. No studies examine combinations of sarin and cyclosarin in NTE toxicity models, and there are no animal studies of repeated exposures similar to those of Husain with sarin (Husain, Vijayaraghavan, et al., 1993)

This limited understanding and information about NTE effects creates uncertainty about whether it can be ignored. The other data create uncertainty that long-term effects can only arise after recognized exposures and that long-term effects from mild exposures cannot occur.

The effects of agents on nonneural tissues (lymphocytes, bone marrow) are poorly understood. There is animal research evidence that sign-free doses of soman permit viruses to enter the brain that would not normally enter. Modification of responses to infection by nerve agents cannot be excluded, although human clinical experience has not noted such effects.

There is little information about interactions of nerve agents with other chemicals at lower levels of exposure. There is some evidence that combined exposure of mustards with nerve agents can increase the toxicity of both. A person taking an atropinelike compound (e.g., an antihistamine drug) might have decreased response to nerve agent—similar to the protective effect seen in animals pretreated with atropine (SIPRI, 1976).

The experience of workers recovered from mild exposures enough to resume work being prone to industrial and motor vehicle accidents deserves mention. The duration of the effect was not well defined, and the observation was not studied in detail. The effect should be kept in mind in analyses of accidents during the war (Writer, DeFraites, and Brundage, 1996) and in accidents of returned veterans (Kang and Bullman, 1996). Of course, many other factors are involved in increased accidents during periods of high operational activity and on return from overseas.

In 1998, a new Russian (Soviet-developed) nerve agent, Novichok—said to be a binary agent and highly toxic—was mentioned in the press (Englund, 1992a, 1992b; Adams, 1996; Tucker, 1996; Uhal 1997; "Russia Dodges . . . ," 1997). A Russian scientist-émigré was said to have indicated that some U.S. detectors might not recognize the agent and that it might have been available to Iraq (Smart, 1997). There are no peer-reviewed or scientific journal references to this agent, although there are some press reports. A Russian scientist, Dr. Vil Mirzaynov, has described a Soviet secret program of nerve agent developments. In an interview posted on the Internet, Dr. Mirzaynov said he was certain that the Soviets and Russia had not sent Novichok to Iraq.

It has been known for a long time that there are anticholinesterase chemicals that are 10 to 100 times more potent than current agents reviewed (SIPRI, 1971). The existence Novichok is scientifically undocumented, and its use has not been mentioned in any of the postwar revelations about Iraqi chemicals. The matter is mentioned here for completeness but does not appear relevant to a scientific review of chemical agents associated with the Gulf War.

RECOMMENDATIONS

The descriptions of the findings in mild nerve agent exposures should be kept in mind in any review of medical records using some of the distinguishing features mentioned in the clinical discussion, as well as the overall pattern and sequence of symptoms. Epidemiology reviews of medical experience in the theater should keep in mind the reports of increased outpatient visits for eye, headache, and respiratory complaints noted in a farm clinic on days when organophosphate pesticides were sprayed nearby.

It may be technically possible to document nerve agent and anticholinesterase exposure using material AFIP possesses. Whether it is practical or desirable to do so is a matter for discussion with the institute and relevant specialists.

Doing a study on a screening basis would be unadvisable, but such studies might be warranted if there is a probability of prior exposure to detectable amounts.

In the ongoing discussions with Japanese clinicians about their follow-up studies, it would be valuable to develop a clearer picture of the long-term outcomes of the many mild cases who did not require treatment.

It is not known what records exist for the occupationally exposed U.S. production workers or what health data on them exists. There would be interest in long-term follow-up of such workers, most of whom would be rather elderly now. Such a study would be difficult and expensive, especially in providing suitable controls and obtaining credible data about other occupational exposures.

The problem of illnesses in veterans of the Gulf War has inspired a large amount of research related to nerve agents, stress, PB, and pesticides. It was not within the scope of this report to survey such activity or to report on work in progress or in unreviewed drafts. Thus, any suggestions about research offered here may be redundant.

Further evaluations of NTE-based delayed effects from nerve agents should examine the effects of sarin-and-cyclosarin combinations. It would be helpful to use animal models of repeated subclinical exposure to replicate the effects Husain reported and to determine the threshold level of exposure that produces the effect. If the effects are consistently observed, it would be important to attempt their replication in some other species such as nonhuman primates, to better judge the hazard to humans from the effects of repeated subclinical exposures. Effects on higher-level brain performance might be examined as well. It is not certain that important combined effects of nerve agents and organophosphate chemicals could not occur. Those working in the field might be asked about experimental designs to look at combined effects that might relate to pesticides to which troops were exposed during the war, if any.

The role of receptor downregulation from sustained subclinical exposures is worth additional research. Some effects of this downregulation may be pathological. The hypothesis that ACh excess and receptor downregulation may produce long-term effects on the brain (Buccafusco et al., 1997; Kaufer et al., 1998) also merits further evaluation, with particular attention to the recovery process and duration of effects. Further documentation of effects from subclinical exposures to military agents and interactions with anticholinesterase pesticides and pretreatments appears to be important. The use of cholinergic drugs acting directly on receptors (e.g., nicotine) will no doubt be pursued, especially by the VA.

The consequences of the Gulf War have brought to light the possibility that humans subject to extreme stress may have alterations in the permeability of their blood-brain barrier, which permits the entry into the brain of molecules normally excluded, as is suspected with PB (Sharabi et al., 1991; Sharma et al., 1991; Friedman et al., 1996). There is also evidence in animals that nerve agents at lower doses may permit the entry of viruses normally excluded by the barrier (Grauer et al., 1996). These phenomena need much more research and documentation in humans.

Regional activity within the brain increases cerebral blood flow to the active region. This in turn may alter the regional distribution to the brain of lipophylic agents and toxins such as nerve agents. The state of cerebral activity at the time of exposure may influence the response to nerve agents and other toxins. This variable might be examined in modeling the effects of agents at lower levels of exposure.

The observation that a variety of cholinergic stimuli (stress, PB, organophosphate pesticides, and nerve agents) can induce the expression of a regulatory gene, c-fos, that is involved in adaptation of the brain to external stimuli appears to be important, but more investigation is needed to understand the duration of the effect and just what end-results occur biochemically and functionally.

Some thought should be given to study in animals of the aggregate effects of stress, PB, organophosphate pesticides, and low-level nerve agent. Longer-term observations, performance effects, and biochemical studies are indicated for these analog exposures, to simulate possible exposures of the Gulf War.

The possibility of a convergent mechanism with a common pathway for several exposures might be kept in mind in epidemiology studies that might develop an aggregate index of exposures of different kinds with which to compare later health effects.

It may well be that nerve agents had nothing to do with illnesses of veterans of the Gulf War, but enough is known—and unknown—about their effects (especially in combination with other factors) not to ignore them.

Chapter Six

CONCLUSIONS AND RECOMMENDATIONS

CONCLUSIONS

Four broad conclusions can be drawn from this review. First, a militarily effective dose of any of the agents considered in this review would not have escaped notice. Such a dose would have produced symptoms requiring treatment or would have killed the soldiers exposed. While there might have been some difficulty identifying a specific agent, no symptoms consistent with exposures to large doses of any of the agents included in this review were reported. One individual was apparently exposed to mustard gas residual.

Second, low-level exposures to many of these agents could have produced symptoms that were simply overlooked or attributed to other, more commonplace sources, such as irritation from dust and sand, upper respiratory infections, gastroenteritis, asthma, or the flu. The possibility of exposures to low levels of more than one agent either simultaneously or in relatively close proximity makes diagnosis difficult. Therefore, on clinical grounds alone, it is not possible to dismiss low-dose exposures to one or more of the agents or the possibility that such exposures contributed to some of the symptoms experienced by the Gulf War veterans. That said, it is difficult to accept that exposures affecting large numbers of troops would have escaped clinical notice. Furthermore, the literature reports no clinical symptoms developing years after exposure, which was the case for about half of the veterans reporting health problems.

Third, the literature suggests that some interaction may occur between chemical warfare agents and other factors. Several factors, such as stress, PB, and anticholinesterase nerve agents, that may contribute to the symptoms seen in the veterans can activate regulatory genes (such as c-fos) in the brains of animals. Because of the potential long-term effects of these genes, this observation may be important. However, the long-term effects in animals and the clinical significance for humans remain to be determined. Epidemiological studies of illnesses in the veterans might consider the possibility of aggregate effects.

Since mustards, trichothecene toxins, and nerve agents also inhibit AChE, it may be useful to examine their effects on regulatory gene expression as well.

Fourth, very little of the literature treats long-term effects of exposures to doses below those that would cause acute clinical symptoms. Considerably more research is needed in this area before even preliminary suppositions can be formulated.

RECOMMENDATIONS

The primary recommendation is that research be conducted to fill the gaps noted here. The most obvious area needing additional research is the heath effects of low-level exposures to agents or toxins. We would note that, since the Gulf War, DoD and the VA have begun to fund a good deal of research. Research in other areas would also be beneficial, including the following:

- understanding the effects of mustard agents on the central nervous system

- long-term follow-up studies on the Japanese exposed to sarin in the subway attack, particularly those exposed to low levels

- better understanding of the acute respiratory toxicity of aflatoxin in non-human primates

- research to determine the long-term effects of converging cholinergic activation of c-fos

- follow-up study of the duration of response of the convergent response mechanism of nerve agent action that Kaufer et al. (1998) described

- extension of the observations pertaining to the downregulation of nicotinic receptors in the brain from low-dose DFP

- making those involved in the epidemiological studies of accidents during and immediately after the Gulf War aware of the observation that sarin workers who had mild exposures were noted to have many industrial and vehicular accidents.

Finally, interactions between the various chemical warfare agents and other chemicals on the battlefield, as well as other psychosocial factors, such as stress, will need to be examined to develop a more complete understanding of the possible health consequences of exposure to chemical and biological warfare agents.

DOSE AND EXPOSURE CHARACTERIZATIONS

SYSTEMIC, ORAL, INTRAVENOUS, AND INTRAPERITONEAL EXPOSURES

Systemic, oral, intravenous, and intraperitoneal exposures are commonly expressed in terms of the weight of the agent (milligrams or micrograms) per kilogram of the weight of the organism dosed.

CUTANEOUS EXPOSURES

Cutaneous exposures may be expressed in terms of a total dose or in terms of the weight of the agent (milligrams or micrograms) per square centimeter times the total area exposed.

The lethal dose (LD) for the organism in question is expressed in one of two ways:

- LD_{50} represents the dose that produces 50-percent mortality in the exposed population of interest.

- LD_{10} represents the dose that produces 10-percent mortality in exposed population of interest.

The incapacitating dose (ID) for the organism in question is similarly expressed:

- ID_{50} is the dose that incapacitates 50 percent of the population of interest.

- ID_{10} is the dose that incapacitates 10 percent of the population of interest.

Incapacitation can vary from moderate (unable to see, breathless) to severe (convulsions).

RESPIRATORY EXPOSURES

Respiratory exposures are expressed in terms of the product of the concentration (C) of the vapor or aerosol, usually expressed as milligrams (or micrograms) per cubic meter (or liter), e.g., 35 mg-min/m3 or 0.13 μg-min/l, and the length of the exposure (T). The resulting value is known as the CT.

Note that CT is an expression of exposure, not the amount inhaled or deposited. The same CT can be produced by varying concentration or exposure time. The effect of a given CT may or may not be the same if T is varied from a few minutes to several hours. For example, a CT of 5 can be obtained by exposure to 0.05 mg/m^3 for 100 minutes or to 5 mg/m^3 for 1 minute. The generalization is not reliable for very short exposures (during which breath might be held) or very long exposures (during which metabolic detoxification may operate).

As above, certain key dosages are of interest[1]:

- **LCT$_{50}$** is the CT required to produce 50-percent mortality in the exposed population.

- **ICT$_{50}$** is the CT required to incapacitate 50 percent of the exposed population.

---

[1]These definitions are also used for vapor or aerosol effects on the skin.

DATA ON NERVE AGENTS

The following tables present detailed information on the chemical and physical properties, as well as additional exposure-effect relations and symptoms from occupational exposures. Much of the latter information is derived from Holmes (1959).

Table B.1

Chemical and Physical Properties of Tabun

Agent	Tabun GA ethyl N,N-dimethylphosphoroamidocyanidate
Chemical structure	

$$CH_3CH_2 - O - \overset{\overset{\displaystyle O}{\|}}{\underset{\underset{\displaystyle CN}{|}}{P}} - N \overset{\diagup CH_3}{\diagdown CH_3}$$

Molecular weight	162.13
Physical state (20°C)	Colorless to brownish liquid giving off a colorless vapor
Vapor density (compared to air)	5.63
Liquid density (g/cc)	1.073 at 25°C
Boiling point (°C, 760 mm Hg)	220–246, with decomposition
Melting point (°C)	–14 to –50
Vapor pressure (mm Hg)	0.07 at 25°C
Volatility (mg/m^3)	400 to 600 at 20°C 610 at 25°C (1/20th of that of water) 858 at 30°C, 90 at O°C
Viscosity (cp at 20°C)	Not found
Surface tension (dynes/cm at 20°C)	Not found
Solubility	Miscible in both polar and nonpolar solvents; 9.8 percent in water at 25°; very soluble in alcohols and other organic solvents
Decomposition temperature (°C)	150 (complete in 3-1/4 hours)
Odor	Almond to faintly fruity; none when pure
Thickening	Possible, but unlikely; has low volatility in any case

SOURCES: U.S. Army (1990); SIPRI (1973); Karakchiev (1973); OSRD (1946); AD Little (1986), Ch. 5.

Table B.2

Chemical and Physical Properties of Sarin

Agent	Sarin
	GB
	Isopropyl methylphosphonofluoridate
	Trilon 46
Chemical structure	

$$H_3C - \underset{\underset{F}{|}}{\overset{\overset{O}{\|}}{P}} - O - \underset{\underset{CH_3}{|}}{\overset{\overset{CH_3}{|}}{CH}}$$

Molecular weight	140.10
Physical state (20°C)	Colorless liquid giving off a colorless vapor
Vapor density (compared to air)	4.86
Liquid density (g/cc)	1.102 at 20°C
Boiling point (°C, 760 mm Hg)	147–158, with decomposition
Melting point (°C)	–56
Vapor pressure (mm Hg)	2.9 at 25°C, 2.10 at 20°C
Volatility (mg/m^3)	4,100 at 0°
	6,091 at 20°
	29,800 at 30°
Viscosity (cp at 20°C)	Not found
Surface tension (dynes/cm at 20°C)	Not found
Solubility	Miscible in both polar and nonpolar solvents
	Infinitely soluble in water at 20°C
	Readily soluble in fats, lipids, and all other organic solvents
Decomposition temperature (°C)	150 (complete in 2-1/2 hours)
Odor	Weak, fruity; almost none in pure state
Thickening	Possible

SOURCES: U.S. Army (1990); SIPRI (1973); Karakchiev (1973); OSRD (1946); AD Little (1986), Ch. 5.

Table B.3

Chemical and Physical Properties of Soman

Agent:	Soman GD 1,2,2-trimethylpropyl methylphosphonofluoridate; Pinacolyl methylphosphonofluoridate Trilon
Chemical structure	

$$H_3C - \overset{\overset{\textstyle O}{\|}}{\underset{\underset{\textstyle F}{|}}{P}} - O - \overset{}{\underset{\underset{\textstyle CH_3}{|}}{CH}} - \overset{\overset{\textstyle CH_3}{|}}{\underset{\underset{\textstyle CH_3}{|}}{C}} - CH_3$$

Molecular weight	182.178
Physical states (20°C)	Colorless liquid giving off a colorless vapor
Vapor density (compared to air)	6.33
Liquid density (g/cc)	1.0222 at 25°C
Boiling point (°C, 760 mm Hg)	197.8 (calculated); 167 (with decomposition)
Melting point (°C)	–30 to –80 (depending on source)
Vapor pressure (mm Hg)	0.40 at 25°C
Volatility (mg/m^3)	2,650 at 20°C; 3,900 at 25°; 5,570 at 30°—comparable to engine oil
Viscosity (cp at 20°C)	Not found
Surface tension (dynes/cm)	24.5 at 26.5°C
Solubility	Miscible in both polar and nonpolar solvents—2.1 percent in water at 20°C, 20 percent at 25°C; readily soluble in fats, lipids and organic solvents; soluble in sulfur mustard
Decomposition temperature (°C)	130 (unstabilized, 4 hours; stabilized, 200 hours)
Odor	With impurities, weak odor of camphor, or pinacolyl alcohol, nutmeg, orange peel; none to weakly fruity in pure state

SOURCES: U.S. Army (1990); SIPRI (1973); Karakchiev (1973); AD Little (1986), Ch. 5.

Table B.4

Chemical and Physical Properties of Cyclosarin

Agent	Cyclosarin GF CMPF O-cyclohexylmethylfluorophosphonate
Chemical structure	

$$\begin{array}{c} O \\ \| \\ H_3C - P - O - \hexagon \\ \| \\ F \end{array}$$

Molecular weight	180.2
Physical state (20°C)	Liquid
Vapor density	6.2
Boiling point (°C)	239
Melting point (°C)	−30
Vapor pressure (mm Hg)	0.044 at 20°C
Volatility (mg/m^3)	438 at 20°C; 581 at 25°C
Viscosity and surface tension	Not found
Solubility	Insoluble in water 0.37 percent at 20°C
Rate of hydrolysis	Very stable, only hydrolyzes when heated or with alkalis
Odor—variable reports	65 percent of subjects detected at 14.8 mg/m^3, but descriptions varied (Marrs et al., 1996)
Evaporates	20 times slower than water

SOURCES: U.S. Army (1990), Marrs et al. (1996).

Table B.5

Chemical and Physical Properties of Thiosarin

Agent	Thiosarin
Chemical Structure	

$$(CH_3)_2 - CH - O - \overset{\overset{\displaystyle S}{\|}}{\underset{\underset{\displaystyle F}{|}}{P}} - CH_3$$

NOTE: The properties can only be speculated upon. It is assumed to be a liquid, with some properties similar to sarin, with hydrolysis of P–F bond expected. Some P=S pesticides require metabolic activation by oxidative enzymes to P=O form for activity. A delayed effect would be expected if this applied to thiosarin. There is reason to doubt this, however, from the slight information available on the analog thiosoman (SIPRI, 1973). This chemical is said to inhibit AChE *in vitro* with a log inhibition constant pI_{50} of 8.9, which is somewhat less potent an inhibitor than soman, whose pI_{50} is 9.2. Since this is an *in vitro* study, there is no ability for metabolic conversion in the usual manner.

Table B.6

Chemical and Physical Properties of VX

Agent	VX V-agents Ethyl-S-diisopropylaminoethylmethylthiosphosphonate;
Chemical structure	
Molecular weight	267.38
Physical state (20°C)	Amber-colored liquid; colorless in pure form
Vapor density (compared to air)	9.2
Liquid density (g/cc)	1.0124 at 20°C
Boiling point (°C, 760 mm Hg)	298.4 (calculated), with decomposition
Melting point (°C)	−39
Vapor pressure (mm Hg)	0.0007 at 20°
Volatility (mg/m^3)	10.5 at 25°C (1/2000 as volatile as sarin)
Viscosity (cp at 20°C)	Not found
Surface tension (dynes/cm at 20°C)	32.011 (extrapolated)
Solubility	Poorly soluble (3 percent) in water at 25°C; very soluble in organic solvents, fats, and lipids
Decomposition temperature (°C)	150 (half-life is 36 hours); 700 to 800
Odor	None in the pure state; with impurities, reminiscent of rotten fish, mercaptanlike

SOURCES: U.S. Army (1990); SIPRI (1971); Karakchiev (1973); AD Little (1986), Ch. 5.

Table B.7

Dermal Exposures to Nerve Agent Required for Lethality to Humans

Agent	Vapor (CT) $(mg\text{-}min/m^3)$	Liquid μg/person	mg/kg
Tabun	20,000–40,000 15,000[a]	1,000–1,500	50–70
Sarin	12,000–15,000 10,000[a]	1,000–1,700	25–50
Soman	10,000 2,500[a]	600 350[a]	5–20
Cyclosarin	15,000 2,500[a]	350	—
VX	600–700 150[a]	3.4–6.0 <5[a]	0.1–0.2

SOURCES: SIPRI (1973), U.S. Army (1990), OSRD (1946), Karakchiev (1973), McNamara et al. (1973), Oberst (1959), NAS (1997).

NOTE: Contact with skin normally provokes sweating for a week or two, but persistence for 95 days has been reported (Freeman et al., 1954).

[a]Revised estimate from NAS (1997).

Table B.8

Dermal Exposures to Nerve Agent: Other Effect Thresholds for Humans

Agent	Threshold
Tabun	No effect at or below 2,000 CT, except for slight changes in plasma and AChE levels
Sarin	ICT_{50} at 8,000; incapacitating liquid dose is 20 mg/person or 0.1 mg/kg; no effect at or below 1.6 mg/person
Soman	Incapacitating liquid dose is 3–6 mg/person

SOURCES: Grob (1953), Neitlich (1965), U.S. Army (1990), Krakow and Fuhr (1949), SIPRI (1973).

Table B.9

**Exposures to Nerve Agent Vapor
Required for Lethality or
Incapacitation of Rhesus Monkeys**

Agent	LCT_{50}	ICT_{50}
Tabun	135–187	102–110
Sarin	42–74	30–60
Cyclosarin	75–130	62–100

SOURCE: Cresthull (1957).
NOTE: Exposures were 2 min and 10 min.

Table B.10

Animal Performance Effects of Nerve Agent Exposures

Agent	Dose	Animal	Effect
Sarin, soman	1/48 to 1/9 of LD_{50}	Rodents or rats	Anxiety and (sarin only) impairment of coordination and balance
Soman	53 µg/kg	Rodents	Impaired performance on sensitive behavioral tests for 50 percent of rodents
Tabun, sarin, soman, VX	0.5–0.9 LD_{50} (48 hr)	Rats, guinea pigs[a]	Soman and VX are more disruptive of avoidance conditioning than tabun or sarin
Soman	4.5 µg/kg	Baboons	Impaired discriminant responses
Sarin	0.5 LD_{50}	Rhesus monkeys	Little disruption

SOURCES: Gause et al. (1985), Sirkka (1990), Hartgraves and Murphy in Somani (1992), Lattal et al. (1971), Mays (1985).

[a]All four were given to rats, but only sarin and soman were given to guinea pigs.

Table B.11

Signs and Symptoms Comparison, Percentage Reduction in AChE Activity

Sign or Symptom	Group B Analysis (356 cases)					Group A Analysis (635 cases)					
	0–25	25–40	40–60	>60	Total	0–10	10–25	25–40	40–60	>60	Total
Miosis	75.5	87.5	88.8	100.0	79.8	75.2	88.9	92.3	97.0	100.0	85.4
Dim or blurred vision	52.5	84.0	80.7	93.7	62.2	44.4	62.0	73.1	69.7	100.0	59.4
Lachrymation	25.0	28.6	27.8	37.5	26.4	29.6	24.2	41.0	48.5	50.0	31.9
Unequal pupils	36.3	53.6	38.9	62.5	40.5						
Photophobia	25.4	41.2	47.3	56.3	31.5						
Eye ache or pain	29.8	48.3	38.9	50.0	34.6	5.9	7.2	11.5	27.3	43.7	10.2
Conjunctivitis	23.8	33.9	52.8	56.3	29.8	8.9	13.1	15.4	33.3	62.5	15.2
Difficulty focusing	22.6	48.3	44.5	75.0	31.2	7.1	13.1	10.3	33.3	43.7	12.9
Cough	63.8	64.4	47.2	87.5	63.3	66.9	61.4	64.1	69.7	50.0	54.3
Distress from smoking	46.0	51.7	38.8	37.5	45.8						
Nausea or anorexia	25.0	34.0	30.6	68.8	29.0	26.0	28.1	30.8	45.4	62.5	30.3
Vomiting	6.5	3.6	2.8	25.0	6.5	5.3	1.3	2.6	21.2	25.2	5.4
Diarrhea	8.9	11.1	2.8	37.5	9.8	3.5	6.5	6.4	6.0	12.5	5.6
Backache	8.9	10.7	16.6	18.7	10.4	4.7	7.8	11.5	6.0	6.2	7.1
Frequency or dysuria	8.1	12.5	11.1	31.1	10.1						
Headache	45.7	57.2	61.0	81.2	50.0	43.2	45.7	61.5	75.7	68.7	50.5
Dizziness	20.6	30.4	27.8	56.3	24.4	11.2	11.8	15.4	30.3	31.3	14.2
Disturbed sleep	27.0	41.2	47.2	75.0	32.4	33.1	27.4	33.3	54.5	75.0	34.4
Dreams	15.7	21.5	16.6	68.7	19.1						
Confusion, grogginess	12.5	21.5	36.2	62.7	18.5						
Impaired memory	8.9	10.7	25.0	31.1	11.8						
Syncope	2.0	1.8	2.8	12.5	2.5						
Rhinorrhea	80.0	84.0	86.0	87.7	81.5	84.0	89.5	85.9	93.9	81.3	87.3

Table B.11—Continued

	Group B Analysis (356 cases)					Group A Analysis (635 cases)					
	0–25	25–40	40–60	>60	Total	0–10	10–25	25–40	40–60	>60	Total
Increased sweating	24.2	32.2	55.7	68.8	30.7	13.0	17.6	29.5	30.3	62.5	20.5
Increased salivation	13.1	12.5	16.7	31.2	14.0						
Impaired taste or smell	14.9	21.5	16.7	31.2	16.8						
Weakness	26.6	26.8	33.3	68.7	29.2						
Fatigability	43.6	42.9	50.0	75.0	45.5	34.3	31.4	32.0	33.3	31.3	32.8
Pallor	2.8	7.2	11.1	43.7	6.2						
Cold or hot extremities	11.3	12.5	35.5	56.3	15.4						
Paresthesia, numbness, or hypesthesia	9.7	17.9	25.0	37.5	13.7	5.9	6.5	11.5	21.2	25.0	9.0
Twitch or fasciculation	11.3	14.3	16.7	50.0	14.0	3.5	3.3	6.4	3.0	25.0	4.7
Sore joints or muscles	10.1	8.9	8.3	18.7	10.1						
Common cold before exposure	24.2	25.1	39.0	12.5	25.2						
Common cold after exposure	27.4	26.8	36.2	0	27.0						
History of hay fever, asthma, or allergy	14.5	8.9	22.2	6.3	14.0						
Duration of signs and symptoms											
1 day	14.5	7.1	8.3	0	12.0	17.9	17.9	9.5	3.1	0	15.9
2 days	19.7	7.1	2.8	0	15.2						
3 days	20.6	12.5	3.8	6.3	18.0	37.7	37.7	33.4	9.4	12.5	35.1
4–7 days	24.5	41.0	36.2	25.0	28.4	15.3	15.3	20.7	18.7	12.5	15.9
7–14 days	3.2	8.9	3.8	12.5	5.6	0.2	0.2	14.3	6.3	25.0	2.5
2 weeks or more	4.4	17.9	25.0	56.3	10.9	0	0	11.1	3.1	31.2	2.0

SOURCE: Holmes (1959).

NOTES: This table compares signs and symptoms in Groups A and B; When group B was started, many additional signs and symptoms were included. These are all mild occupational exposures to sarin. Groups A and B were studied at different times using somewhat different recording methods. This is the largest compendium of clinical data on sarin exposures of humans found. Note that the prevalence of findings increases at greater levels of cholinesterase inhibition, but there are many findings at the lowest levels. Note the cases of sore joints and muscles. At the bottom of the table is information about duration of symptoms and relationship to degree of cholinesterase inhibition. Although more inhibition relates to longer duration, some low-inhibition cases were prolonged.

SURVEY OF C-FOS

C-fos is one of a family of intermediate early genes (IEGs), identified as a proto-oncogene in virology research. These genes are present in many tissues but under basal conditions usually at very low levels. Varied stimuli initiate increased levels of c-fos messenger RNA within minutes that persist for minutes to weeks. The FOS protein c-fos produces is a regulatory protein that forms dimer complexes with another IEG product of c-Jun (a family of JUN proteins), which in turn activates an inducible transcription factor, P1, which binds to a DNA that controls target gene expression. The means by which such mechanisms convert external stimuli into longer-term changes within the cell have been a matter of great scientific interest (some 8,000 titles relating to c-fos were published in the past three to four years.) (Chiasson, 1997; Bozas, 1997, Lane et al., 1998; Inada, 1998).

In some cases, the effects of c-fos expression are protective (Kaina, 1997; Giovanelli, 1998), but they are also implicated in cell death via apoptosis (Inada, 1998).

The study of the effects within the nervous system of inducible transforming factors has been intense and varied. These studies can be expected to improve understanding of the longer-term effects of military agents on the nervous system—eventually. The physiological consequences of acutely or chronically altering the expression of IEG transforming factors in humans or freely behaving animals remains largely unknown (Chiasson, 1997).

Physical (Patronas et al., 1998), physiological (Minson et al., 1997) and pharmacological (Giovanelli, 1998) stimuli presented once or on multiple occasions can alter the "normal" functioning of the brain for the long term (Chiasson, 1997).

Stimuli, such as neurotransmitter-receptor interactions, can be coupled to gene action, leading to changes in neuronal function lasting minutes to a lifetime. Early studies showed that drug-induced seizures, kindled seizures, and noxious stimulation showed regional activation of IEGs within the brain and spinal cord (Chiasson, 1997; Harris, 1997).

IEGs regulate the expression of varied neuropeptides and trophic molecules, such as nerve growth factor or cholineacetyl transferase, suggesting an important role in neuroplasticity: the adapting of the brain to changed circumstances (Chiasson, 1997; Pongrac and Rylett, 1998). There are growing indications that c-fos and other messenger RNAs may have effects in addition to translation (Chiasson, 1997).

C-fos and other IEGs are substantially involved in stress responses, with definite regional differences noted for different forms of stress (Chiasson, 1997; Rachman, 1998; Martinez, Phillips, and Herbert, 1998; Serova et al., 1998; Bozas, 1997, Schreiber, 1991).

Cholinergic mechanisms are often involved in activating c-fos, which in turn can regulate neurotransmitter abundance (Bernard et al., 1993; Pongrac and Rylett, 1998; Cook, 1998; Bucci, 1998).

C-fos is increased when seizures occur (White and Price, 1993) and may play a role in protection from further seizures (Rocha and Kaufman, 1998), although other data using antisense analogs of c-fos suggest the reverse is so in other models (Lu et al., 1997). It has been shown that, with soman-induced seizures in rats, increases in c-fos are later reflected by an increase in a heat shock protein, hsp70, which generally reflects neuronal "distress," while antisense versions of c-fos prevent the appearance of hsp70 (Baille et al., 1997).

Although c-fos and c-Jun are insufficient alone to produce apoptosis, studies in hypoxia-injured animals show that they are saliently involved in selectively vulnerable cells in switching on target genes (APP751) that induce apoptosis (Walton et al., 1998) and tumor necrosis factor. After unilateral mechanical injury to the hippocampus in mice, there is widespread expression of c-fos throughout the brain, followed within 24 hours by the production of interleukin 1 alpha and tumor necrosis factor alpha lasting 6 to 15 days. These factors are also induced in invading macrophages and glial cells. Similar effects do not arise from lesions in striatum or cortex. The physiological significance is unknown (Tchelingerian, 1997).

There are other indications of a role for c-fos in the elusive communications between immune and nervous systems. Vagal afferent neurons are activated following systemic administration of endotoxin, while administration of the interleukin IL 1-beta systemically induces in experimental animals expression of c-fos in afferent vagus neurons, providing an avenue for immune system signaling to the brain (Goehler et al., 1998). Although the focus of this survey has been the central nervous system, the fact that peripheral tissues also demonstrate considerable IEG activity in response to environmental changes should be kept in mind.

Abend Y, Goland S, Evron E, Sthoeger ZM, and Geltner D, "Acute Renal Failure Complicating Organophosphate Intoxication," *Ren Fail*, 16, 1994, pp. 415–417.

Abou-Donia MB, "Organophosphorus Ester-Induced Delayed Neurotoxicity," *Ann Rev Pharmacol Toxicol*, 1981, pp. 511–548.

Abou-Donia MB, Wilmarth KR, Jensen KF, Oehme FW, and Kurt TL, "Neurotoxicity Resulting from Coexposure to PB, Deet, and Permethrin Implications of Gulf War Chemical Exposures," *J Toxicol Environ Health*, 48, 1996, pp. 35–56.

American Thoracic Society, "Guidelines as to What Constitutes an Adverse Respiratory Health Effect, with Special Reference to Epidemiologic Studies of Air Pollution," *Am Rev Respir Dis*, 131, 1985, pp. 666–668.

Aponte JA et al., *Dimencopal Opthalmic Content Testing*, ADB0136251, 1975.

Arthur D Little, Inc., Phosgene Oxime, personal communication from Richard Taylor, 1983.

_____, *Chemical Casualty Treatment Protocol Development, Phase I: Treatment Approaches*, Brooks Air Force Base, Texas: Aerospace Medical Division, Air Force Systems Command, September 1986. (NOTE: Each of the seven chapters of this report was published as a separate volume.)

Adams DJ, "Biological Substances as Possible Percutaneous Hazards," *Agents of Biological Origin Symposium*, 1989.

Adams, JR, "Russia's Toxic Threat," *The Wall Street Journal*, April 30, 1996, p. A18.

Albuquerque EX, Boyne AF, Brookes N, Burt DR, and Deshpande SS, *Molecular and Behavioral Studies of Anticholinesterase Agents on Various Receptor Targets in the Peripheral and Central Nervous System: Acute and Chronic Studies Using Biophysical, Biochemical, Histological, and Therapeutics Approaches*, Baltimore, Md.: Maryland University, Baltimore School of Medicine, 1983.

Albuquerque EX, Deshpande SS, Kawabuchi M, Aracava Y, Idriss M, Rickett DL, and Boyne AF, "Multiple Actions of Anticholinesterase Agents on Chemosensitive Synapses: Molecular Basis for Prophylaxis and Treatment of Organophosphate Poisoning," *Fund Appl Toxicol*, 5, 1985, pp. S182–S203.

Aleksandrov VN, *Toxic Agents*, Joint Publications Research Service, 48748, 1969.

Allen SJ, Wild CP, Wheeler JG, et al., "Aflatoxin Exposure, Malaria and Hepatitis B Infection in Rural Gambian Children," *Trans R Soc Trop Med Hyg*, 86, 1992, pp. 426–430.

Anderson DR, Harris LW, Woodard CL, and Lennox WJ, "The Effect of PB Pretreatment on Oxime Efficacy Against Intoxication by Soman or VX in Rats," *Drug Chem Toxicol*, 15, 1992, pp. 285–294.

Anderson RJ, and Chamberlain WL, "Changes in Nerve Membrane Polarization Following Repeated Exposure to Soman," *J Toxicol Environ Health*, 24, 1988, pp. 121–128.

Ankrah NA, Addo PG, Abrahams CA, Ekuban FA, and Addae MM, "Comparative Effects of Aflatoxins G1 and B1 at Levels Within Human Exposure Limits on Mouse Liver and Kidney," *West Afr J Med*, 12, 1993, pp. 105–109.

Anzueto A, deLemos RA, Seidenfeld J, et al., "Acute Inhalation Toxicity of Soman and Sarin in Baboons," *Fund Appl Toxicol*, 14, 1990, pp. 676–687.

Ariens A, Meeter E, Wolthuis OL, and Van Benthem RMJ, "Reversible Necrosis at the End-Plate Region in Striated Muscles of the Rat Poisoned with Cholinesterase Inhibitors," *Experimentia*, 25, 1969, pp. 57–59.

Assad A, Wilhelmsen C, Kokes J, Bavari S, Pitt L, and Wade J, Effect of Neutrophil Depletion on the Pathogenesis of Ricin-Induced Acute Pulmonary Toxicity in Rats, abstract, Ft. Detrick, Md.: U.S. Army Medical Research Institute of Infectious Diseases, 1996.

Asset G, and Finklestein D, "Informal Note No. 14 on Some Aspects of the Chemical Corps Work on Aerosols," Army Chemical Center, Md.: Research and Engineering Division, Field Office, Chief Chemical Officer, DTIC AD310–461, 1951.

Aulerich RJ, Bursian SJ, and Watson GL, "Effects of Sublethal Concentrations of Aflatoxins on the Reproductive Performance of Mink," *Bull Environ Contam Toxicol*, 50, 1993, pp. 750–756.

Autrup H, and Seremet T, "Evidence of Human Antibodies That Recognize Aflatoxin Epitope in Groups with High and Low Exposure to Aflatoxins," *Archives of Environmental Health*, 45, 1990, pp. 31–36.

Autrup JL, Schmidt J, and Autrup H, "Exposure to Aflatoxin B1 in Animal-Feed Production Plant Workers," *Environ Health Perspect*, 99, 1993, pp. 195–197.

Azizi F, Amini M, and Arbab P, "Time Course of Changes in Free Thyroid Indices, rT3, TSH, Cortisol and ACTH Following Exposure to Sulfur Mustard," *Exp Clin Endocrinol*, 101, 1993, pp. 303–306.

Baille V, Lallement G, Carpentier P, Foquin A, Pernot-Marino I, and Rondouin G, "C-fos Antisense Oligonucleotide Prevents Delayed Induction of hsp70 mRNA After Soman-Induced Seizures," *NeuroReport*, 8, 1997, pp. 1819–1822.

Baladi M, "Clinical and Laboratory Findings in Iranian Fighters with Chemical Gas Poisoning," in Heyndrickx (1984), pp. 254–259.

Balint GA, "Further Analysis of Ricin's Pyrogenic Effect," *Exp Toxicol Pathol*, 45 (5–6), 1993, pp. 303–304.

Babarsky R, "Khamisiyah Plume Analysis," *Conference Proceedings*, Conference on Federally Sponsored Gulf War Veterans' Illnesses Research, June 17–19, 1998, 1998, p. 81.

Bartholomew PM, Gainutsos G, Cohen SD, "Differential Cholinesterase Inhibition and Muscarinic Receptor Changes in Cd-1 Mice Made Tolerant to Malathion," *Toxicol Appl Pharmacol*, 81, 1985, pp. 147–55.

Baxter CS, Wey HE, and Burg WR, "A Prospective Analysis of the Potential Risk Associated with Inhalation of Aflatoxin-Contaminated Grain Dusts," *Food Genetic Toxicol*, 19, 1981, pp. 765–769.

Baze WB, "Soman-Induced Morphological Changes: An Overview in the Non-Human Primate," *J Appl Toxicol*, 13, 1993, pp. 173–177.

Bell IR, Miller CS, and Schwartz GE, "An Olfactory-Limbic Model of Multiple Chemical Sensitivity Syndrome: Possible Relationships to Kindling and Affective Spectrum Disorders," *Biol Psychiatry*, 32, 1992, pp. 218–42.

Bell, IR, Warg-Damiani L, Baldwin CM, Walsh ME, and Schwartz GER, "Self-Reported Chemical Sensitivity and Wartime Chemical Exposures in Gulf War Veterans With and Without Decreased Global Health Ratings," *Military Medicine*, 163 (11), 1998, p. 725.

Belt RJ, Haas CD, Joseph U, Goodwin W, Moore D, and Hoogstraten B, "Phase I Study of Anguidine Administered Weekly," *Cancer Treat Rep*, 63, 1979, pp. 1993–1995.

Benschop HP, Berends F, and de Jong LPA, "GLC-Analysis and Pharmacokinetics of the Four Stereoisomers of Soman," *Fund Appl Toxicol*, 1, 1981, pp. 177–182.

Benschop HP, Konings CAG, Genderen JV, and de Jong LPA, "Isolation, In Vitro Activity, and Acute Toxicity in Mice of the Four Stereoisomers of Soman," *Fund Appl Toxicol*, 4, 1984, pp. S84–S95.

Bernard V, Dumartin B, Lamy E, and Bloch B, "Fos Immunoreactivity After Stimulation or Inhibition of Muscarinic Receptors Indicates Anatomical Specificity for Cholinergic Control of Striatal Efferent Neurons and Cortical Neurons in the Rat," *Eur J Neurosci*, 5 (9), September 1, 1993, pp. 1218–1225.

Bertoncin D, Russolo A, Caroldi S, and Lotti M, "Neuropathy Target Esterase in Human Lymphocytes," *Arch Env Health*, 40, 1985, pp. 139–144.

Binenfeld Z, *New Military Neurotoxins—Yugoslavia*, JPRS 43014, Washington, D.C.: U.S. Department of Commerce, 1967.

Blank IH, Griesemer RD, and Gould E, "The Penetration of an Anti-cholinesterase Agent (Sarin) into Skin," *J Invest Dermatol*, 29, 1957, pp. 299–309.

Blick DW, Miller SA, Brown GC, and Murphy MR, "Behavioral Toxicity of Anti-cholinesterases in Primates: Chronic Physostigmine and Soman Interactions," *Pharmacol Biochem Behav*, 45, 1993, pp. 677–683.

Bonomi A, Quarantelli A, Zambin EM, et al., "Effects of Aflatoxin B1 Contaminated Rations on Productive and Reproductive Efficiency in Swine (Experimental Contribution)," *Rivista Di Scienza Dell'Alimentazione*, 24, 1995, pp. 361–384.

Boskovic B, and Kusic R, "Long-Term Effects of Acute Exposure to Nerve Gases upon Human Health," in *Chemical Weapons: Destruction and Conversion*, New York: Crane Russak Co. (dist.), 1980, pp. 113–115.

Boter HL, Dijk C van, "Stereospecificity of Hydrolytic Enzymes in Reaction with a Symmetric Organophosphorus Compound: The Inhibition of Acetyl-cholinesterase and Butyrylcholinesterase by Enantiomeric Forms of Sarin," *Biochem Pharmacol*, 18, 1969, p. 2,403-2,407.

Bouldin TW, Earnhardt TS, and Goines ND, "Sequential Changes in the Permeability of the Blood-Nerve Barrier over the Course of Ricin Neuronopathy in the Rat," *Neurotoxicol*, 11, 1990, pp. 23–34.

Bourgeois C, Olson L, Comer D, Evans H, et al., "Encephalophy and Fatty Degeneration of the Viscera: A Clinicopathologic Analysis of 40 Cases," *Am J Clin Pathol*, 56, 1971, pp. 558–571.

Bourgeois C, Shank RC, Grossman RA, Johnsen DO, and Wooding WL, Chandavimol P, "Acute Aflatoxin B1 Toxicity in the Macaque and Its Similarities to Reye's Syndrome," *Lab Invest*, 24, 1971, pp. 206–16.

Bowers M, Goodman E, and Sim VM, "Some Behavioral Changes in Men Following Anticholinesterase Administration," *J Nerv Ment Dis*, 138, 1964, pp. 383–389.

Bozas E, Tritos N, Phillipidis H, and Stylianopoulou F, "At Least Three Neurotransmitter Systems Mediate a Stress-Induced Increase in c-fos mRNA in Different Rat Brain Areas," *Cellular and Molecular Neurobiology*, 17 (2), 1997.

Bramwell, et al., "Human Exposure to VS," Porton Down, Wiltshire, UK., Porton Technical Paper 830, 1963.

Brody EG, and Gammill JF, *Seventy-Five Cases of Accidental Nerve Agent Poisoning at Dugway Proving Ground*, Salt Lake City: Dugway Proving Ground, DTIC AD48826, 1954.

Brookes P, "The Early History of the Biological Alkylating Agents 1918–1990," *Mutat Res*, 233, 1990, pp. 3–14.

Brooks F, Xenakis S, Ebner D, and Balson P, "Psychological Reactions During Chemical Warfare Training," *Military Medicine*, 148, 1983, pp. 232–235.

Broomfield CA, "A Purified Recombinant Organophosphorus Acid Anhydrase Protects Mice Against Soman," *Pharmacol Toxicol*, 70, 1992, pp. 65–6.

Buccafusco JJ, Prendergast MA, Pauly JR, Terry AV, Goldstein BD, and Shuster LC, "A Rat Model for Gulf War Illness-Related Selective Memory Impairment and the Loss of Hippocampal Nicotinic Receptors," abstract, *Soc Neurosci Abstr*, 23, 1997, pp. 316.

Bucci DJ, Rosen DL, and Gallagher M, "Effects of Age on Pilocarpine-Induced c-fos Expression in Rat Hippocampus and Cortex," *Neurobiol Aging*, 19 (3), May–June 1998, pp. 227–32.

Bucci TJ, Parker RM, and Gosnell PA, "Toxicity Studies on Agents GB and GD (Phase 2): 90-Day Subchronic Study of GD (Soman) in CD-Rats," Jefferson, Ark.: National Center for Toxicological Research, DTIC ADA258180, March 1992a.

_____, "Toxicity Studies on Agents GB and GD (Phase 2): Delayed Neuropathy Study of Sarin, Type I, in SPF White Leghorn Chickens," Jefferson, Ark.: National Center for Toxicological Research, DTIC ADA258664, April 1992b.

_____, "Toxicity Studies on Agents GB and GD (Phase 2): Delayed Neuropathy Study of Sarin, Type II, in SPF White Leghorn Chickens," Jefferson, Ark.: National Center for Toxicological Research, DTIC ADA257357, April 1992c.

_____, "Toxicity Studies on Agents GB and GD (Phase 2): Delayed Neuropathy Study of Soman in SPF White Leghorn Chickens," Jefferson, Ark.: National Center for Toxicological Research, DTIC ADA258643, May 1992d.

Buck WB, Beasley VR, and Swanson SP, *Toxicologic and Analytical Studies with T-2 and Related Trichothecene Mycotoxins*, Ft. Detrick, Md.: U.S. Army Medical Research and Development Command, DTIC ADA172207, 1983.

Bukowski R, Vaughn C, Bottomley R, and Chen T, "Phase II Study of Anguidine in Gastrointestinal Malignancies: A Southwest Oncology Group Study," *Cancer Treat Rep*, 66, 1982, pp. 381–383.

Bullman TA, and Kang HK, "The Effects of Mustard Gas, Ionizing Radiation, Herbicides, Trauma, and Oil Smoke on U.S. Military Personnel: The Results of Veteran Studies," *Annu Rev Public Health*, 15, 1994, pp. 69–90.

Bunner D, *Trichothecene Mycotoxins Intoxications: Signs, Symptoms, Pathophysiology, and Management (Based On Initial Laboratory Animal Studies and Review of Phase I Trails as Anticancer Agents in Man*, Ft. Detrick, Md.: U.S. Army Medical Research Institute of Infectious Diseases, 1983.

Bunner D, Wannemacher R, Neufeld H, Hessler C, Parker G, Cosgriff T, and Dinterman R, "Pathophysiology of Acute T-2 Intoxication in the Cynomolgus Monkey and Comparison to the Rat as Model," Ft. Detrick, Md.: U.S. Army Medical Research Institute of Infectious Diseases, DTIC ADA135983, 1983.

Bunner DL, Neufeld HA, Brennecke LH, Campbell YG, Dinterman RE, and Pelosi JG, *Clinical and Hematologic Effects of T-2 Toxin in Rats*, Ft. Detrick, Md.: U.S. Army Medical Research Institute of Infectious Diseases, DTIC ADA158874, 1985.

Burchfiel JL, "Persistent Effect of Sarin and Dieldrin on the Electroencephalogram of Monkey and Man," *Toxicol Appl Pharmacol*, 35, 1976, pp. 365–379.

Burchfiel JL, and Duffy FH, "Organophosphate Neurotoxicity: Chronic Effects of Sarin on the Electroencephalogram of Monkey and Man," *Neurobehav Toxicol Teratol*, 4, 1982, pp. 767–778.

Busby WF, and Wogan GN, "Food Borne Mycotoxins and Alimentary Mycotoxicosis," in Rieman H and Bryan FL, eds., *Food Borne Infections and Intoxications*, 2nd ed., New York: Academic Press, 1979, pp. 515–599.

Cadigan FC, and Chipman M, "The Effects of Acute and Chronic Low-Dose Exposure to Anticholinesterase," in Ernsting J, ed., *Maintenance of Air Operations While Under Attack with Chemical Weapons*, Aerospace Medical Panel's Specialists' Meeting, Brussels, Belgium, 1979.

Callaway E, "An Accident Involving Exposure to a Nerve Gas," DTIC Quarterly Report No. 2, DTIC AD144023, 1950.

Callaway S, and Blackburn JW, *A Comparative Assessment of the Vapour Toxicities of GB, GD, GF, T2132, T2137 and T2146 to Male and Female Rats*, Arlington, Va.: Armed Services Technical Information Agency, Porton Technical Paper 404, DTIC AD31119, 1954.

Calvet JH, Jarreau PH, Levame M, D'ortho, MP, Lorino H, Harf A, and Macquin-Mavier I, "Acute and Chronic Respiratory Effects of Sulfur Mustard Intoxication in Guinea Pig," *J Appl Physiol*, 76, 1994, pp. 681–688.

Cappa M, Grossi A, Benedetti S, Drago F, Loche S, and Ghigo E, "Effect of the Enhancement of the Cholinergic Tone by PB on the Exercise-Induced Growth Hormone Release in Man," *J Endocrin Invest*, 16, 1993, pp. 421–424.

Carter B, and Cammermeyer M, "Biopsychological Responses of Medical Unit Personnel Wearing Chemical Defense Ensemble in a Simulated Chemical Warfare Environment," *Military Medicine*, 150, 1985, pp. 239–249.

_____, "Human Responses to Simulated Chemical Warfare Training in U.S. Army Reserve Personnel," *Mil Med*, 154, 1989, pp. 281–288.

Cecchine G, Golomb BA, Hilborne L Spector D, and Anthony CR, *A Review of the Scientific Literature as It Pertains to Gulf War Illnesses*, Vol. 8: *Pesticides*, Santa Monica, Calif.: RAND, MR-1018/8-OSD, 2000.

Central Intelligence Agency, *Modeling the Chemical Agent Release at the Khamisiyah Pit*, Washington DC, 1997.

_____, Briefing to the Presidential Advisory Committee, July 9, 1996.

Chan PKC, and Gentry PA, "LD50 Values and Serum Biochemical Changes induced by T-2 Toxin Rats and Rabbits," *Toxicol Appl Pharmacol*, 73, 1984, pp. 402–410.

Chao TC, "Perak, Malaysia, Mass Poisoning: Tale of the Nine Emperor Gods and Rat Tail Noodles," *Am J Forensic Med Pathol*, 13, 1992, pp. 261–263.

Chao TC, Maxwell SM, Lyen K, Wang D, and Chia HK, "Mass Poisoning in Perak, Malaysia or the Tale of the Nine Emperor Gods and Rat Tail Noodles," *J Forensic Sci Soc*, 31, 1991, pp. 283–288.

Chemical Research, Development & Engineering Center, *Proceedings for the Symposium on Agents of Biological Origin*, Laurel, Md.: Kossiakoff Center Applied Physics Laboratory, Johns Hopkins University, March 21–23, 1989.

Cherkes AI, ed., *Handbook of Toxicology of Toxic Agents*, Washington, D.C.: U.S. Department of Commerce, Clearinghouse for Federal Scientific and Technical Information, 1965.

Cherniack MG, "Organophosphorus Esters and Polyneuropathy," *Ann Intern Med*, 104, 1986, pp. 264–266.

Chiasson BJ, Hong MG, and Robertson HA, "Putative Roles for the Inducible Transcription Factor c-fos in the Central Nervous System: Studies with Antisense Oligonucleotides," *Neurochem Int*, 31 (3), September 1997, pp. 459–475.

Chippendale TJ, Zawolkow GA, Russell RW, and Overstreet DH, "Tolerance to Low Acetylcholinesterase Levels: Modification of Behavior Without Acute Behavioral Change," *Psychopharmacologia*, 26, 1972, pp. 127–139.

Christiansen VJ, Hsu CH, and Robinson CP, "The Effects of Ricin on the Sympathetic Vascular Neuroeffector System of the Rabbit," *J Biochem Toxicol*, 9, 1994, pp. 219–223.

Churchill L, Pazdernik TL, Jackson JL, Nelson SR, Samson FE, and McDonough JHJ, "Topographical Distribution of Decrements and Recovery in Muscarinic Receptors from Rat Brains Repeatedly Exposed to Sublethal Doses of Soman," *J Neurosci*, 4, 1984, pp. 2069–2079.

CIA—*see* Central Intelligence Agency.

Clancy T, and Franks F, Jr., *Into the Storm: A Study in Command*, New York: G.P. Putnam's Sons, 1997.

Clark G, "Organophosphate Insecticides and Behavior: A Review," *Aerosp Med*, 42, 1971, pp. 735–740.

Clement JG, "Hormonal Consequences of Organophosphate Poisoning," *Fund Appl Toxicol*, 5, 1985, pp. S61–S77.

Clement JG, "Efficacy of Various Oximes Against GF (cyclohexylmethyl-phosphonofluoridate) Poisoning in Mice," *Arch Toxicology*, 66, 1992, pp. 143–144.

Clement JG, "Toxicity of the Combined Nerve Agents GB/GF in Mice: Efficacy of Atropine and Various Oximes as Antidotes," *Arch Toxicol*, 68, 1994, pp. 64–66.

Clement JG, and Copeman HT, "Soman and Sarin Induce a Long-Lasting Naloxone-Reversible Analgesia in Mice," *Life Sci*, 34, 1984, pp. 1415–1422.

Cogan DG, "Lewisite Burns of the Eye," *JAMA*, 122, 1943, pp. 435–436.

Colardyn F, and De Bersaques J, "Clinical Observations and Therapy of Injuries and Vesicants," in Heyndrickx (1984), pp. 298–301.

Coleman JL, Little PE, Putton GE, Bannara KA, "Cholinolytics in the Treatment of Anticholinesterase Poisoning, IV: The Effects of Binary Combinations with Oxime Therapy," *Canadian Journal of Physiology and Pharmacology*, 44, 1966, pp. 745–764.

Conference on Federally Sponsored Gulf War Veterans' Illnesses Research, *Program and Abstract Book*, June 17–19, 1998.

Cook AA, "Illness and Injury Among U.S. Prisoners of War from Operation Desert Storm," *Mil Med*, 159, 1994, pp. 437–53.

Cook DF, Wirtshafter D, "Quinpirole Attenuates Striatal c-fos Induction by 5-HT, Opioid and Muscarinic Receptor Agonists," *European Journal of Pharmacology*, 349, 1998, pp. 41–47.

Coombs AY, Freeman G, *Observations of the Effects of GB on Intellectual Function in Man*, Army Chemical Center, Md.: Chemical Corps, Medical Laboratories, DTIC AD43035, 1954.

Coppock RW, Gelberg HB, Hoffmann I, and Buck WB, "The Acute Toxicopathy of Intravenous Diacetoxyscirpenol (Anguidine) Administration in Swine," *Fund Appl Toxicol*, 5, 1985, pp. 1034–1049.

Cordesman AH, and Wagner AR, *The Lessons of Modern War*, Vol. II: *The Iran-Iraq War*, Boulder, CO: Westview Press, 1990.

_____, *The Lessons of Modern War*, Vol. III: *The Afghan and Falklands Conflicts*, Boulder, CO: Westview Press, 1991.

Cosgriff TM, Bunner DL, Wannemacher RW, Jr., Hodgson LA, and Dinterman RE, "The Hemostatic Derangement Produced by T-2 Toxin in Cynomolgus Monkeys," *Toxicol Appl Pharmacol*, 82, 1986, pp. 532–539.

Costa LG, Schwab BW, and Murphy SD, "Tolerance to Anticholinesterase Compounds in Mammals," *Toxicology*, 25, 1982, pp. 79–97.

Coulombe RA, Jr., "Symposium: Biological Action of Mycotoxins," *J Dairy Sci*, 76, 1993, pp. 880–891.

Coulombe RAJ, Huie JM, Ball RW, Sharma RP, and Wilson DW, "Pharmacokinetics of Intratracheally Administered Aflatoxin B1," *Toxicol Appl Pharmacol*, 109, 1991, pp. 196–206.

Cowan DN, Gray GC, DeFraites RF, "Counterpoint: Responding to Inadequate Critique of Birth Defects Paper," *Am J Epidem*, 146, 1998, pp. 326–327.

Cowan FM, Broomfield CA, and Smith WJ, "Sulfur Mustard Exposure Enhances Fc Receptor Expression on Human Epidermal Keratinocytes in Cell Culture: Implications for Toxicity and Medical Countermeasures," *Cell Biol Toxicol*, 14 (4), August 1998, pp. 261–266.

Craig AB, and Freeman G, "Clinical Observations on Workers Accidentally Exposed to G Agents," Army Chemical Center, Md.: Department of Defense, DTIC AD3398, 1953.

Craig AB, Woodson GS, and Fales JT, "Observations on the Effects of Exposure to Nerve Gas, I. Clinical Observations and Cholinesterase Depression," *Am J Med Sci*, 238, 1959, pp. 13–17.

Creasia DA, Thurman JD, Jones LJI, et al., "Acute Inhalation Toxicity of T-2 Mycotoxin in Mice," *Fund Appl Toxicol*, 8, 1987, pp. 230–235.

Cresthull P, Koon WS, McGrath FP, and Oberst F, "Inhalation Effects (Incapacitation and Mortality) for Monkey Exposed to GA, GB and GF

Vapors," Army Chemical Center, Md.: Chemical Warfare Laboratory, Report 2179, DTIC AD145581, 1957.

Cresthull P, Koon WS, Musselman NP, Bowers M, and Oberst FW, *Percutaneous Exposure of the Arm or the Forearm of Man to VX Vapor*, Army Chemical Center, Md.: Chemical Warfare Laboratory, DTIC AD145587, 1963.

Cresthull P, Williams L, Crook JW, Graf CH, Christiensen MK, and Oberst FW, *Cumulative Toxic Effects of Repeated Doses of Inhaled GB Vapor in Dogs*, Edgewood Arsenal, Md.: Chemical Corps Laboratory, DTIC AD236945, 1960.

Crocker GB, "The Evidence of Chemical and Toxin Weapon Use in Southeast Asia and Afghanistan," in *First World Congress: New Compounds in Biological Warfare: Toxicological Evaluation, Proceedings*, Ghent, Belgium: State University of Ghent and National Science Foundation, 1984.

Croft WA, Jarvis BB, and Yatawara CS, "Airborne Outbreak of Trichothecene Toxicosis," *Atmos Environ*, 20, 1986, pp. 549–552.

Crossland A, and Townsend A, "Observations, Impressions, Pitfalls and Recommendations from Field CBW Research Among Refugees in Southeast Asia," in *First World Congress: New Compounds in Biological Warfare: Toxicological Evaluation, Proceedings*, Ghent, Belgium: State University of Ghent and National Science Foundation, 1984.

Crowell J, Parker R, Bucci T, and Dacre J, "Neuropathy Target Esterase in Hens after Sarin and Soman," *Journal of Biochemical Toxicology*, 4, 1989, pp. 15–20.

Cukrova V, Langrova E, and Akao M, "Effects of Aflatoxin B1 on Myelopoiesis in Vitro," *Toxicology*, 70, 1991, pp. 203–212.

Cullen MR, "The Worker with Multiple Chemical Sensitivities: An Overview," *Occup Med*, 2, 1987, pp. 655–661.

Cysewski SJ, Wood RL, Pier AC, and Baetz AL, "Effects of Aflatoxin on the Development of Acquired Immunity to Swine Erysipelas," *Am J Vet Res*, 39, 1978, pp. 445–8.

Dacre JC, "Toxicology of Some Anticholinesterases Used in Chemical Warfare Agents: A Review," in *Cholinesterases, Fundamental and Applied Aspects*, New York: Walter De Gruyter & Co., 1984, pp. 415–426.

_____, "Toxicological Studies on Chemical Agents GA, GB, GD, VX, HD, and L," in *Proceedings of Third International Symposium on Protection Against Chemical Warfare Agents*, abstract, 1989, p. 179.

Dacre JC, and Goldman M, "Toxicology and Pharmacology of the Chemical Warfare Agent Sulfur Mustard," *Pharmacol Rev*, 48, 1996, pp. 289–326.

Daniels JM, Liu L, Stewart RK, and Massey TE, "Biotransformation of Aflatoxin B1 in Rabbit Lung and Liver Microsomes," *Carcinogenesis*, 11, 1990, pp. 823–827.

Dannenberg AM, Jr., Pula PJ, Liu LH, et al., "Inflammatory Mediators and Modulators Released in Organ Culture from Rabbit Skin Lesions Produced In Vivo by Sulfur Mustard," *Am J Pathol*, 121, 1985, pp. 15–27.

Daughters D, Zackheim SH, and Maibach H, "Urticaria and Anaphylactoid Reactions After Topical Applications of Mechlorethamine," *Arch Dermatol*, 107, 1973, pp. 429–430.

Davies DR and Holland P, "Effect of Oximes and Atropine Upon the Development of Delayed Neuropathy in Chickens Following Poisoning by DFP and Sarin," *Biochemcial Pharmacology*, 21, 1972, pp. 3,145–3,151.

Davies H, Richter R, Keifer M, Broomfield C, Stowalla J, and Furlong C, "The Effect of Human Serum Paraoxonase Polymorphism Is Reversed with Diazoxon, Soman and Sarin," *Nature Genetics*, 14, 1996, pp. 334–336.

De Bisschop HC, Mainil JG, and Willems JL, "In Vitro Degradation of the Four Isomers of Soman in Human Serum," *Biochem Pharmacol*, 34, 1985, pp. 1895–1900.

De Jong LPA, *Aging and Stereospecific Reactivation of Soman-Inhibited Acetylcholinesterases from Various Species*, Rijswijk, Netherlands: Prins Maurits Lab, DMC 1987–28, 1987.

De la Cruz RR, Pastor AM, and Delgado-Garcia JM, "The Neurotoxic Effects of Ricinus Communis Agglutinin-II," *J Toxicol—Toxin Revs*, 14, 1995, pp. 1–46.

De Bruyn EJ, Corbett GK, and Bonds AB, "Depression of the Cat Cortical Visual Evoked Potential by Soman," *Life Sciences*, 48, pp. 1269–1276, January 1991.

Defense Intelligence Agency, Iraqi Chemical Warfare Data, declassified document file 970613-092596, 1997.

Defense Science Board, *Report of the Defense Science Board Task Force on Persian Gulf War Health Effects*, Washington, D.C.: Office of the Undersecretary of Defense for Acquisition and Technology, 1994.

Deneauve-Lockhart C, Sauvaget P, Touron C, and Chariot P, "Acute Occupational Exposure to Mustard Gas," abstract, *Arch Mal Prof Med Trav Secur Soc*, 53, 1992, pp. 121–124.

Denning DW, Quiepo SC, Altman DG, et al., "Aflatoxin and Outcome from Acute Lower Respiratory Infection in Children in the Philippines," *Ann Trop Paediat*, 15, 1995, pp. 209–216.

Department of the Army, "Assay Techniques for Detection of Exposure to Sulfur Mustard, Cholinesterase Inhibitors, Sarin, Soman, GF, and Cyanide," Washington, D.C., Technical Bulletin MED 296, May 1996.

DeRobertis E, "Molecular Biology of Synaptic Receptors," *Science*, 171, 1971, pp. 963–971.

DeRoetth A Jr., Dettbarn WD, Rosenberg P, Wilensky JG, and Wong A, "Effect of Phospholine Iodide on Blood Cholinesterase Levels of Normal and Glaucoma Subjects," *Am J Ophthal*, 1965, pp. 586–92.

Dettbarn WD, "Nerve Agent Toxicity and its Prevention at the Neuromuscular Junction: An Analysis of Acute and Delayed Toxic Effects in Extraocular and Skeletal Muscle," Nashville, Tenn.: Vanderbilt University, Department of Pharmacology, DTIC ADA144972, 1984.

DHHS—*see* U.S. Department of Health and Human Services.

Di Paolo N, Guarnieri A, Gariso G, Sacchi G, Mangiarotti AM, and Di Paolo M, "Inhaled Mycotoxins Lead to Acute Renal Failure," *Nephrol Dial Transplan*, 9, 1994, pp. 116–120.

Diggs CH, Scoltock MJ, and Wiernik PH, "Phase II Evaluation of Anguidine (NSC-141537) for Adenocarcinoma of the Colon or Rectum," *Cancer Clin Trials*, Winter 1978, pp. 297–299.

Dille S, and Smith PW, "Central Nervous System Effects of Chronic Organophosphate Insecticides," *Aerosp Med*, 35, 1964, pp. 475–478.

Dimitri RA, and Gabal MA, "Immunosuppressant Activity of Aflatoxin Ingestion in Rabbits Measured by Response to Mycobacterium Bovix Antigen, I. Cell Mediated Immune Response Measured by Skin Test Reaction," *Vet Hum Toxicol*, 38, 1996, pp. 333–6.

Dirnhuber P, French MC, Green DM, Leadbeater L, and Stratton JA, "The Protection of Primates Against Soman Poisoning by Pretreatment with PB," *J Pharmacol*, 31, 1979, pp. 295–299.

Doebler JA, Wiltshire ND, Mayer TW, et al., "The Distribution of [125I]ricin in Mice Following Aerosol Inhalation Exposure," *Toxicology*, 98, 1995, pp. 137–149.

Drewes LR, "Electroencephalographic Studies of Soman's Action in the Cat," *Fifth Annual Chemical Defense Bioscience Review*, Columbia, Md.: Johns Hopkins University Applied Physics Laboratory, 1985.

Drody BB, and Gammill JF, *Seventy-Five Cases of Accidental Nerve Gas Poisoning at Dugway Proving Ground*, Dugway Proving Ground, Md.: Medical Investigation Branch, December 10, 1954.

DSB—*see* Defense Science Board.

Duffy FH, and Burchfiel JL, "Long-Term Effects of the Organophosphate Sarin on EEGs in Monkeys and Humans," *Neurotox*, 1, 1980, pp. 667–689.

Dugyala RR, Kim YW, et al., "Effects of Aflatoxin B1 and T-2 Toxin on the Granulocyte-Macrophage Progenitor Cells in Mouse Bone Marrow Cultures," *Immunopharmacol*, 27, 1994, pp. 57–65.

Dulaney MD, Jr., Hoskins B, and Ho IK, "Studies on Low Sub-Acute Administration of Soman, Sarin and Tabun in the Rat," *Acta Pharmacol Toxicol*, 57, 1985, pp. 234–241.

Dunn MA, Hackley BE, Jr., and Sidell FR, "Pretreatment for Nerve Agent Exposure," in Sidell FR, Takafuji ET, Franz DR, eds., *Textbook of Military Medicine: Medical Aspects of Chemical and Biological Warfare*, Washington, D.C.: Borden Institute, Walter Reed Medical Center, 1997, pp. 181–196.

Dunn P, "The Chemical War: Journey to Iran," *NBC Defense and Technology Int*, 1986, p. 1.

Ehrenberg L, and Osterman-Golkar S, "Alkylation of Macromolecules for Determining Mutagenic Agents," *Terat Cargino Mut*, 1, 1980, pp. 105–127.

Ehrlich JP, and Burleson GR, "Enhanced and Prolonged Pulmonary Influenza Virus Infection Following Phosgene Inhalation," *J Toxicol Environ Health*, 34, 1991, pp. 259–273.

Eldefrawi M, Valdes JJ, and Schweizer G, "Interactions of Organophosphate Nerve Agents with the Nicotinic Acetylcholine Receptor," abstract, *Proceedings of the Fifth Annual Chemical Defense Bioscience Review*, Aberdeen Proving Ground, Md.: U.S. Army Medical Research, Institute of Chemical Defense, 1985.

Elsmore TF, "Circadian Susceptibility to Soman Poisoning," *Fund Appl Toxicol*, 1, 1981, pp. 238–241.

Elson E, "Report on Possible Effects of Organophosphate 'Low-Level' Nerve Agent Exposure," *Health Affairs*, 1996.

Englund W, "Ex-Soviet Scientist Says Gorbachev's Regime Created New Nerve Gas in '91," *Baltimore Sun*, September 16, 1992a, p. 3A.

_____, "Russia Still Doing Secret Work on Chemical Arms," *Baltimore Sun*, October 18, 1992b, p. 1A.

Eyring H, *Advantages of Two-Component Chemicals in Munitions, in Binary Weapons and the Problem of Chemical Disarmament*, Washington, D.C.: American Chemical Society, 1976, pp. 13–14.

Fairhurst S, Maxwell SA, Scawin JW, and Swanston DW, "Skin Effects of Tri-chothecenes and Their Amelioration by Decontamination," *Toxicology*, 46, 1987, pp. 307–319.

Fang Y, *Chemical Agents Development in USSR*, trans. from Chinese, Alexandria, Va.: Defense Technical Information Center, 1983.

Fernandez A, Ramos JJ, Saez T, Sanz MC, and Verde MT, "Changes in the Coagulation Profile of Lambs Intoxicated with Aflatoxin in Their Feed," *Vet Res*, 26, 1995, pp. 180–184.

Fernandez A, Verde MT, Gomez J, Gascon M, and Ramos JJ, "Changes in the Prothrombin Time, Haematology and Serum Proteins During Experimental Aflatoxicosis in Hens and Broiler Chickens," *Res Vet Sci*, 58, 1995, pp. 119–122.

Filbert MG, Dochterman LW, Smith CD, Forster JS, Phann S, and Cann FJ, "Effect of Mannitol Treatment on Soman-Induced Brain and Heart Lesions in the Rat," *Drug Dev Res*, 30, 1993, pp. 45–53.

Fine DR, Shepherd HA, Griffiths GD, and Green M, "Sub-Lethal Poisoning by Self-Injection with Ricin," *Med Sci Law*, 32, 1992, pp. 70–72.

Finesinger JE, Callaway E, and Seed JC, "Psychological Studies on the Effects of CW Agents," Edgewood Arsenal, Md.: Chemical Warfare Laboratories, DTIC AD144023, 1950.

Fleisher JH, Harris LW, and Berkowitz PT, "Metabolism of P32 Isopropyl Methylphosphonofluoridate (Sarin) in Dogs," Edgewood Arsenal, Md.: Department of the Army, DTIC AD692841, 1969.

Fodstad O, Kvalheim G, Godal A, et al., "Phase I Study of the Plant Protein Ricin," *Cancer Res*, 44, 1984, pp. 862–865.

Fonnum F, Aas P, Sterri S, and Kelle B, "Modulation of the Cholinergic Activity of Bronchial Muscle During Inhalation of Soman," *Fundamental and Applied Toxicology*, 4, 1984, pp. S52–57.

Fonnum F, and Sterri SH, "Factors Modifying the Toxicity of Organophospho-rous Compounds Including Soman and Sarin," *Fund Appl Toxicol*, 1, 1981, pp. 143–147.

Fonseca MI, Lunt GG, and Aguilar JS, "Inhibition of Muscarinic Cholinergic Receptors by Disulfide Reducing Agents and Arsenicals: Differential Effect on Locust and Rat," *Biochem Pharmacol*, 41, 1991, pp. 735–742.

Fontelo PA, Beheler J, Bunner DL, and Chu FS, "Detection of T-2 Toxin by an Improved Radioimmunoassay," *Appl Environ Microbiol*, 45, 1983, pp. 640–643.

Forgacs J, "Stachybotrytoxicosis," in Kadis et al., eds., *Microbial Toxins VIII*, New York: Academic Press, 1972, pp. 294–298.

Foxwell BMJ, Detre SI, Donovan TA, and Thorpe PE, "The Use of Anti-Ricin Antibodies to Protect Mice Intoxicated with Ricin," *Toxicology*, 34, 1985, pp. 79–88.

Franke S, *Manual of Military Chemistry*, Vol. 1: *Chemistry of Chemical Warfare Agents*, trans. from German, Cameron Station, Va.: Defense Technical Information Center, 1967.

Franke S, *Bacterial, Animal and Plant Toxins as Combat Agents, Manual of Military Chemistry*, Vol. 2, Berlin: Militaerverlag der DDR., 1976, pp. 484–485, 488–496.

Franz DR, and Jaax NK, "Ricin Toxin," in Sidell FR, Takafuji ET, Franz DR, eds., *Textbook of Military Medicine: Medical Aspects of Chemical and Biological Warfare*, Washington, D.C.: Borden Institute, Walter Reed Medical Center, 1997, pp. 631–642.

Fredriksson T, "Hydrolysis of Soman and Tabun (Two Organophosphorous Cholinesterase Inhibitors) in Cutaneous Tissues," *Acta Derm-venerol*, 49, 1969, pp. 490–492.

Freeman G, Clements J, Moore J, Inbody J, Clanton B, Luisman E, Berman B, Craig A, Cornblath M, and Johnson R, *Observations of the Effects of Low Concentrations of GB on Man in Rest and Exercise*, Army Chemical Center, Md: Medical Laboratories, DTIC AD04561, 1952.

Freeman G, Hilton KC, and Brown ES, *V Poisoning in Man*, Edgewood Arsenal, Md.: U.S. Government Printing Office, DTIC AD151549, 1956.

Freeman G, Marzulli FN, Craig AB, and Trimble JR, *The Toxicity of Liquid GA Applied to the Skin of Man*, Army Chemical Center, Md., 1954.

Fricke RF, "Decreased Toxicity of T-2 Mycotoxicosis in Mice Pre-Treated with Microsomal Enzyme Inducers," Abstract #1955, *Fed Proc*, 42, 1993, p. 626.

Friedman A, Kaufer D, Shemer J, Hendler I, Soreq H, and Tur-Kaspa I, "Pyridostigmine Brain Penetration Under Stress Enhances Neuronal Excitability and Induces Early Immediate Transcriptional Response," *Nature Medicine*, 2, 1996, pp. 1382–1385.

Funk, D, "Pentagon Admits Gulf War Vet Likely Exposed to Toxin," *Army Times*, January 9, 1997.

Gall P, "The Use of Therapeutic Mixtures in the Treatment of Cholinesterase Inhibition," *Fundam Appl Toxicol*, 1, 1981, pp. 214–216.

GAO—*see* U.S. General Accounting Office.

Gaon MD, and Werne J, *A Study of Human Exposure to GB*, Denver, Colo.: Rocky Mountain Arsenal, 1955.

Garland FN, "Combat Stress Control in the Post-War Theater: Mental Health Consultation During the Redeployment Phase of Operation Desert Storm," *Mil Med*, 158, 1993, pp. 334–338.

"Gas Exposure in Gulf War Revisited," *The Washington Post*, July 24, 1997, p. A28.

Gause EM, Hartmann RJ, Leal BZ, and Geller I, "Neurobehavioral Effects of Repeated Sublethal Soman in Primates," *Pharmacol Biochem Behav*, 23 (6), December 1985, pp. 1003–1012.

Gershon S, and Shaw FH, "Psychiatric Sequelae of Chronic Exposure to Organophosphorous Insecticides," *Lancet*, 1, 1961, pp. 1371–1374.

Gibbons R, Gardner J, Cunnion S, Gackstetter G, and Kroenke K, "Identifying New Causes of Disease: Historical Examples and the Dilemma of Illnesses in Gulf War Veterans," *Conference on Federally Sponsored Gulf War Veterans' Illnesses Research—Program and Abstract Book*, June 1998.

Gilchrist HL, *A Comparative Study of World War Casualties from Gas and Other Weapons*, Edgewood Arsenal, Md.: U.S. Government Printing Office, 1928.

Gill DM, "Bacterial Toxins: A Table of Lethal Amounts," *Microbiol Revs*, 46, 1982, pp. 86–94.

Gilman AG, Rall T, Mies A, Taylor, P, *Goodman and Gilman's The Pharmacological Basis of Therapeutics*, 8th ed., New York: Pergamon Press, 1990.

Giovannelli L, Casamenti F, and Pepeu G, "C-fos Expression in the Rat Nucleus Basalis Upon Excitotoxic Lesion with Quisqualic Acid: A Study in Adult and Aged Animals, Department of Preclinical and Clinical Pharmacology, University of Florence, Italy, *J Neural Transm*, 105 (8–9), 1998, pp. 935–48.

Goehler LE, Gaykema RP, Hammack SE, Maier SF, and Watkins LR, "Interleukin-1 Induces c-Fos Immunoradioactivity in Primary Afferent Neurons of the Vagus Nerve," *Brain Res*, 804 (2), September 7, 1998, pp. 306–310.

Goldenberg GJ, et al., "Evidence for a Transport Carrier of Nitrogen Mustard in Nitrogen Mustard Sensitive and Resistant L5178Y Lymphocytes," *Cancer Research*, 30, 1970, pp. 2,285–2,291.

Goldman M, and Dacre JC, "Lewisite: Its Chemistry, Toxicology, and Biological Effects," *Rev Environ Contam Toxicol*, 110, 1989, pp. 75–115.

Goldman M, Klein AK, Kawakami TG, and Rosenblatt LS, *Toxicity Studies on Agents GB and GD*, Davis, Calif.: University of California, Laboratory for Energy-Related Health Research, DTIC ADA187841, 1987.

Goldstein BD, Kiser BD, and Pincher DR, *Physiology of Peripheral Sensory Receptors Following Sub-Acute Administration of Soman*, Augusta, Ga.: Department of Pharmacology & Toxicology, Medical College of Georgia, 1985.

Golomb BA, *A Review of the Scientific Literature as It Pertains to Gulf War Illnesses*, Vol. 2: *Pyridostigmine Bromide*, Santa Monica, Calif.: RAND, MR-1018/2-OSD, 1999a.

_____, *A Review of the Scientific Literature as It Pertains to Gulf War Illnesses*, Vol. 2: *Pyridostigmine Bromide Executive Summary*, Santa Monica, Calif.: RAND, MR-1018/2/1-OSD, 1999b.

_____, *A Review of the Scientific Literature as It Pertains to Gulf War Illnesses*, Vol. 3: *Immunizations*, Santa Monica, Calif.: RAND, MR-1018/3-OSD, 2000.

Goodwin W, Stephens R, McCracken JD, and Groppe C, "Therapy for Advanced Colorectal Cancer with a Combination of 5FU and Anguidine: A Southwest Oncology Group Study," *Cancer Treat Rep*, 65, 1981, p. 359.

Gordon JJ, Inns RH, Johnson MK, et al., "The Delayed Neuropathic Effects of Nerve Agents and Some Other Organophosphorus Compounds," *Arch Toxicol*, 52, 1983, pp. 71–82.

Gordon JJ, Leadbeater L, and Maidment MP, "The Protection of Animals Against Organophosphate Poisoning by Pretreatment with a Carbamate," *Toxicol Appl Pharmacol*, 43, 1978, pp. 207–216.

Goshorn I, Wilkins M, Peters W, and Zelkind S, *Protection Afforded by M11 Canister Against Mixtures of Phosgene Oxime and GA or GB*, Army Chemical Center, Md.: Chemical Warfare Laboratories, DTIC AD127130, 1956.

Goyal RK, Muscarinic Receptor Subtypes, "Physiology and Clinical Implications," *New Engl J Med*, 321, 1989, pp. 1022–1028.

Grasso P, Sharratt M, Davies DM, and Irvine D, "Neurophysiological and Psychological Disorders and Occupational Exposure to Organic Solvents," *Food Chem Toxicol*, 22 (10), October 1984, pp. 819–852.

Grauer E, Ben Nathan D, Lustig S, Kapon J, and Danenberg HD, "Cholinesterase Inhibitors Increase Brain-Blood Barrier (BBB) Permeability: Neuroinvasion of a Noninvasive Sindbis Virus as a Marker for BBB Integrity," in King JM, ed., *1996 Medical Defense Bioscience Review, Proceedings*, Vol. I, Ft. Detrick, Md.: U.S. Army Medical Research and Materiel Command, May 12–16, 1996, pp. 1202–1209.

Gray GC, Coate BD, Anderson CM, et al., "The Postwar Hospitalization Experience of U.S. Veterans of the Persian Gulf War," *N Engl J Med*, 335, 1996, pp. 1505–1513.

Gray GC, Knoke JD, Berg SW, Wagnall FS, and Garrett CE, "Counterpoint: Responding to Suppositions and Misunderstandings," *Am J. Epidem*, 143, 1998, pp. 326–333.

Gray GC, Smith TC, Knoke JD, and Heller JM, "Hospitalization Risk After Possible Exposure to Iraqi Chemical Munitions Destruction During the Persian Gulf War," *Conference on Federally Sponsored Gulf War Veterans' Illnesses Research—Program and Abstract Book*, Washington D.C., June 1998.

_____, "The Postwar Hospitalization of Gulf War Veterans Possibly Exposed to Chemical Munitions Destruction at Khamisiya, Iraq," *Am J Epidemiol*, 150 (5), September 1, 1999, pp. 532–540.

Griffiths GD, Allenby AC, Bailey SC, Hambrook JL, Rice P, and Upshall DG, *The Inhalation Toxicity of Ricin Purified 'In-House' from the Seeds of Ricinus Communis Var, Zanzibariensis*, Porton Down, Salisbury, UK: Ministry of Defense, 1994.

Griffiths GD, Lindsay CD, Allenby AC, et al., "Protection Against Inhalation Toxicity of Ricin and Abrin by Immunization," *Hum Exp Toxicol*, 14, 1995, pp. 155–164.

Griffiths BB, Rea WJ, Johnson AR, and Ross GH, "Mitogenic Effects of Mycotoxins on T_4 Lymphocytes," *Microbios*, 86, 1996, pp. 127–134.

Grob D, "Manifestations and Treatment of Nerve Gas Poisoning in Man," *U.S. Armed Forces Med J*, 7, 1956, pp. 781–789.

Grob D, and Harvey AM, "The Effects and Treatment of Nerve Gas Poisoning," *Am J Med*, 14, 1953, pp. 52–55.

Grob D, and Harvey JC, "Effects in Man of the Anticholinesterase Compound Sarin (Isopropyl Methylphosphonofluoridate)," *J Clin Invest*, 37, 1958, pp. 350–68.

Grob D, Harvey AM, Langworthy OR, et al., "The Administration of Di-Isopropyl Fluorophosphate (DFP) to Man," *Bull Johns Hopkins Hosp*, 81, 1947, pp. 257–266.

Grob D, and Johns RJ, "Use of Oximes in the Treatment of Intoxication by Anticholinesterase Compounds in Normal Subjects," *Am J Med*, 24, 1958, pp. 497–511.

Grob D, Ziegler B, Saltzer CA, and Johnston GI, *Further Observations on the Effects in Man of Methyl Isopropyl Fluorophosphonate (GB): Effects of Percutaneous Absorption through Intact and Abraded Skin*, Edgewood, Md.: Chemical Warfare Laboratory, DTIC AD25222, 1953.

Groopman JD, Scholl P, and Wang JS, "Epidemiology of Human Aflatoxin Exposures and Their Relationship to Liver Cancer," *Prog Clin Biol Res*, 395, 1996, pp. 211–222.

Gross CL, Meier HL, Papirmeister B, Brinkley FB, and Johnson JB, "Sulfur Mustard Lowers Nicotinamide Adeninedinucleotide Concentrates in Human Skin Grafted to Athymic Nude Mice," *Toxicol Appl Pharmacol*, 81, 1985, pp. 85–90.

Grunnet E, "Contact Urticaria and Anaphylactoid Reaction Induced by Topical Application of Nitrogen Mustard," *Br J Dermatol*, 94, 1976, pp. 101–103.

Guengerich FP, Johnson WW, et al., "Involvement of Cytochrome P450 Glutathione S-Transferase and Epoxide Hydrolase in the Metabolism of Aflatoxin B1 and Relevance to Risk of Human Liver Cancer," *Environ Health Perspect*, 104 (Suppl 3), 1996, pp. 557–562.

Gupta RC, Patterson GT, and Dettbarn WD, "Acute Tabun Toxicity: Biochemical and Histochemical Consequences in Brain and Skeletal Muscles of Rat," *Toxicology*, 46, 1987a, pp. 329–341.

_____, "Biochemical and Histochemical Alterations Following Acute Soman Intoxication in the Rat," *Fund Appl Pharmacol*, 87, 1987b, pp. 393–402.

Guttu M, Terry AM, Pauly J, and Buccafusco J, "Memory Impairment in Spontaneously Hypertensive Rates—Role of Central Nicotinic Receptors," Abstract 90.17. *Society for Neuroscience*, 23, 1997.

Haber LF, *The Poisonous Cloud*, Oxford: Clarendon Press, 1986.

Hackley BE, Jr., Steinberg GM, and Lamb JC, "Formation of Potent Inhibitors of AChE by Reaction of Pyridinaldoximes with Isopropyl Methylphosphonofluoridate (GB)," Army Chemical Center, Md.: Chemotherapy Branch, U.S. Army Chemical Warfare Laboratories, January 1958.

Hackman J, Note in *Chemisch Wochbald*, No. 31, 1934, p. 366.

Haddad LM, and Wincester JF, *Clinical Management of Poisoning and Drug Overdose*, Philadelphia: W.B. Saunders Co., 1983.

Haggerty GC, Kurtz PJ, and Armstong RD, "Duration and Intensity of Behavioral Change After Sublethal Exposure to Soman in Rats," *Neurobehavioral Toxicology*, 8, 1986, pp. 695–702.

Haig AM, Jr., *Chemical Warfare in Southeast Asia and Afghanistan*, Washington, D.C.: U.S. Department of State, 1982.

Haldane JBS, *Callinicus: A Defence of Chemical Warfare*, London: Kegan Paul, Trench, Trubner & Co., Ltd., 1925.

Haley RW, "Point: Bias from the 'Healthy-Warrior Effect' and Unequal Follow-up in Three Government Studies of Health Effects of the Gulf War," *American J of Epidemiology*, 148 (4), August 15, 1998a, pp. 315–323.

_____, "Selection Bias from the 'Healthy-Warrior Effect' and Unequal Follow-up in Federally Sponsored Surveys of Gulf War Veterans," *Conference on Federally Sponsored Gulf War Veterans' Illnesses Research—Program and Abstract Book*, June 1998b.

Haley RW, Armitage R, Bonte FJ, Bryan, WW, Cullum CM, Fleckenstein JL, Frohman EM, Hoffman RF, Hom J, Maddrey AM, Marshall W, Orsulak PJ, Petty F, Roland PS, Shoup AG, Trivedi MH, Van Ness PC, Victor RG, Vongpatanasin W, and Wolfe GI, "Gulf War–Associated Neurological Syndrome in a Decorated Special Forces Officer Compared with His Monozygotic Twin," *Conference on Federally Sponsored Gulf War Veterans' Illnesses Research—Program and Abstract Book*, June 1998.

Haley RW, Horn J, Roland PS, et al., "Evaluation of Neurologic Function in Gulf War Veterans," *JAMA*, 277, 1997, pp. 223–230.

Haley RW, and Kurt TL, "Self-Reported Exposure to Neurotoxic Chemical Combinations in the Gulf War, A Cross-Sectional Epidemiologic Study," *JAMA*, 277, 1997, pp. 231–237.

Haley RW, Kurt TL, and Horn J, "Is There a Gulf War Syndrome? Searching for Syndromes by Factor Analysis of Symptoms," *JAMA*, 277, 1997, pp. 215–222.

Hallman W, Kipen H, Diefenbach M, Kang H, Wartenberg D, Fielder N, and Natelson B, "Defining Gulf War Illness: Self-Reported Health Status Among VA Registry Veterans," *Conference on Federally Sponsored Gulf War Veterans' Illnesses Research—Program and Abstract Book*, June 1998.

Harris JA, "Using C-fos as a Neural Marker of Pain," *Brain Research Bulletin*, 45 (1), 1998, pp. 1–8.

Harris R, and Paxman J, *A Higher Form of Killing, The Secret Story of Chemical and Biological Warfare*, New York: Hill and Wang, 1982.

Harrison JC, and Garner RC, "Immunological and HPLC Detection of Aflatoxin Adducts in Human Tissues After an Acute Poisoning Incident in S.E. Asia," *Carcinogenesis*, 12, 1991, pp. 741–743.

Harrison, RJ, *Textbook of Medicine: With Relevant Physiology and Anatomy*, New York: Wiley, 1997.

Hartgraves SL, and Murphy MR, "Behavioral Effects of Low-Dose Nerve Agents," in Somani (1992).

Harvey RB, Edrington TS, Kubena LF, Elissalde MH, Corrier DE, and Rottinghaus GE, "Effect of Aflatoxin and Diacetoxyscirpenol in Ewe Lambs," *Bull Environ Contam Toxicol*, 54, 1995, pp. 325–330.

Hassett CC, *Study of Long-Term Human and Ecological Effects of Chemical Weapons Systems*, DTIC AD406297, 1963.

Hatta K, Miura Y, Asukai N, and Hamabe Y, "Amnesia from Sarin Poisoning," *Lancet*, 347 (9011), 1996, p. 1343.

Hayes WJ, Jr., *Pesticides Studied in Man*, Baltimore, Md.: Williams & Wilkins, 1982.

Hayward IJ, Wall HG, and Hixson CJ, *The Effects of Repeated Intramuscular Low-Doses of Soman in Rhesus Monkeys*, Aberdeen Proving Ground, Md.: U.S. Army Medical Research Institute of Chemical Defense, 1990.

Helm U, and Weger N, "Grundzuge der Wehrtoxikologie," in *Wehrmedizin: Ein kurzes Handbuch mit Beitragen zur Katastrophenmedizin*, Munich: Urban & Scharzenberg, 1980, pp. 245–285.

Helmkamp JD, "United States Military Casualty Comparisons During the Persian Gulf War," *JOM*, 36, 1994, pp. 609–615.

Hendry KM, and Cole EC, "A Review of Mycotoxins in Indoor Air," *J Toxicol Environ Health*, 38, 1993, pp. 183–198.

Henriksson J, Johannisson A, Bergqvist PA, and Norrgren L, "The Toxicity of Organoarsenic-Based Warfare Agents: In Vitro and In Vivo Studies," *Arch Environ Contam Toxicol*, 30, 1996, pp. 213–219.

Heyndrickx A, ed., *First World Congress: New Compounds in Biological and Chemical Warfare: Toxicological Evaluation, Proceedings*, Ghent, Belgium: State University of Ghent and the National Science Foundation of Belgium, 1984.

Hilborne LH, and Golomb BA, *A Review of the Scientific Literature as It Pertains to Gulf War Illnesses*, Vol. 1: *Infectious Diseases*, Santa Monica, Calif.: RAND, MR-1018/1-OSD, 2000.

Himuro K, Murayama S, Nishiyama K, Shinoe T, Iwase H, Nagao M, Takatori T, and Kanazawa I, "Distal Sensory Axonopathy After Sarin Intoxication," *Neurology*, 51 (4), 1998, pp. 1195–1197.

Hines FJ, "A Comparison of Clinical Diagnoses Among Male and Female Soldiers Deployed During the Persian Gulf War," *Mil Med*, 158, 1993, pp. 99–101.

Hinshaw DB, Dabrowska MI, Becks LL, Levee MG, and Lelli JL, Jr, "Sulfur Mustard Induces Apoptosis and Necrosis in Endothelial Cells," in King JM, ed.,

1996 Medical Defense Bioscience Review Proceedings, Volume II, Columbia, Md.: Johns Hopkins University, May 12–16, 1996.

Hirsch W, *Soviet BW and CW Capabilities 1939–45*, 1950; provided to U.S. Senate at a hearing on March 30, 1982.

Hirshberg A, Lerman Y, "Clinical Problems in Organophosphate Insecticide Poisoning: The Use of a Computerized Information System," *Fundam Appl Toxicol*, 4 (2 Pt 2), April 1984, pp. S209–S214.

Hoffman JL, "Mustard Gas: Detoxification by Methlyation and Retrospective Analysis of Exposure," *Conference on Federally Sponsored Gulf War Veterans' Illnesses Research—Program and Abstract Book*, June 1998.

Holmes JH, *Exposure to GB*, Final Report for Edgewood Arsenal, Denver: University of Colorado Medical School, DTIC AD218636, 1959.

Holmes and Gaon, 1956, in Jamal (1995b).

Hom J, Haley RW, and Kurt TL, "Neuropsychological Correlates of Gulf War Syndrome," *Arch Clin Neuropsych*, 12, 1997, pp. 531–44.

Horvath D, Deptartment of Veterans Affairs, talk given at a meeting of the Association of Military Surgeons of USA (AMSUS), in Nashville, Tenn., November 1997.

Hoskins B, *A Physiological and Biochemical Basis for the Action of Soman and Related Agents in the Acetylcholine Receptor*, Chicago: Illinois Institute of Technology, Department of Biology, DTIC ADA110841, 1982.

House—*See* U.S. House of Representatives.

Hu H, Cook-Degan R, and Shukri A, "The Use of Chemical Weapons," *JAMA*, 262, 1989, pp. 640–643.

Huff WE, Harvey RB, Kubena LF, Rottinghause GE, "Toxic Synergism Between Aflatoxin and T-2 Toxin in Broiler Chickens," *Poult Sci*, 67 (10), October 1988, pp. 1418–1423.

Hughes JN, and Lindsay CD, "Morphology of Ricin and Abrin Exposed Endothelian Cells Is Consistent with Apoptotic Cell Death," *Hum Exp Toxicol*, 15, 1996, pp. 443–451.

Husain K, Kumar P, Vijayaraghavan R, Singh R, and Das Gupta S, "Influence of Pretreatment of Carbamates on Dynamic Pulmonary Mechanics in Rats Exposed to Sarin Aerosols," *Ind J Physiol Pharmacol*, 37, 1993, pp. 249–251.

Husain K, Pant SC, Vijayaraghavan R, and Singh R, "Assessing Delayed Neurotoxicity in Rodents After Nerve Gas Exposure," *Def Sci J*, 44, 1994, pp. 161–164.

Husain K, Vijayaraghavan R, Pant SC, Raza SK, and Pandey KS, "Delayed Neurotoxic Effect of Sarin in Mice After Repeated Inhalation Exposure," *J Appl Toxicol*, 13, 1993, pp. 143–145.

Hyams KC, Wignall FS, and Roswell R, "War Syndromes and Their Evaluation: From the U.S. Civil War to the Persian Gulf War," *Ann Intern Med*, 125, 1996, pp. 398–405.

Inada S, Hiragun K, Seo K, Yamata T, "Multiple Bowens Disease Observed in Former Workers of a Poison Gas Factory in Japan," *Journal of Dermatology*, 5, 1978, pp. 49–60.

Inada K, Okada S, Phuchareon J, Hatano M, Sugimoto T, Moriya H, and Tokuhisa T, "c-Fos Induces Apoptosis in Germinal Center B Cells," *J Immunol*, 161 (8), October 15, 1998, pp. 3853–3861.

Infield GB, *Disaster at Bari*, New York, NY: Ace Books, 1971.

Inoue N, "Psychiatric Symptoms Following Accidental Exposure to Sarin, "*Fukuoka Acta Medica*, 86, 1995, pp. 373–377.

Institute of Medicine, *Evaluation of the Department of Defense Persian Gulf Comprehensive Clinical Evaluation Program*, Washington D.C.: National Academy Press, 1996.

_____, *Adequacy of the Comprehensive Clinical Evaluation Program, Nerve Agents*, Washington, D.C.: National Academy Press, 1997.

IOM—*see* Institute of Medicine.

"Iraq May Have Moved Chemical Weapons into Southern Kuwait," *Financial Times*, August 9, 1990, p. 2.

"Iraq: How Iraq is Defying the World Concerning the Alleged Use of Chemical Weapons by its Armed Forces against the Kurdish Population," *Financial Times*, August 81988, p. 20.

"Iraqi Threat of Chemical Warfare with Israel," *Financial Times*, April 3, 1990, p. 22.

Ishiguro M, Tanabe S, Matori Y, and Sakakibara R, "Biochemical Studies on Oral Toxicity of Ricin: IV, a Fate of Orally Administered Ricin in Rats," *J Pharmacobio Dyn*, 15, 1992, pp. 147–156.

Jacobson KH, Christensen MK, DeArmon IA, and Oberst FW, "Studies of Chronic Exposures of Dogs to GB (Isopropyl Methyphosphonofluoridate) Vapor," *Arch Indust Health*, 19, 1959, p. 5.

Jagadeesan V, Rukmini C, Vijayaraghavan M, and Tulpule PG, "Immune Studies with T-2 Toxin Effect of Feeding and Withdrawal in Monkeys," *Food Chem Toxicol*, 20 (1), February 1982, pp. 83–87.

Jakab GJ, Hmieleski RR, Zarba A, Hemenway DR, and Groopman JD, "Respiratory Aflatoxicosis: Suppression of Pulmonary and Systemic Host Defenses in Rats and Mice," *Toxicol Appl Pharmacol*, 125, 1994, pp. 198–205.

Jamal GA, "Long Term Neurotoxic Effects of Chemical Warfare Organophosphate Compounds (Sarin)," editorial, *Adverse Drug React Toxicol Rev*, 14, 1995, pp. 83–84.

_____, "Long Term Neurotoxic Effects of Organophosphate Compounds," *Adverse Drug React Toxicol Rev*, 14, 1995, pp. 85–99.

Jamal GA, Hansen S, Apartopoulous F, and Peden A, "The Gulf War Syndrome: Is There Evidence of Dysfunction in the Nervous System?" *J Neurol Neurosurg Psychiatry*, 60, 1996, pp. 449–451.

Jarvis BB, "Tricothecene Mycotoxins: Preparation, Analysis, and Chemical Reactivity," College Park, Md.: University of Maryland, 1985.

Joffe MH, et al., "Effects of Aqueous Solution of Cutaneous Applied Phosgene Oxime in Humans," DTIC AD35624, 1954.

Johanson WG, Jr., Anzueto A, et al., "Etiology of Respiratory Failure in Organophosphate Intoxication in Nonhuman Primates," *Fifth Annual Chemical Defense Bioscience Review*, 1985, p. 82.

Johns RJ, "The Effects of Low Concentrations of GB on the Human Eye," Army Chemical Center, Md., ABD 9548421, 1952.

Johnsen H, Edden E, Lie O, Johnsen BA, and Fonnum F, "Metabolism of T-2 Toxin by Rat Liver Carboxytesterase," *Biochem Pharmacol*, 35, 1986, pp. 1469–1473.

Johnson DE, *Pathophysiology of Soman and Sarin*, Aberdeen Proving Ground, Md.: U.S. Army Institute of Chemical Defense and the U.S. Air Force, DAMD17-83-C-3080, 1985.

Johnson DE, Anzueto A, Hamil HF, et al., *Studies of the Effects of Organophosphorous Exposure on the Lung*, San Antonio TX: Southwest Research Institute, 1988.

Johnson MK, "The Delayed Neuropathy Caused by Some Organophosphorous Esters: Mechanisms and Challenge," *CRC Crit Rev Toxicology*, 3, 1975, pp. 289–316.

Johnson MK, "Molecular Events in Delayed Neuropathy: Experimental Aspects of Neuropathy Target Esterase," in Baillyntyne and Marrs, eds., *Clinical and Experimental Toxicology of Organophosphates and Carbamates*, London: Butterworth and Heinemann, 1992.

Johnson MK, and Read DJ, "The Influence of Chirality on the Delayed Neuropathic Potential of Some Organophosphorus Esters: Neuropathic and Prophylactic Effects of Stereoisomeric Esters of Ethyl Phenylphosphonic acid (EPN Oxon and EPN) Correlate with Quantities of Aged and Unaged Neuropathy Target Esterase In Vivo," *Toxicol Appl Pharmacol*, 90, 1987, pp. 103–115.

Johnson MK, Read D, and Benschop H, "Interaction of the Four Stereoisomers of Soman with Acetylcholinesterase and Neuropathy Target Esterase of Hen Brain," *Biochemical Pharmacology*, 34, 1985, pp. 1945–1951.

Johnson MK, Willems JL, DeBisschop HC, Read DJ, and Benschop HP, "Can Soman Cause Delayed Neuropathy?" *Fund Appl Toxicol*, 5, 1985, pp. S180–S181.

Joseph SC, "A Comprehensive Clinical Evaluation of 20,000 Persian Gulf War Veterans," *Mil Med*, 162, 1997, pp. 149–155.

Joy R, and Goldman R, "Microenvironments, Modern Equipment and the Mobility of Soldiers," in *Symposium on Medical Aspects of Stress in the Military Climate*, Washington, D.C.: Walter Reed Army Medical Center, 1964, pp. 101–124.

Kadar T, Cohen G, Sahar R, Alkalai D, and Shapira S, "Long-Term Study of Brain Lesions Following Soman, in Comparison to DFP and Metrazol Poisoning," *Hum Exp Toxicol*, 11, 1992, pp. 517–523.

Kadar T, Shapira S, Cohen G, Sahar R, Alkalai D, and Reveh L, "Sarin-Induced Neuropathy in Rats," *Hum Exp Toxicol*, 14, 1995, pp. 252–259.

Kaina B, Haas S, and Kappes H, "A General Role for c-Fos in Cellular Protection Against DNA-Damaging Carcinogens and Cytostatic Drugs," *Cancer Res*, 57 (13), July 1, 1997, pp. 2,721–2,731.

Kang HK, and Bullman TA, "Mortality Among U.S. Veterans of the Persian Gulf War," *New Engl J Med*, 335, 1996, pp. 1,496–1,504.

Kang HK and Bullman TA, "Counterpoint: Negligible 'Healthy-Warrior Effect' on Gulf War Veterans Mortality," *Am J Epidem*, 146, 1998, pp. 324–325.

Kant GJ, Shih TM, Bernton EW, Fein HG, Smallridge RC, and Mougey EH, "Effects of Soman on Neuroendocrine and Immune Function," *Neurotox Teratol*, 13, 1991, pp. 223–228.

Kaplan JG, Kessler J, Rosenberg N, Pack D, and Schaumburg HH, "Sensory Neuropathy Associated with Dursban (Chlorpyrifos) Exposure," *Neurology*, 43, 1993, pp. 2193–2196.

Karakchiev NI, "Toxicology of Chemical Warfare Agents and Defense Against Weapons of Mass Destruction," trans. from Russian, Charlottesville, Va.: Department of the Army, 1973.

Karczmar AG, "Acute and Long Lasting Central Actions or Organophosphorous Agents," *Fundam Appl Toxicol*, 4, 1984, pp. S1–S17.

Kassa J and Bajgar J, "Comparison of the Efficacy of HI-6 and Obidoxime Against Cyclohexylmethyl-phosphonofluoridate (GF) in Rats," *Human and Environmental Toxicology*, 14, 1995, pp. 923–928.

Kato T, and Hamanaka T, "Ocular Signs and Symptoms Caused by Exposure to Sarin Gas," *Am J Ophthalmol*, 121, 1996, pp. 209–210.

Kaufer D, Friedman A, Seidman S, and Soreq H, "Acute Stress Facilitates Long-Lasting Changes in Cholinergic Gene Expression," *Nature*, 393, 1998, pp. 373–377.

Kaulla E, et al., "Changes Following Anticholinesterase Exposure," *Arch Environ Health*, 2, 1961, pp. 168–177.

Kaur C, and Ling EA, "Induced Hydrocephalus in Postnatal Rats Following an Intracerebral Injection of Ricin," *J Hirnforsch*, 34, 1993, pp. 493–501.

Keenan WF, "Non-Surgical Medical Care of Enemy Prisoners of War During Operation Desert Storm," *Mil Med*, 156, 1991, pp. 648–650.

Kelly SS, Mutch E, Williams FM, and Blain PG, "Electrophysiological and Biochemical Effects Following Single Doses of Organophosphates in the Mouse," *Arch Toxicol*, 68 (7), 1994, pp. 459–466.

Kemppainen BW, Riley RT, Pace JG, and Hoerr FJ, "Effects of Skin Storage Conditions and Concentration of Applied Dose on [3H]T-2 Toxin Penetration Through Excised Human and Monkey Skin," *Fund Chem Toxic*, 24, 1986, pp. 221–227.

Kemppainen BW, Riley RT, Pace JG, Hoerr FJ, and Joyave J, "Evaluation of Monkey Skin as a Model for in Vitro Percutaneous Penetration and Metabolism of [3H]T-2 Toxin in Human Skin," *Fund Appl Toxicol*, 7, 1986, pp. 367–375.

Kimbrough TD, Llewellyn GC, and Weekley LB, "The Effect of Aflatoxin B1 Exposure on Seratonin Metabolism," *Metabolic Brain Disease*, 1992, pp. 175–182.

King JR, Peters BP, and Monteiro-Riviere NA, "Laminin in the Cutaneous Basement Membrane as a Potential Target in Lewisite Vesication," *Toxicol Appl Pharmacol*, 126, 1994, pp. 164–173.

King JR, Riviere JE, and Monteiro-Riviere NA, "Characterization of Lewisite Toxicity in Isolated Perfused Skin," *Toxicol Appl Pharmacol*, 116, 1992, pp. 189–201.

Kisby GE, Springer N, and Spencer SP, "A Novel and Sensitive Method for Detecting Mustard-Induced DNA Adducts," *Conference on Federally Sponsored Gulf War Veterans' Illnesses Research—Program and Abstract Book*, June 1998.

Klain GJ, and Jaeger JJ, *Castor Seed Poisoning in Humans: A Review*, San Francisco, CA: Letterman Army Institute of Research, Presidio of San Francisco, 1990, p. 205.

Klaassen CD, ed., *Casarett and Doull's Toxicology: The Basic Science of Poisons*, 5th ed., New York: McGraw Hill, 1996.

Klein AK, Nasr ML, and Goldman M, "The Effects of In Vitro Exposure to the Neurotoxins Sarin (GB) and Soman (GD) on Unscheduled DNA Synthesis by Rat Hepatocytes," *Toxicol Lett*, 38, 1987, pp. 239–249.

Knudson GB, "Operation Desert Shield: Medical Aspects of Weapons of Mass Destruction," *Mil Med*, 156, 1991, pp. 267–271.

Koelle GB, "Pharmacology of Organophosphates," *J Appl Toxicol*, 14, 1994, pp. 105–109.

Kokes J, Assaad A, Pitt L, Estep J, Mcanulty E, and Parker G, "Acute Pulmonary Response of Rats Exposed to a Sublethal Dose of Ricin Aerosol," *FASEB Journal*, 8 (4–5), 1994.

Koplovitz I, Gresham VC, Dochterman LW, Kaminskis A, and Stewart JR, "Evaluation of the Toxicity, Pathology, and Treatment of Cyclohexyl-methylphosphonofluoridate (CMPF) Poisoning in Rhesus Monkeys," *Arch Toxicol*, 66, 1992, pp. 622–628.

Korenyi-Both AL, and Juncer DJ, "Al Eskan Disease: Persian Gulf Syndrome," *Mil Med*, 162, 1997, pp. 1–13.

Korpela M, and Tahti H, "Effects of Organic Solvents on Erythrocyte Membrane Acetylcholine Esterase Activity," *Arch Toxicol*, 8, Suppl, 1985, pp. 148–151.

_____, "Effect of Organic Solvents on Human Erythrocyte Membrane Acetylcholinesterase Activity In Vitro," *Arch Toxicol*, 9, Suppl 1986a, pp. 320–323.

_____, "The Effect of Selected Organic Solvents on Intact Human Red Cell Membrane Acetylcholinesterase In Vitro," *Toxicol Appl Pharmacol*, 85 (2), September 1986b, pp. 257–262.

_____, "The Effect of In Vitro and In Vivo Toluene Exposure on Rat Erythrocyte and Synaptosome Membrane Integral Enzymes," *Pharmacol Toxicol*, 63 (1), July 1988, pp. 30–32.

Korsak RJ, and Sato MM, "Effects of Chronic Organophosphate Pesticide Exposure on the Central Nervous System," *Clin Toxicol*, 11, 1977, pp. 83–95.

Koshes RJ, and Rothberg JM, "Ambulatory Mental Health Services at a U.S. Army Combat Support Post: The Effects of the Persian Gulf War," *Mil Med*, 160, 1995, pp. 507–513.

Koster R, "Synergisms and Antagonisms Between Physostigmine and Di-Isopropyl Fluorophosphate in Cats," *J Pharmacol, Exp Ther*, 88, 1946, pp. 39–49.

Kovacs KJ, "C-Fos as a Transcription Factor: A Stressful (Re)view from a Functional Map," *Neurochem Int*, 33 (4), October 1998, pp. 287–297.

Krakow EH and Fuhr I, "Toxicity of GA Vapor by Cutaneous Absorption for Monkey and Man," Army Chemical Center, Md.: Chemical Corps, Medical Division, DTIC AD491 578, 1949.

Kroenke K, Koslowe P, and Roy M, "Symptoms in 18, 495 Persian Gulf War Veterans, Latency of Onset and Lack of Association with Z-Reported Exposures," *J Occup Environ Med*, 40 (6), June 1998, pp. 520–528.

Krustanov L, "Changes in Serum Cholinesterase in the Case of Combined Mustard Gas—Tabun Intoxications," *Voenno-meditinska* [Bulgarian], 17, DTIC AD909889L, 1962, pp. 26–29.

Kundiev YI, Krasnyuk EP, and Viter VP, "Specific Features of the Changes in the Health Status of Female Workers Exposed to Pesticides in Greenhouses," *Toxicol Lett*, 33, 1986, pp. 85–89.

LaBlanc FN, Benson BE, and Gilg AD, "A Severe Organophosphate Poisoning Requiring the Use of an Atropine Drip," *Clin Toxicol*, 24, 1986, pp. 69–76.

LaBorde JB, Bates HK, Dacre JC, and Young JF, "Developmental Toxicity of Sarin in Rats and Rabbits," *J Toxicol Environ Health*, 47 (3), February 23, 1996, pp. 249–265.

Lane SJ, Adcock IM, Richards D, Hawrylowicz C, Barnes PJ, and Lee TH, "Corticosteroid-Resistant Bronchial Asthma Is Associated with Increased c-fos Expression in Monocytes and T Lymphocytes," *J Clin Invest*, 102 (12), December 15, 1998, pp. 2156–2164.

Larsson P, and Tjalve H, "Bioactivation of Aflatoxin B1 in the Nasal and Tracheal Mucosa in Swine," *J An Sci*, 74, 1996, pp. 1672–1680.

Lattal K, Maxey G, and Wilbur E, "The Effects of Serial 1/2 LD50 Doses of GB upon Delayed Response and Conditioned Avoidance Response Tests," Edgewood8 Arsenal, Md., Technical Report 2289, DTIC AD723394, 1971.

Lee SC, Beery JT, and Chu FS, "Immunoperoxidase Localization of T-2 Toxin," *Appl Pharmacol*, 72, 1984, pp. 228–235.

Leek M, Griffiths G, et al., "Pathological Aspects of Ricin Toxicity in Mammalian Lymph Node and Spleen," *Med Sci Law*, 30, 1990, pp. 141–148.

Lees-Haley PR, and Brown RS, "Biases in Perception and Reporting Following a Perceived Toxic Exposure," *Percept Mot Skills*, 75, 1992, pp. 531–544.

Lenz DE, Maxwell DM, and Austin CW, "Development of a Rat Model for Subacute Exposure to the Toxic Organophosphate VX," *Journal of the American College of Toxicology*, 15, Supp. 2, S69–77, 1996.

Li BY, Frankel AE, and Ramakrishnan S, "High-Level Expression and Simplified Purification of Recombinant Ricin A Chain," *Protein Expr Purif,* 3, 1992, pp. 386–394.

Li Q, Minami M, Clement JG, and Boulet CA, "Elevate Frequency of Sister Chromatid Exchanges in Lymphocytes of Victims of the Tokyo Sarin Disaster and in Experiments Exposing Lymphocytes to By-Products of Sarin Synthesis," *Toxicol Lett*, 98 (1–2), 1998, pp. 95–103.

Lipton SA, and Rosenberg PA, "Excitatory Amino Acids as a Final Common Pathway for Neurologic Disorders," *New Engl J Med*, 330, 1994, pp. 613–622.

Loewenstein-Lichtenstein Y, Schwarz M, Glick D, Norgaard-Pedersen B, and Zakut H, "Genetic Predisposition to Adverse Consequences of Anti-Cholinesterases in 'Atypical' BCHE Carriers," *Nat Med*, 1 (10), October 1995, pp. 1082–1085.

Lohs K, *Delayed Toxic Effects of Chemical Warfare Agents*, Stockholm: Almqvist & Wiksell International, 1975.

Longmire AW, "The Medical Care of Iraqi Enemy Prisoners of War," *Mil Med*, 156, 1991, pp. 645–647.

Lotti M, "The Pathogenesis of Organophosphate Polyneuropathy," *Crit Rev Toxicol*, 21, 1991, pp. 465–487.

Lotti M, "A. M. Cholinergic Symptoms and Gulf War Syndrome," *Nature Med*, 1, 1995, pp. 1225–1226.

Lu XC, Tortella FC, Ved HS, Garcia GE, and Dave JR, "Neuroprotective Role of c-fos Antisense Oligonucleotide: In Vitro and In Vivo Studies," *Neuroreport*, 8 (13), September 1997, pp. 2925–2929.

Ludlum DB, and Austin-Ritchie P, "Detection of Sulfur Mustard-Induced DNA Modifications," abstract, *Chem Biol Interact*, 91, 1994, pp. 39–49.

Lutsky I, Mor N, Yagen B, and Joffe AZ, "The role of T-2 Toxin in Experimental Alimentary Toxic Alcukia: A Toxicity Study in Cats," *Toxic Appl Pharmacol*, 43, 1978, pp. 111–124.

Lye MS, Ghazali AA, Mohan J, Alwin N, and Nair RC, "An Outbreak of Acute Hepatic Encephalopathy Due to Severe Aflatoxicosis in Malaysia," *Am J Tropical Medicine & Hygeine*, 53, 1995, pp. 68–72.

Macilwain C, "Study Proves Iraq Used Nerve Gas," *Nature*, 363, 1993, p. 3.

Maizlish N, Schenker M, Weisskopf C, Seiber J, and Samuels S, "A Behavioral Evaluation of Pest Control Workers with Short-Term, Low-Level Exposure to the Organophosphate Diazinon," *Am J Ind Med*, 12 (2), 1987, pp. 153–172.

Malatesta P, Bianchi B, and Malatesta C, "A Contribution to the Study of Urticant Substances," *Bollettino Chimico Farmaceutico*, 122, 1983, pp. 96–103.

Marrs TC, Maynard RL, and Sidell FR, *Chemical Warfare Agents, Toxicology and Treatment*, NY: John Wiley & Sons, 1996.

Marshall E, "Bracing for a Biological Nightmare," *Science*, 1997, 275, pp. 745.

Marshall F, and Gass A, "Gulf War Diseases: A Critical Review of 400 Examinations," *Conference on Federally Sponsored Gulf War Veterans' Illnesses Research—Program and Abstract Book*, June 1998.

Marshall GN, Davis LM, and Sherbourne CD, *A Review of the Scientific Literature As It Pertains to Gulf War Illnesses*, Vol. 4: *Stress*, Santa Monica, Calif.: RAND, MR-1018/4-OSD, 1999.

Martinez M, Phillips PJ, and Herbert J, "Adaptation in Patterns of c-fos Expression in the Brain Associated with Exposure to Either Single or Repeated Social Stress in Male Rats," *Eur J Neurosci*, 10 (1), January 1998, pp. 200–233.

Massey TE, "Cellular and Molecular Targets in Pulmonary Chemical Carcinogenesis: Studies with Aflatoxin B1," *Can J Physiol Pharmacol*, 74, 1996, pp. 621–628.

Masuda N, Takatsu M, Morinari H, Ozawa T, Nozaki H, and Aikawa N, "Sarin Poisoning in Tokyo Subway," *Lancet*, 345, 1995, pp. 1446–1447.

Matsuda Y, Nagao M, Takatori T, Niijima H, Nakajima M, Iwase H, Kobayashi M, and Iwadate K, "Detection of the Sarin Hydrolysis Product in Formalin-Fixed Brain Tissues of Victims of the Tokyo Subway Terrorist Attack," *Toxicology and Applied Pharmacology*, 150 (2), 1998, pp. 310–320.

Maxwell DM, *Specificity of Carboxylesterase Protection Against the Toxicity of Organophosphorous Compounds*, abstract, Aberdeen Proving Ground, Md.: Army Medical Research Institute of Chemical Defense, DTIC ADA258091/8, 1992.

Maxwell DM, and Brecht KM, "Quantitative Structure-Activity Analysis of Acetylcholinesterase Inhibition by Oxono and Thiono Analogues of Organophosphorus Compounds," *Chem Res Toxicol*, 5 (1), 1992, pp. 66–71.

Maxwell DM, et al., "The Effect of Blood Flow and Detoxification on in vivo Cholinesterase inhibition by Soman in the Rat," *Toxicol and Appl Pharm*, 88, 1987, pp. 66–67.

Mayer CF, "Endemic Panmyelotoxicosis in the Russian Grain Belt, Part One: The Clinical Aspects of Alimentary Toxic Aleukia (ATA): A Comprehensive Review," *Mil Surg*, 113, 1953a, pp. 173–189.

_____, "Endemic Panmyelotoxicosis in the Russian Grain Belt, Part Two: The Botany, Phytopathology and Toxicology of Russian Cereal Food," *Mil Surg*, 113, 1953b, pp. 295–315.

Mays MZ, "Performance on a One-Way Avoidance Conditioning Task Following Nerve Agent Intoxication," *Proceedings of the Fifth Annual Chemical Defense Bioscience Review*, Aberdeen Proving Ground, Md.: U.S. Army Medical Research Institute of Chemical Defense, 1985.

McAdams AJ, and Joffe MH, *A Toxico-Pathologic Study of Phosgene Oxime*, Army Chemical Center, Md.: Medical Laboratories, Research Report 381, 1955.

McDiarmid MA, Jacobson-Kram D, Koloder K, et al., "Increased Frequencies of Sister Chromatid Exchange to Soldiers Deployed to Kuwait," *Mutagenesis*, 10, 1995, pp. 263–265.

McDonough JH, Jr., Dochterman LW, Smith CD, and Shih TM, "Protection Against Nerve Agent–Induced Neuropathology, but not Cardiac Pathology, Is Associated with the Anticonvulsant Action of Drug Treatment," *Neurotoxicology*, 16, 1995, pp. 123–132.

McDonough JH, Jaax NK, Crowley RA, Mays MZ, and Modrow HE, "Atropine and/or Diazepam Therapy Protects Against Soman-Induced Neural and Cardiac Pathology," *Fund Appl Toxicol*, 13, 1989, pp. 256–276.

McKenzie JE, and Ballamy RF, *Cholinergic Induced Coronary Vasospasm: Treatment of Organophosphate Toxicity*, abstract, Bethesda, Md.: Uniformed Services University of the Health Sciences, 1993.

McLean M, and Dutton MF, "Cellular Interactions and Metabolism of Aflatoxin: An Update," *Pharmacol Ther*, 65, 1995, pp. 163–192.

McLeod CG, Jr., "Pathology of Nerve Agents: Perspectives on Medical Management," *Fund Appl Toxicol*, 5, 1985, pp. S10–S16.

McNamara BP, Leitnaker FC, and Vocci FJ, "Proposed Limits for Human Exposure to VX Vapor in Military Operations," DTIC AD770434, 1973.

McNamara BP, Owens EJ, Christensen MK, Vocci FJ, Ford DF, and Rozimarek H, *Toxicological Basis for Controlling Levels of Mustard in the Environment*, Edgewood Arsenal, Md.: Department of the Army, DTIC ADA011260, 1975.

McNamara BP, Owens EJ, Crook JW, et al., *Long-Term Airborne Exposure to Methylphosphonic Difluoride (DF) Vapor in Animals*, Defense Technical Information Center, ARCSL-TR-78023, 1979.

Medical Economics Company, *Physicians Desk Reference*, 52 ed., Medical Economics Company, 1998.

Meier HL, Gross CL, and Papirmeister B, "The Release of Histamine from Human Basophil Appears to Be Regulated by an Esterase and a Muscarinic-Like Receptor," abstract, *Proceedings of the Fifth Annual Chemical Defense Bioscience Review*, Aberdeen Proving Ground, Md.: U.S. Army Medical Research Institute of Chemical Defense, 1985.

Metcalf DR, and Holmes JH, "EEG, Physiological and Neurological Alterations in Humans with Organophosphorous Exposure," *Ann NY Acad Sci*, 160, 1969, pp. 357–365.

Meyn RE, "Cell Cycle Effects of Alkylating Agents," *Pharm Ther*, 24, 1984, pp. 147–163.

Meyn RE, and Murray D, "Cell Cycle Effects of Alkylating Agents," *Pharmacol Ther*, 24, 1984, pp. 147–163.

Mierzejewski J, "The Immune Processes in Animals Poisoned with Methylfluorphosphoric Acid Isopropyl Ester (MfAIE): Effect of Poisoning on Certain Immunological Indices," *Med Dosw Mikrobiol*, 22, 1970a, pp. 293–299.

Mierzejewski J, "The Immune Processes in Animals Poisoned with Methylfluorphosphoric Acid Isopropyl Ester (MfAIE): Effect of Multiple Poisoning on Some Immunological Indices," *Med Dosw Mikrobiol*, 22, 1970b, pp. 387–394.

Miller J, "The Inspectors: New Expert Panels Say Iraq Still Withholds Gas Data," *The New York Times*, February 14, 1998, p. 112.

Minami M, Hui DM, Wang Z, Katsumata M, Inagaki H, Li Q, Inuzuka S, Mashiko K, Yamamoto Y, Otsuka T, and Boulet CA, Clement JG, "Biological Monitoring of Metabolites of Sarin and Its By-Products in Human Urine Samples," *J Toxico Sci*, 23 Suppl 2, 1998, pp. 250–254.

Minson JB, Llewellyn-Smith IJ, Chalmers JP, Pilowsky PM, and Arnolda LF, "c-fos Identifies GABA-Synthesizing Barosensitive Neurons in Caudal Ventrolateral Medulla," *Neuroreport*, 8 (14), September 29, 1997, pp. 3015–3021.

Mirocha CJ, Pawlosky RJ, and Chatterjee K, "Analytical Methodology, Detection of Trichothecenes from Southeast Asian Samples and Their Residue in Animal Tissue," *First World Congress: New Compounds in Biological Warfare: Toxicological Evaluation, Proceedings*, Ghent, Belgium: State University of Ghent and National Science Foundation, 1984.

MMWR—*see* Morbidity and Mortality Weekly Report

Morbidity and Mortality Weekly Report, Recommendations for Protecting Human Health Against Potential Adverse Effects of Long-Term Exposure to Low-Doses of Chemical Warfare Agents, MMWR, 37, 1988, pp. 72–79.

Modrow HE, and McDonough JH, "Change in Atropine Dose Effect Curve After Subacute Soman Administration," *Pharmacology Biochemistry & Behavior*, 24, 1986, pp. 845–848.

Mol MAE, Wolthuis OL, "An In Vitro Assay for Dermatotoxicity Using Cultured Human Epidermal Cells," *Lab Appl Sci Res*, 1987.

Momeni AZ, and Amindjavaheri M, "Skin Manifestations of Mustard Gas in a Group of 14 Children and Teenagers: A Clinical Study," *Int J Dermatol*, 33, 1994, pp. 184–187.

Momeni AZ, Enshaeih S, Meghdadi M, and Amindjavaheri M, "Skin Manifestations of Mustard Gas: A Clinical Study of 535 Patients Exposed to Mustard Gas," *Arch Dermatol*, 128, 1992, pp. 775–780.

Morino H, Sakakibara R, and Ishiguro M, "The Binding of Ricin to Its Receptor Is Not Required for the Expression of Its Toxicity," *Biol Pharm Bull*, 18, 1995, pp. 1770–1772.

Morita H, Yanagisawa N, Nakajima T, et al., "Sarin Poisoning in Matsumoto, Japan," *Lancet*, 346, 1995, pp. 290–293.

Morris D, "Investigations of Incidents and Exposures Relevant to the Potential Causes of Gulf War Illnesses," Conference on Federally Sponsored Gulf War Veteran's Illness Research, June 1998.

Mougey EH, Pennington LL, Kant CJ, Leu JR, and Raslear TG, "Effects of Organophosphate DFP on Hormonal Rhythms in the Rat," *Fifth Annual Chemical Defense Bioscience Review*, Aberdeen Proving Ground, Md.: U.S. Army Medical Research, Institute of Chemical Defense, 1985.

Mumford SA, "Physiological Assessment of the Nerve Gasses," Porton, Wilks, U.K.: Chemical Defence Research Establishment, Memorandum No. 39, 1950.

Murata K, Araki S, Yokoyama K, Okumura T, Ishimatsu S, Takasu N, and White RF," Asymptomatic Sequelae to Acute Sarin Poisoning in the Central and Autonomic Nervous System 6 Months after the Tokyo Subway Attack," *J Neurol*, 244, 1997, pp. 601–606.

Murayama S, "Peripheral Nerve Disorders: Clinical Pathological Approaches," *Rinsho Shinkeigaku*, 37 (12), 1997, pp. 1103-1104.

Murphy WK, Burgess MA, Valdivieso M, Livingston RB, and Bodey GP, Freireich EJ, "Phase I Clinical Evaluation of Anguidine," *Cancer Treat Rep*, 62, 1978, pp. 1497–1502.

Mutch E, Blain PG, and Williams FM, "Interindividual Variations in Enzymes Controlling Organophosphate Toxicity in Man," *Hum Exp Toxicol*, 11, 1992, pp. 109–161.

Nakajima T, Ohta S, Morita H, Midorikawa Y, Mimura S, and Yanagisawa N, "Epidemiological Study of Sarin Poisoning in Matsumoto City, Japan," *J Epidemiol*, 8 (1), March 1998, pp. 33–41.

Nakajima T, Sasaki K, Ozawa H, Sekijima Y, Morita H, Fukushima Y, and Yanagisawa N, "Urinary Metabolites of Sarin in a Patient of the Matsumoto Sarin Incident," *Archives of Toxicology*, 72 (9), 1998, pp. 601–603.

Nakajima T, Sato S, Morita H, and Yanagisawa N, "Sarin Poisoning of a Rescue Team in the Matsumoto Sarin Incident in Japan," *Occup Environ Med*, 54 (10), October 1997, pp. 697–701.

Namba T, Nolte CT, Jackrel J, and Grob D, "Poisoning Due to Organophosphate Insecticides: Acute and Chronic Manifestations," 50, *Am J Med*, 1971, pp. 475–492.

Narang U, Anderson GP, Ligler FS, and Burans J, "Fiber Optic-Based Biosensor for Ricin," *Biosens Biolelectron*, 12, Nos. 9–10, 1997, pp. 937–945.

National Academy of Sciences, *Protection Against Trichothecene Mycotoxins*, Washington, D.C.: National Academy Press, 1983.

National Academy of Sciences, National Research Council, Committee on Toxicology, *Possible Long-Term Health Effects of Short-Term Exposure to Chemical Agents*, Vol. 1: *Anticholinesterases and Anticholinergics*, Washington, D.C.: National Academy Press, 1982.

_____, National Research Council, Committee on Toxicology, *Possible Long-Term Health Effects of Short-Term Exposure to Chemical Agents*, Vol. 2: *Cholinesterase Reactivators, Psychochemicals, Irritants, and Vesicants*, Washington, D.C.: National Academy Press, 1982.

_____, National Research Council, Committee on Toxicology, *Possible Long-Term Health Effects of Short-Term Exposure to Chemical Agents*, Vol. 2:

Cholinesterase Reactivators, Psychochemicals, and Irritants and Vesicants, Washington, D.C.: National Academy Press, 1984.

_____, National Research Council, Committee on Toxicology, *Possible Long-Term Health Effects of Short-Term Exposure to Chemical Agents*, Vol. 3: *Final Report: Current Health Status of Subjects*, Washington, D.C.: National Academy Press, 1985.

_____ National Research Council, Committee on Toxicology, Subcommittee on Guidelines for Military Field Drinking-Water Quality, *Guidelines for Chemical Warfare Agents in Military Field Drinking Water*, Washington, D.C.: National Academy Press, 1995.

_____, National Research Council, Committee on Toxicology, Subcommittee on Toxicity Values for Selected Nerve and Vesicant Agents, *Review of Acute Human-Toxicity Estimates for Selected Chemical-Warfare Agents*, Washington, D.C.: National Academy Press, 1997.

National Institutes of Health, Technology Assessment Workshop Panel, "The Persian Gulf Experience and Health," *JAMA*, 272, 1994, pp. 391–396.

NAS–*see* National Academy of Sciences.

NATO—*see* North Atlantic Treaty Organization.

Neitlich HW, *Effect of Percutaneous GD on Human Subjects*, DTIC AD471794, 1965.

Newman JM, Rindler JM, Bergfeld WF, and Brydon JK, "Stevens-Johnson Syndrome Associated with Topical Nitrogen Mustard Therapy," *J Am Acad Dermatol*, 36, 1997, pp. 112–114.

Newman-Taylor AJ, and Morris AJ, "Experience with Mustard Gas Casualties," letter, *Lancet*, 337, 1991, pp. 242.

Newmark J, and Clayton WL, "Persian Gulf War Illness: Preliminary Neurological Impressions," *Mil Med*, 160, 1995, pp. 505–507.

Nieminen SA, Lecklin A, Heikkinen O, and Ylitalo P, "Acute Behavioral Effects of the Organophosphates Sarin and Soman in Rats," *Pharmacol Toxicol*, 67, 1990, pp. 36–40.

Nigam SK, Ghosh SK, and Malaviya R, "Aflatoxin, Its Metabolism and Carcinogenesis—A Historical Review," *J Toxicol Toxin Rev*, 13, 1994, pp. 179–203.

NIH—*see* National Institutes of Health.

Nohara M, and Segawa K, "Ocular Symptoms Due to Organophosphorus Gas (Sarin) Poisoning in Matsumoto," *Br J Ophthalmol*, 80, 1996, p. 1023.

Nolan RJ, Rick DL, Freshour NL, and Saudners JH, "Chlorpyrifos: Pharmacokinetics in Human Volunteers," *Toxicol Appl Pharmacol*, 73, 1984, pp. 8–15.

Noort D, Fidder A, Van der Schans GP, et al., "Dosimetry of Exposure to Sulfur Mustard: Immunochemical and Mass Spectrometric Detection of Sulfur Mustard Adducts to DNA and Proteins," in King JM, ed., *1996 Medical Defense Bioscience Review, Proceedings*, Vol. II, Columbia, Md.: Johns Hopkins University, May 12–16, 1996.

Nordberg A and Svensson AL, "Cholinesterase Inhibitors in the Treatment of Alzheimer's Disease: A Comparison of Tolerability and Pharmacology," *Drug Safety*, 6, 1998, pp. 465–480.

North Atlantic Treaty Organization, *NATO Handbook on the Medical Aspects of NBC Defensive Operations*, Part III, *Chemical*, Washington, D.C.: Departments of the Army, the Navy, and the Air Force, August 1973.

Northup SW, McKenzie W, Thurston R, Hess R, and Kilburn K, Aflatoxin "Effects on Airway Cells in Rodents," abstract, *Fed Proc*, 34, 1995, p. 839.

Nozaki H, and Aikawa N, "Sarin Poisoning in Tokyo Subway," *Lancet*, 345, 1995, pp. 1446–1447.

Nozaki H, Aikawa N, Fujishima S, et al., "A Case of VX Poisoning and the Difference from Sarin," *Lancet*, 346, 1995, pp. 698–699.

Nukajima T, Sato S, Morita H, and Yanagisawa N, *Sarin Poisoning of a Rescue Team in Tao Matsumoto Sarin Incident in Japan*, Los Angeles: Biomedical Library of the University of California at Los Angeles, May 7, 1997.

Oberst FW, Crook JW, Christensen MK, Cresthull P, Koon WS, and Freeman G, *Inhaled GB Retention Studies in Man at Rest and During Activity*, Army Chemical Center, Md.: Chemical Corps Research and Development Command, DTIC AD226805, 1959.

Oberst FW, Koon WS, Christensen MK, Crook JW, Cresthull P, and Freeman G, "Retention of Inhaled Sarin Vapor and Its Effect on Red Blood Cell Cholinesterase Activity in Man," *Clin Pharm Ther*, 9, 1968, pp. 421–427.

Office of the Special Assistant for Gulf War Illnesses, Chemical Warfare Experience in Iran/Iraq War: Iranian Experience (last accessed February 15, 2000 at http://www.gulflink.osd.mil/declassdocs/dia/19970129/123096 _8061115_mic_0001.html) undated a.

_____, CW Use in Iran-Iraq War (last accessed February 15, 2000 at http://www.gulflink.osd.mil/declassdocs/cia/19960702/070296_cia_72566_7 2566_01.html), undated b.

_____, Czech CW Report: Intelligence Assessment of Chemical and Biological Warfare in the Gulf (last accessed February 15, 2000 at http://

www.gulflink.osd.mil/declassdocs/dia/19950925/950925_0401pgf_93.html), undated c.

_____, Factors That Affect the Use of Toxic Chemical Agents (last accessed February 15, 2000 at http://www.gulflink.osd.mil/declassdocs/dia/19950825/950825_22tr3340_143.html), undated d.

_____, Study on IZ Abilities to Conduct Chemical Warfare (last accessed February 15, 2000 at http://www.gulflink.osd.mil/declassdocs/dia/19961031/961031_950825_0150pgv_91d.html), undated e.

_____, Chemical Mines [Iraq] (last accessed February 22, 2000 at http://www.gulflink.osd.mil/declassdocs/dia/19970613/970613_23400458_91d_txt_0001.html), undated f.

_____, Armed Forces Medical Intelligence Center Special Weekly Wire 32–90(A) (last accessed February 15, 2000 at http://www.gulflink.osd.mil/declassdocs/dia/19970613/970613_ww32_90a_90_txt_0001.html), 1990.

_____, Information Paper: Chemical Agent Exposure Operation Desert Storm (last accessed February 15, 2000 at http://www.gulflink.osd.mil/declassdocs/army/19970908/970815_sep96_decls32_0001.html), September 1996.

_____, Case Narrative: U.S. Demolition Operations at Khamisiyah Ammunition Storage Point (last accessed February 15, 2000 at http://www.gulflink.osd.mil/khamisiyah), April 14, 1997a.

_____, Case Narrative: U.S. Marine Corps Minefield Breaching (last accessed February 15, 2000 at http://www.gulflink.osd.mil/marine), July 29, 1997b.

_____, Information Paper: The FOX/NBC Reconnaissance Vehicle (last accessed February 15, 2000 at http://www.gulflink.osd.mil/foxnbc), July 29, 1997c.

_____, Case Narrative: Reported Mustard Agent Exposure: Operation Desert Storm (last accessed February 15, 2000 at http://www.gulflink.osd.mil/fisher), August 27, 1997d.

_____, Case Narrative: Fox Detections in an ASP/Orchard (last accessed February 15, 2000 at http://www.gulflink.osd.mil/asporchard), September 23, 1997e.

_____, Information Paper: M8A1 Automatic Chemical Agent Alarm (last accessed February 15, 2000 at http://www.gulflink.osd.mil/m8a1alarms), October 30, 1997f.

_____, Case Narrative: Kuwaiti Girls' School (last accessed February 15, 2000 at http://www.gulflink.osd.mil/kuwaiti_school/), March 19, 1998a.

_____, Case Narrative: Czech and French Reports of Possible Chemical Agent Detections (last accessed February 15, 2000 at http://www.gulflink.osd.mil/czech_french), July 29, 1998b.

_____, Case Narrative: An Nasiriyah Southwest Ammunition Storage Point: Final Report (last accessed February 19, 2000 at http://www.gulflink.osd.mil/an_nasiriyah_ii/), January 10, 2000.

_____, personal communication on detector alarms, 1999.

Office of Scientific Research and Development, *Chemical Warfare Agents and Related Chemical Problems*, Parts I-II, Washington, D.C.: Office of Scientific Research and Development, National Defense Research Committee, 1946.

Ohtomi S, Takase M, and Kumagai F, Sarin poisoning in Japan, "A Clinical experience in Japan Self Defense Force (JSDF) Central Hospital," *Revue Internationale des Services de Sante des Forces Armées*, 69, 1996, pp. 97–102.

Oken BS, and Chiappa KH, "Statistical Issues Concerning Computerized Analysis of Brainwave Topography," *Ann Neurol*, 19, 1986, pp. 493–497.

Okumura T, Takasu N, Ishimatsu S, et al., "Report on 640 Victims of the Tokyo Subway Sarin Attack," *Ann Emer Med*, 28, 1996, pp. 129–135.

Olajos EJ, DeCaprio AF, and Rosenblum I, "Central and Peripheral Neurotoxic Esterase Activity and Dose-Response Relationship in Adult Hens After Acute and Chronic Administration of Diisopropylfluorophosphate," *Ecotoxicol Environ Saf*, 3–4, 1978, pp. 383–399.

Olney JW, *Cholinergic Neurotoxicity: Mechanisms and Prevention*, St. Louis, MO: Washington University School of Medicine, 1990.

O'Neill JJ, "Non-Cholinesterase Effects of Anticholinesterases," *Fund Appl Toxicol*, 1, 1981, pp. 154–160.

OSRD—see Office of Scientific Research and Development.

OSAGWI—see Office of the Special Assistant on Gulf War Illnesses.

Otto S, *The Ocular Action of Dichlorethyl Sulfide (Mustard Gas) in Man, as Seen at Edgewood Arsenal, Edgewood, Maryland*, DTIC AD495 508, 1946.

PAC—*see* Presidential Advisory Committee on Gulf War Illnesses.

Pace JG, Watts MR, Burrows EP, et al., Fate and Distribution of 3H-Labeled T-2 Mycotoxin in Guinea Pigs, *Toxicol Appl Pharmacol*, 80, 1985, pp. 377–385.

Pant SC, Vijayaraghavan R, and Das Gupta S, "Sarin Induced Lung Pathology and Protection by Standard Therapy Regime," *Biomed Environ Sci*, 6, 1993, pp. 103–111.

Paparello SF, Bourgeois AL, Garst P, and Hyams KC, "Diarrheal and Respiratory Disease Aboard the Hospital Ship USNS Mech T-AH 19 During Operation Desert Shield," *Mil Med*, 158, 1993, pp. 392–395.

Papirmeister B, Feister AJ, Robinson SI, and Ford RD, *Medical Defense Against Mustard Gas: Toxic Mechanisms and Pharmacological Implications*, Boca Raton, FL: CRC Press, 1991, pp. 13–42.

Papirmeister B, Gross CL, Meier HL, Petrali JP, and Johnson JB, "Molecular Basis for Mustard-Induced Vesication," *Fund Appl Toxicol*, 5, 1985, pp. S134–49.

Pasternack MS, and Eisen HN, "A Novel Serine Esterase Expressed by Cytoxic t-Lymphocytes," *Nature*, 314, 1985, pp. 743–745.

Patronas P, Horowitz M, Simon E, and Gerstberger R, Differential Stimulation of c-fos Expression in Hypothalamic Nuclei of the Rat Brain During Short-Term Heat Acclimation and Mild Dehydration," *Brain Res*, 798 (1–2), July 6, 1998, pp. 127–139.

Pauser G, Aloy A, Carvana M, et al., "Lethal Intoxication by War Gases on Iranian Soldiers, Therapeutic Interventions on Survivors of Mustard Gas and Mycotoxin Immersion," in Heyndrickx (1984), pp. 341–351.

Pazdernik TL, Churchill L, Nelson SR, and Samson FE, "Muscarinic Receptor Maps Reveal Selective Brain Damage in Soman-Exposed Rats; Diazepam Prevents This Selective Damage," *Proceedings of the Fifth Medical Chemical Defense Bioscience Review*, Aberdeen Proving Ground, Md.: U.S. Army Medical Research Institute of Chemical Defense, August 1986.

Pazdernik TL, Nelson SR, Cross R, and Samson FE, "Chemical-Induced Seizures: Free Radicals as a Final Common Pathway," abstract, Baltimore, Md.: *Medical Defense Bioscience Review*, 1996.

PDR—*Physician's Desk Reference*; see Medical Economics Company.

Pechura CM, and Rall DP, eds., *Veterans at Risk: The Health Effects of Mustard Gas and Lewisite*, Washington, D.C.: National Academy Press, 1993.

Penman AD, Tarver RS, and Currier MM, "No Evidence of Increase in Birth Defects and Health Problems Among Children Born to Persian Gulf War Veterans in Mississippi," *Mil Med*, 161, 1996, pp. 1–6.

Peoples RW, Spratto GR, Akbar WJ, and Fletcher HP, "Effect of Repeated Administration of Soman on Selected Endocrine Parameters and Blood Glucose in Rats," *Fund Appl Toxicol*, 11, 1988, pp. 587–593.

Perrotta DM, *Long-Term Health Effects Associated with Sub-Clinical Exposures to GB and Mustard*, Washington, D.C.: Environment Committee Armed Forces Epidemiological Board, 1996.

Petrali JP, Maxwell DM, Lenz DE, and Mills KR, "A Study on the Effects of Soman on the Rat Blood-Brain Barrier," *Fourth Annual Chemical Defense Bioscience Review*, Aberdeen Proving Ground, Md.: U.S. Army Medical Research Institute of Chemical Defense, 1984.

Petras JM, "Brain Pathology Induced By Organophosphate Poisoning with the Nerve Agent Soman," *Fourth Annual Chemical Defense Bioscience Review*, Aberdeen Proving Ground, Md.: U.S. Army Medical Research Institute of Chemical Defense, 1984, pp. 407–412.

Pfeifer R, and Irons R, "Mechanisms of Sulfhydryl Dependent Immunotoxicity," in Dean JH, et al., eds., *Immunotoxicology and Immunopharmacology*, New York: Raven Press, 1985, pp. 255–262.

Pierce PF, "Physical and Emotional Health of Gulf War Veteran Women," *Aviat Space Environ Med*, 68, 1997, pp. 317–321.

Polhuijs M, Langenberg JP, and Benschop HP, "New Method for Retrospective Detection of Exposure to Organophosphate Organophosphorous Anti-cholinesterases: Application to Alleged Sarin Victims of Japanese Terrorists," *Toxicology and Applied Pharmacology*, 146 (1), 1997, pp. 156–161.

Pongrac JL, and Rylett RJ, "Molecular Mechanisms Regulating NGF-Mediated Enhancement of Cholinergic Neuronal Phenotype: c-Fos Trans-Activation of the Choline Acetyltransferase Gene," *J Mol Neurosci*, 11 (1), 1998, pp. 79–83.

Pope CN, and Padilla S, "Potentiation of Organophosphorous-Induced Delayed Neurotoxicity by Phenylmethylsulfonyl Fluoride," *J Toxicol Environ Health*, 31, 1990, pp. 261–273.

Pour-Jafari H, "Secondary Sex Ratios in Progenies of Iranian Chemical Victims," *Vet Hum Toxicol*, 36, 1994, pp. 475–76.

Pour-Jafari H, and Moushtaghi AA, "Alterations of Libido in Gassed Iranian Men," *Vet Hum Toxicol*, 34, 1992, p. 547.

Prendergast MA, Terry AV, Jr., and Buccafusco JJ, "Chronic, Low-Level Exposure to Diisopropylfluorophosphate Causes Protracted Impairment of Spatial Navigation Learning," *Psychopharmacology (Berl)*, 129 (2), January 1997, pp. 183–191.

_____, "Effects of Chronic, Low-Level Organophosphate Exposure on Delayed Recall, Discrimination, and Spatial Learning in Monkeys and Rats," *Neurotoxicol Teratol*, 20 (2), March–April 1998, pp. 115–122.

Presidential Advisory Committee on Gulf War Veterans' Illnesses, *Special Report*, Washington, D.C.: U.S. Government Printing Office, October 1997.

_____, *Interim Report*, Washington, D.C.: U.S. Government Printing Office, February 1996a.

_____, *Final Report*, Washington, D.C.: U.S. Government Printing Office, December 1996b.

Prioux-Guyonneau M, Coudray-Lucas C, Coq HM, Cohen Y, and Wepierre J, "Modification of Rat Brain 5-hydroxytryptamine Metabolism by Sublethal Doses of Organophosphate Agents," *Acta Pharmacol et Toxicol*, 51, 1982, pp. 278–284.

Proctor NH and Hughes JP, *Chemical Hazards of the Workplace*, Philadelphia, J.B. Lippincott Company, 1978.

Pshenichnova AA, "Effects of Cholinesterase Inhibitors on Vascular Permeability in Rabbit Eye," abstract, trans. from Russian, *Leningrad Fiziologicheskiy Zhurnal SSR*, 81, 1985, p. 63.

Quin NE, "The Impact of Diseases on Military Operations in the Persian Gulf," *Mil Med*, 147, 1982, pp. 728–734.

Rachman IM, Unnerstall JR, Pfaff DW, and Cohen RS, "Estrogen Alters Behavior and Forebrain C-fos Expression in Ovariectomized Rats Subjected to the Forced Swim Test," *Proc Natl Acad Sci USA*, 95 (23), November 10, 1998, pp. 13941–13946.

Raisuddin S, Singh KP, Zaidi SI, Paul BN, and Ray PK, "Immunosuppressive Effects of Aflatoxin in Growing Rats," *Mycopathologia*, 124, 1993, pp. 189–194.

Rajendran MP, Sundararajan S, Chennakesavalu M, Charles YS, Sundararaj A, Clinicopathology of Aflatoxin Toxicity in Cattle, *Indian Vet J*, 69 (?), 1992, pp. 115–117.

Rall DP, and Pechura CM, "Effects on Health of Mustard Gas," *Nature*, 366, 1993, pp. 398–399.

Raskova, H, ed., *Pharmacology and Toxicology of Naturally Occurring Toxins*, Vols. I and II, London: Pergamon Press, 1971.

Rebentisch E, and Dinkloh H, *Wehrmedizin: Ein kurzes Handbuch mit Beitr. Zur Katastrophenmedizin*, [*Military Medicine: A Short Handbook with Articles About Emergency Medicine*], München, Wien, Baltimore: Urban and Schwarzenberg, 1980.

Rengstorff RH, "Vision and Ocular Changes Following Accidental Exposure to Organophosphates," *J Appl Toxicol*, 14, 1994, pp. 115–118.

Requena L, Requena C, Sanchez M, et al., "Chemical Warfare, Cutaneous Lesions from Mustard Gas," *J Am Acad Dermatol*, 19, 1988, pp. 529–536.

"Researcher Claims Iraq Fired Chemical Weapons During Gulf War," *Army Times*, 1997, p. 18.

Richard JL, and Thurston JR, "Effect of Aflatoxin on Phagocytosis of Aspergillus Fumigatus Spores by Rabbit Alveolar Macrophages," *Appl Microbiol*, 30, 1975, pp. 44–47.

Richter ED, Rosenvald Z, Kasp L, Levy S, and Gruener N, "Sequential Cholinesterase Tests and Symptoms for Monitoring Organophosphate Absorption in Field Workers and in Persons Exposed to Pesticide Spray Drift," *Toxicol Lett*, 33, 1986, pp. 25–35.

Rickett DL, "Soman Produced Respiratory Arrest: Differentiation of Brain Stem and Neuromuscular Actions," abstract, USAMRDC Chemical Progress Review, Ft. Detrick, Md., June 8–9, 1981.

Riegle DW, Jr., and D'Amato AM, *U.S. Chemical and Biological Warfare-Related Dual Use Exports to Iraq and Their Possible Impact on the Health Consequences of the Persian Gulf War*, Washington, D.C.: U.S. Senate, 1994.

Rocha L, and Kaufman DL, "In Vivo Administration of c-Fos Antisense Oligonucleotides Accelerates Amygdala Kindling," *Neurosci Lett*, 241 (2–3), January 30, 1998, pp. 111–114.

Rodnitzky RL, "Occupational Exposure to Organophosphate Pesticides: A Neurobehavioral Study," *Arch Environ Health*, 30 (2), February 1975, pp. 98–103.

Root WS, and Hofmann FG, eds., *Physiological Pharmacology, A Comprehensive Treatise*, New York: Academic Press, 1967.

Rosen RT, and Rosen JD, "Presence of Four Fusarium Mycotoxins and Synthetic Material in Yellow Rain, Evidence for the Use of Chemical Weapons in Laos," *Biomed Mass Spectrom*, 9, 1982, pp. 443–450.

Rosenstock L, Keifer M, Daniell I, McConnell R, and Claypoole K, "Chronic Central Nervous System Effects of Acute Organophosphate Pesticide Intoxication," The Pesticide Health Effects Study Group, *Lancet*, 338, July 27, 1991, pp. 223–227.

Ross RK, Yuan J, Yu MC, et al., "Urinary Aflatoxin Biomarkers and Risk of Hepatocellular Carcinoma," *Lancet*, 339, 1992, pp. 943–946.

Rubin L, and Goldberg M, "Effect of Sarin on Dark Adaptation in Man: Threshold Changes," *J Appl Physiol*, 2, 1957b, pp. 439–444.

Rubin LS, and Goldberg MN, The Effect of GB on Dark Adaptation in Man: "The Effect of Tertiary and Quaternary Atropine Salts on Absolute Scotopic Threshold Changes Engendered by GB," DTIC AD139052, 1957a.

Rubin LS, Krop S, and Goldberg MN, "Effect of Sarin on Dark Adaptation in Man: Mechanism of Action," *J Appl Physiol*, 11, 1957, pp. 445–449.

Rukmini C, Prasad JS, and Rao K, "Effects of Feeding T-2 Toxin to Rats and Monkeys," *Food Cosmet Toxicol*, 18, 1980, pp. 267–269.

Russell RW, Booth RA, Lauretz SD, Smith CA, and Jenden DJ, "Behavioral, Neurochemical and Physiological Effects of Repeated Exposures to Subsymptomatic Levels of the Anticholinesterase, Soman," *Neurobehav Toxicol Teratol*, 8 (6), November–December 1986, pp. 675–685.

Russell RW, Overstreet DH, Cotman CW, Carson VG, Churchill L, Dalglish FW, and Vasques BJ, "Experimental Tests of Hypotheses About Neurochemical Mechanisms Underlying Behavioral Tolerance to the Anticholinesterase, Diisopropyl Fluorophosphate," *J Pharm Exp Ther*, 192, 1975, pp. 73–85.

"Russia Dodges Chemical Arms Ban: New Nerve Agent Hard to Uncover," *Washington Times*, February 4, 1997.

Rutman RJ, "Binary Chemical Weapons: Details, Difficulties, and Dangers," in American Chemical Society, Committee on Chemistry and Public Affairs, *Binary Weapons and the Problem of Chemical Disarmament*, Washington, D.C.: American Chemical Society, 1976, pp. 1–7.

Sack D, Linz D, Shukla R, et al., "Health Status of Pesticide Applicators: Postural Stability Assessments," *J Occup Med*, 35, 1993, pp. 1196–1202.

Saidkarimov SK, Khalikov TR, Vaysbrot VV, and Tadzhiyev BA, "Modeling Disseminated Myocardial Necroses by Organophosphorous Pesticide Basudin," abstract, trans. from Russian, *Tashkent Meditsinskiy Zhurnal Uzbekistana*, 12, 1985, pp. 73–75.

Sajan MP, Satav JG, et al., Activity of Some Respiratory Enzymes and Cytochrome Contents in Rat Hepatic Mitochondria Following Aflatoxin B1 Administration, *Toxicol Lett*, 80, 1995, pp. 55–60.

Sanches ML, Russell CR, and Randolph CL, *Chemical Weapons Convention (CWC) Signatures Analysis: Technical Analysis*, Alexandria, Va.: Defense Nuclear Agency, B171-788, 1993.

Sanchez-Yus E, and Suarez ME, "Uritacria de Contacto y Reaccion Anifilactoide Inducidas por Aplicacion Topica de Mostaza Nirogenada," *Actas Derm Sif*, 68, 1977, pp. 39–44.

Sandvig K, and Van Deurs B, "Endocytosis Intracellular Transport and Cytoxic Action of Shiga Toxin and Ricin," *Physiol Rev*, 76, 1996, pp. 949–966.

Sasser LB, Cushing JA, Mellick PW, Kalkwarf DR, and Dacre JC, "Subchronic Toxicity Evaluation of Lewisite in Rats," *J Toxicol Environ Health*, 47, 1996, pp. 321–334.

Sastry BVR, and Sadavongvivad C, "Cholinergic Systems in Non-Nervous Tissues," *Pharm Rev*, 30, 1979, pp. 65–132.

Savage EP, Keefe TJ, Mounce LM, Heaton RK, Lewis JA, and Burcar PJ, "Chronic Neurological Sequelae of Acute Organophosphate Pesticide Poisoning," *Arch Environ Health*, 43, 1988, pp. 38–45.

Savage EP, Keefe TJ, Mounce LM, Lewis JA, Heaton RK, and Parks LH, *Chronic Neurological Sequelae of Acute Organophosphate Pesticide Poisoning: An Epidemiologic Study*, Boulder, Co.: U.S. Environmental Protection Agency, PB86-17982, 1982.

Schafer DF, and Sorrell MF, "Power Failure, Liver Failure," *New Engl J Med*, 336, 1997, pp. 1173–1174.

Schiefer HB, "Systemic Effects of Topical Application of Trichothecenes in Rodents," *First World Congress: New Compounds in Biological Warfare: Toxicological Evaluation, Proceedings*, Ghent, Belgium: State University of Ghent and National Science Foundation, 1984.

Schiefer HB, and Hancock DS, "Systemic Effects of Topical Application of T-2 Toxin in Mice," *Toxicol Appl Pharmacol*, 76, 1984, pp. 464–472.

Schnurr PP, Friedman MJ, and Green BL, "Post-Traumatic Stress Disorder Among World War II Mustard Gas Test Participants," *Mil Med*, 161, 1996, pp. 131–160.

Schreiber SS, Tocco G, Shors TJ, and Thompson RF, "Activation of Immediate Early Genes After Acute Stress," *Neuroreport*, 2 (1), January 1991, pp. 17–20.

Schultz GP, *Chemical Warfare in Southeast Asia and Afghanistan: An Update*, Washington, D.C.: U.S. Department of State, 1982.

Schwab BW, Costa LG, and Murphy SD, "Muscarinic Receptor Alterations as a Mechanism of Anticholinesterase Tolerance," *Toxicol Appl Pharmacol*, 71, October 1983, pp. 14–23.

Schwab BW, Hand H, Costa LG, and Murphy SD, "Reduced Muscarinic Receptor Binding in Tissues of Rats Tolerant to the Insecticide Disulfoton," *Neurotoxicology*, 2 (4), December 1981, pp. 635–647.

Schwab BW, and Murphy SD, "Induction of Anticholinesterase Tolerance in Rats with Doses of Disulfoton that Produce No Cholinergic Signs," *J Toxicol Environ Health*, 8, 1981, pp. 199–204.

Schwartz WJ, "Understanding Circadian Clocks: From c-Fos to Fly Balls," *Neurological Progress*, 41 (3), 1997, pp. 289–297.

Scremin OU, and Jenden DJ, "Cholinergic Control of Cerebral Flow in Stroke, Trauma, and Aging," *Life Sci*, 58, 1996, pp. 2011–2018.

Scremin OU, Shih TM, and Corcoran KD, "Cerebral Blood Flow-Metabolism Coupling After Administration of Soman at Non-Toxic Levels," *Brain Res Bull*, 26, 1991, pp. 353–356.

Seagrave S, *Yellow Rain: A Journey Through the Terror of Chemical Warfare*, New York: M. Evans and Company, Inc., 1981.

Seed JC, "An Accident Involving Vapor Exposure to a Nerve Gas," DTIC Quarterly Report No. 2, 1950, DTIC AD144023, 1952.

Segal R, Milo I, Joffe A, and Yogen B, "Tricothecene Induced Hemolysis," *Toxicology and Applied Pharmacology*, 70, 1983, p. 343.

Senanayake N, and Karalliedde L, "Neurotoxic Effects of Organophosphorous Insecticide, An Intermediate Syndrome," *New Engl J Med*, 316, 1987, pp. 761–763.

Senate—*See* U.S. Senate.

Serova LI, Saez E, Spiegelman BM, and Sabban EL, "c-Fos Deficiency Inhibits Induction of mRNA for Some, but Not All, Neurotransmitter Biosynthetic Enzymes by Immobilization Stress," *J Neurochem*, 70v(5), May 1998, pp. 1935–1940.

Sharabi Y, Danon YL, Berkenstadt H, Almog S, Mimouni-Bloch A, Zisman A, Dani S, and Atsmon J, "Survey of Symptoms Following Intake of PB During the Persian Gulf War," *Isr J Med Sci*, 27, Nos. 11–12, November–December 1991, pp. 656–658.

Sharma HS, Cervos-Navarro J, and Dey PK, "Increased Blood-Brain Barrier Permeability Following Short-Term Swimming Exercise in Conscious Normotensive Young Rats," *Neurosci Res*, 10, 1991, pp. 211–221.

Shays C, Statement of Rep. Christopher Shays, Washington, D.C.: U.S. Congress House of Representatives, Committee on Government Reform and Oversight, Subcommittee on Human Resources, 1997.

Shen HM, Shi CY, Lee HP, and Ong CN, "Aflatoxin B-1 Induced Lipid Peroxidation in Rat Liver," *Toxicol Appl Pharmacol*, 127 (1), 1994, pp. 145–150.

Shih ML, McMonagle JD, Dolzine TW, and Gresham VC, "Metabolite Pharmacokinetics of Soman, Sarin and GF in Rats and Biological Monitoring of Exposure to Toxic Organophosphorus Agents," *J Appl Toxicol*, 14, 1994, pp. 195–199.

Shih TM, Penetar DM, McDonough JH Jr. et al., "Age-Related Differences in Soman Toxicity and in Blood and Brain Regional Cholinesterase Activity," *Brain Res Bull*, 24, 1990, pp. 429–436.

Shipley MT, Nickell WT, Drake RL, and Frydel B, "Long-Term Reduction of AChE in Cortical Cholinergic Target Sites After a Single Soman Challenge," abstract, Proceedings of the Fifth Annual Chemical Defense Bioscience Review, Aberdeen Proving Ground, Md.: U.S. Army Medical Research, Institute of Chemical Defense, 1985.

Sidell FR, *Human Responses to Intravenous VX*, Edgewood, Md.: U.S. Army Medical Research Institute of Chemical Defense, DTIC AD811991, 1967.

_____, *Sarin and Soman: Observations on Accidental Exposures*, DTIC AD769737, 1973.

_____, "Soman and Sarin Clinical Manifestations and Treatment of Accidental Poisoning by Organophosphates," *Clin Toxicol*, 7, 1974, pp. 1–17.

_____, "Nerve Agents," in Sidell, Takafuji, and Franz (1997), pp. 129–179.

Sidell FR, and Groff WA, "The Reactivability of Cholinesterase Inhibition by VX and Sarin in Man," *Toxicol Appl Pharmacol*, 74, 1974, pp. 241–252.

Sidell FR, and Hurst CG, "Long-Term Health Effects of Nerve Agents and Mustard," in Sidell, Takafuji, and Franz (1997), pp. 229–246.

Sidell FR, Takafuji ET, and Franz DR, eds., *Textbook of Military Medicine*, Part I: *Warfare, Weaponry, and the Casualty*, Vol. 3.: *Medical Aspects of Chemical and Biological Warfare*, Washington, D.C.: Borden Institute, Walter Reed Medical Center, 1997.

Sidell, F.R., Urbanetti, J.S., Smith, W.J., Hurst, C.G., "Vesicants," in Sidell, Takafuji, and Franz (1997).

Sim VM, *Effect on Pupil Size of Exposure to GB Vapour*, Porton Down: Chemical Defence Establishment, U.K. Ministry of Defence, 1956.

_____, *Variability of Different Intact Human Skin Sites to the Penetration of VX*, Edgewood, Md.: CRDLC, Department of Defense, DTIC AD271163, 1962.

Sim VM, Duffy FH, Burchfiel JL, and Gaon MD, *Nerve Agents and Pesticides: Value of Computer Analysis of Electroencephalograms in the Diagnosis of Exposure to Organophosphates and Chlorinated Hydrocarbons*, Edgewood Arsenal, Md., DTIC AD785679, 1971.

Sim VM, McClure C, Vocci FJ, Feinsilver L, and Groff WA, *Tolerance of Man to VX Contaminated Water*, Army Chemical Center, Edgewood, Md.: CRDLC, Department of Defense, DTIC AD449722, 1964.

Simpson JC, Roberts LM, and Lord JM, "Free Ricin, A Chain Reaches an Early Compartment of the Secretory Pathway Before It Enters the Cytosol," *Exp Cell Res*, 229, 1996, pp. 447–451.

Singer AW, Jaax NK, and McLeod CG, "Cardiomyopathy in Soman and Sarin Intoxicated Rats," *Toxicol Lett*, 36, 1987, pp. 243–249.

SIPRI—*see* Stockholm International Peace Research Institute.

Sirkka U, Nieminen SA, and Ylitalo P, "Neurobehavioral Toxicity with Low-Doses of Sarin and Soman," *Meth Find Exp Clin Pharmacol*, 12, 1990, pp. 245–250.

Smart JK, History of "Chemical and Biological Warfare: An American Perspective," in Sidell, Takafuji, Franz (1997), pp. 9–86.

Smith KJ, Hurst CG, Moeller RB, Skelton HG, and Sidell FR, Sulfur "Mustard: Its Continuing Threat as a Chemical Warfare Agent, the Cutaneous Lesions Induced, Progress in Understanding Its Mechanism of Action, Its Long-Term Health Effects, and New Developments for Protection and Therapy," *J Am Acad Derm*, 32, 1995, pp. 765–766.

Smith TC, Gray GC, and Knoke JD, "Post-War Non-Federal Hospitalization Experience of U.S. Veterans of the Persian Gulf War," *Conference on Federally Sponsored Gulf War Veterans' Illnesses Research, Conference Proceedings*, June 17–19, 1998, p. 48.

Smith WJ, and Dunn MA, "Medical Defense Against Blistering Chemical Warfare Agents," *Arch Dermatol*, 127, 1991, pp. 1207–1213.

Smoragiewicz W, Cossette B, Boutard A, and Krzystyniak K, "Trichothecene Mycotoxins in the Dust of Ventilation Systems in Office Buildings," *Int Arch Occup Environ Health*, 65, 1993, pp. 113–117.

Snider TH, Wientjes MG, Joiner RL, and Fisher GL, "Arsenic Distribution in Rabbits After Lewisite Administration and Treatment with British Anti-Lewisite (BAL)," *Fundam Appl Toxicol*, 14, 1990, pp. 262–272.

Sohrabpour H, "Clinical Manifestations of Chemical Agents on Iranian Combatants During Iran-Iraq Conflict," in Heyndrickx (1984), pp. 291–297.

Solberg VB, Broski FH, Dinterman RE, and George DT, "Penetration of Tritiated T-2 Mycotoxin Through Abraded and Intact Skin and Methods to Decontaminate Tritiated T-2 Mycotoxin from Abrasions," *Toxicol*, 28, 1990, pp. 803–812.

Somani SM, *Chemical Warfare Agents*, New York: Academic Press, Inc., 1992.

_____, *Gulf War Syndrome: Potential Effects of Low-Level Exposure to Sarin and/or PB Under Conditions of Physical Stress*, Hearing Before the Subcommittee on Human Resources, Committee on Government Reform and Oversight, U.S. House of Representatives, 1997.

Sparks PJ, Daniell W, Black DW, et al., "Multiple Chemical Sensitivity Syndrome: A Clinical Perspective, I. Case Definition, Theories of Pathogenesis, and Research Needs," *J Occup Med*, 36, 1994, pp. 718–730.

Specter A, chairman, Committee on Veterans' Affairs, U.S. Senate, 105th Congress, *Report of the Special Investigation Unit on Gulf War Illnesses*, Washington, D.C.: U.S. Government Printing Office, 1998.

Spektor DM, *A Review of the Scientific Literature As It Pertains to Gulf War illnesses*, Vol. 6: *Oil Well Fires*, Santa Monica, Calif.: RAND, MR-1018/6-OSD, 1998.

Speigleberg U, "Psychopathological and Neurological Aftereffects and Permanent Damage from Industrial Intoxication by Phosphoric Acid Esters (Alkyl Phosphates)," *Proceedings of the 14th International Congress of Occupational Health*, Madrid, Spain 1963.

Stabile DE, *The Effect of Modified Steroid Levels on GD and GB Toxicity*, Edgewood Arsenal, Md.: Department of the Army, Research Laboratories, Edgewood Arsenal Technical Memorandum 112-7, 1967.

Stade K, Pharmacology and Clinical Aspects of Synthetic Poisons, AD477552, 1964.Stahl CJ, Green CC, and Farnum JB, "The Incident at Tuol Chrey: Pathologic and Toxicologic Examinations of a Casualty After Chemical Attack," *J Foren Sci*, 30, 1985, pp. 317–337.

Steenland K, Jenkins B, Ames RG, O'Malley M, Chrislip D, and Russo J, "Chronic Neurological Sequelae to Organophosphate Pesticide Poisoning," *Am J Public Health*, 84 (5), May 1994, pp. 731–736.

Stephens R, Spurgeon A, and Berry H, "Organophosphates: The Relationship Between Chronic and Acute Exposure Effects," *Neurotoxicol Teratol*, 18, 1996, pp. 449–453.

Steyn PS, "Mycotoxins, General View, Chemistry and Structure," *Toxicol Lett*, 82–83, 1995, pp. 843–845.

Stockholm International Peace Research Institute, *The Problem of Chemical and Biological Warfare*, 1: *The Rise of CB Weapons*, Stockholm: Almqvist and Wiksell, 1971.

_____, *The Problem of Chemical and Biological Warfare*, 2: *CB Weapons Today*, Stockholm: Almqvist and Wiksell, 1973.

_____, *Medical Protection Against Chemical Warfare Agents*, Stockholm: Almqvist and Wiksell, 1976.

_____, *Chemical Weapons: Destruction and Conversion*, London: Taylor & Francis, Ltd., 1980.

Stremmel D, *Present Day Status of Research on Organophosphate Antidotes*, DTIC ADB013082, 1972.

Stretch PH, Bliese PD, Marlow DH, Wright KM, Knudson KH, and Hoover CH, "Physical Health Symptomatology of Gulf War–Era Service Personnel from the States of Pennsylvania and Hawaii," *Mil Med*, 1995, 160, pp. 131–136.

Suzuki T, Morita H, Ono K, et al., "Sarin Poisoning in Tokyo Subway," (1), *Lancet*, 345, 1995, pp. 980–981.

Taher AA, "Cleft Lip and Palate in Tehran," *Cleft Palate Craniofac J*, 29, 1992, pp. 15–16.

Tabershaw IR, and Cooper WC, "Sequelae of Acute Organic Phosphate Poisoning," *J Occup Med*, 8, 1966, pp. 5–20.

Taylor HL, and Orlansky J, "The Effects of Wearing Protective Chemical Warfare Combat Clothing on Human Performance," *Aviat Space Environ Med*, 63, 1993, pp. A1–A41.

Taylor JE, El-Fakahony E, and Richelson E, "Long-Term Regulation of Muscarinic Acetylcholine Receptors on Cultured Nerve Cells," *Life Sci*, 25, 1979, pp. 2181–2187.

Taylor RF, Phosgene Oxime, memorandum to W. Augerson, July 1983.

Tchelingerian J, Le Saux F, Pouzet B, and Jacque C, "Widespread Neuronal Expression of c-Fos Throughout the Brain and Local Expression in Glia Following a Hippocampal Injury," *Neuroscience Letters*, 226, 1997, pp. 175–178

Teitlebaum A, and Goldman R, "Increased Energy Cost of Multiple Clothing Layers," *J Appl Physiol*, (32), 1972, pp. 743–744.

Thigpen JT, Vaughn C, and Stuckey WJ, "Phase II Trial of Anguidine in Patients with Sarcomas Unresponsive to Prior Chemotherapy: A Southwest Oncology Group Study," *Cancer Treat Rep*, 65, 1981, pp. 881–882.

Thompson AR, *Inhibition of Thrombin by Sarin*, DTIC AD695618, 1969.

Thompson WL, and Wannemacher RW, Jr., "Detection and Quantification of T-2 Mycotoxin with a Simplified Protein Synthesis Inhibition Assay," *Appl Environ Microbiol*, 1984, pp. 1176–1180.

Thurman JD, Creasia DA, Johnson AJ, "Adrenal Cortical Necrosis Caused by T-2 Mycotoxicosis in Female, but Not Male, Mice," *Am J Vet Res*, 47, 1986, pp. 1122–1124.

Tokuoka S, Hayashi Y, Inai K, et al., "Early Cancer and Related Lesions in the Bronchial Epithelium in Former Workers of Mustard Gas Factory," *Acta Pathol Jpn*, 36, 1986, pp. 533–542.

Trask CH, Christensen MK, Cresthull P, Oberst FW, and McNamara BP, *An Estimation of the Per Cent Military Effectiveness of Soldiers with Various Degrees of Incapacitation from BG Vapor in Various Tactical Situations*, DTIC AD225136, 1959.

Traub K, Bernier J, Olson K, Pindzola M, and Spencer L, "Autoradiography Shows Compartmental Distribution of 14-C (3, 3-dimethyl-2-butoxy)-methylphosphorylfluoride (Soman) in the CNS of Rats," abstract, *Proceedings of the Fifth Annual Chemical Defense Bioscience Review*, Aberdeen Proving Ground, Md.: U.S. Army Medical Research Institute of Chemical Defense, 1985.

Trusal, LR, "Stability of T-2 Mycotoxin in Aqueous Media," *Applied and Environmental Microbiology*, November 1985, pp. 1311–1312.

Tsutsumi N, and Miyazaki K, "Enhancing Effect of Ethanol on Aflatoxin B1-Induced DNA Damage in Glutathione-Depleted Rat Hepatocytes," *Int J Oncol*, 4, 1994, pp. 123–127.

Tucker, Johnathan, "Converting Former Soviet Chemical Warfare Plants," *Non-Proliferation Review*, 4, Fall 1996.

Tuovinen K, Kaliste-Korhonen E, and Hanninen O, "Gender Differences in Activities of Mouse Esterase and Sensitivities to DFP and Sarin Toxicity," *General Pharmacology*, 29 (3), 1997, pp. 333–335.

Tutelyan VA, and Kravchenko LV, *New Data on Metabolism and Action Mechanism of Mycotoxins*, Vestnik Akademii Meditsinskikh Nauk SSSR, trans. from Russian, 1981, pp. 88–89.

Tyler-Smith MS, Gray GC, and Knoke JD, "The Postwar Non Federal Hospitalization Experience of U.S. Veterans of The Persian Gulf War," *Conference on Federally Sponsored Gulf War Veterans' Illnesses Research—Program and Abstract Book*, June 1998.

Uhal HT, Soviet Chemical Warfare Agents Novichok and Substance 33: Were they Used During the Persian Gulf War? undated (last accessed March 8, 2000 at http://www.trillium.net/norenvironmental/novi_1.htm).

Ueno Y, *Developments in Food Science 4, Trichothecenes—Chemical, Biological, and Toxicological Aspects*, Tokyo: Kodansha, Ltd., 1983.

Ueno Y, "Toxicological Features of T-2 Toxins and Related Tricothecenes," Fundamental and Applied Toxicology, 4, 1984, pp. S124–S132.

Ueno Y, Muto A, and Kobayashi J, Toxicological Properties of T-2 Toxin and Related Trichothecenes, in Heyndrickx (1984), pp. 160–172.

Umeuchi H, Kikuchi C, Matsuoka Y, Sunagane N, Uruno T, and Kubota K, "T-2 Toxin a Mycotoxin from Fusarium Fungi Effect on Learning Ability of Mice" (abstract), *Jpn J Pharmacol*, 71 (Suppl 1), 1996, pp. 102P.

United Nations, *Use of Chemical Weapons by Iraqi Regime Report of the Specialists Appointed by the Secretary-General to Investigate Allegations by the Islamic Republic of Iran Concerning the Use of Chemical Weapons*, New York, NY: United Nations, 1984.

United Nations Special Commission, *Report to the Security Council*, New York: United Nations, 1991.

_____, *Report to the Security Council*, New York: United Nations, 1992.

_____, *Report to the Security Council*, New York: United Nations, 1995.

UNSCOM—*see* United Nations Special Commission.

USAMRIID—*see* U.S. Army Medical Research Institute of Infectious Diseases.

U.S. Army, *Potential Military Chemical/Biological Agents and Compounds*, FM 3-9, NAVFAC P-467, AFR 355-7, December 12, 1990.

U.S. Army Command and General Staff College, *Chemical and Biological Weapon Employment*, Ft. Leavenworth, KS: U.S. Army Command and General Staff College, 1963.

U.S. Army Medical Research Institute of Chemical Defense, *Medical Management of Chemical Casualties Handbook*, Aberdeen Proving Ground, Md., 1995.

U.S. Army Medical Research Institute of Infectious Diseases, "Information Sheet: Trichothecene Mycotoxins: Intoxications and Experimental Therapy," Ft. Detrick, Md., 1983.

U.S. Army, XVIII Corps, Dusty Agents Implications for Chemical Warfare Protection (last accessed February 18. 2000, at http://www.gulflink.osd.mil/declassdocs/army/19970107/970107_apr96_decls13_0001.html), January 27, 1998.

U.S. Department of Health and Human Services, "Final Recommendation for Protecting the Health and Safety Against Potential Adverse Effects of Long-Term Exposure to Low Doses of Agents GA, GB, VX, and Mustard Agent (H, HD, HT) and Lewisite (L)," *Federal Register*, 53, 1988, p. 8,504.

U.S. Department of Health and Human Services, Public Health Service, Agency for Toxic Substances and Disease Registry, *Toxicological Profile for Mustard "Gas,"* Atlanta, Ga., September 1992.

U.S. General Accounting Office, *Illnesses in Gulf War Veterans, Improved Monitoring of Clinical Progress and Reexamination of Research Emphasis are Needed*, Washington, D.C.: United States General Accounting Office, 1997.

U.S. House of Representatives, *Use of Chemical Agents in Southeast Asia Since the Vietnam War*, Hearing Before the Subcommittee on Asian and Pacific Affairs, Washington, D.C.: U.S. Government Printing Office, 1979.

U.S. House of Representatives, *Foreign Policy and Arms Control Implications of Chemical Weapons*, Hearings Before the Subcommittee on International Security and Scientific Affairs and on Asian and Pacific Affairs of the Committee of Foreign Affairs, House of Representatives, 97th Congress, March 30 and July 13, 1982, Washington D.C.: U.S. Government Printing Office, 1982.

U.S. House of Representatives, *Status of Efforts to Identify Gulf War Syndrome*, Hearing Before the Subcommittee on Human Resources, Committee on Government Reform and Oversight, Washington, D.C.: U.S. Government Printing Office, April 24, 1997.

U.S. Senate, *Is Military Research Hazardous to Veterans' Health? Lessons from World War II, The Persian Gulf, and Today*, Hearings Before the Committee on Veteran's Affairs, U.S. Senate, Washington, D.C.: U.S. Government Printing Office, 1994.

Utgoff, V, personal communication, Comments on the History of Chemical Warfare, June 1998.

Valdes JJ, Chester NA, Menking D, Shih T, and Whalley C, "Regional Sensitivity of Neuroleptic Receptors to Sub-Acute Soman Intoxication, *Brain Res Bull*, 14, 1985, pp. 117–21.

Vale JA, and Scott GW, "Organophosphorous Poisoning," *Guys Hosp Reps*, 123, 1974, pp. 13–25.

Van Helden H, Berends F, and Wolthuis O, *On the Existence of a Soman Depot, Cholinesterases*, Berlin: Walter de Gruyter Co., 1984, pp. 375–88.

Van Helden HPM, and Wolthuis OL, "Evidence for an Intramuscular Depot of the Cholinesterase Inhibitor Soman in the Rat," *Eur J Pharmacol*, 89, 1983, pp. 271–274.

Van Meter WG, Karczmar AG, Fiscus RR, "CNS Effects of Anticholinesterases in the Presence of Inhibited Cholinesterases," *Arch Int Pharm*, 231, 1978, pp. 249–60.

Vedder EB, *The Medical Aspects of Chemical Warfare*, Baltimore, Md.: Williams & Wilkins Co., 1925.

Venturini MC, Quiroga MA, Risso MA, Lorenzo CD, Omata Y, Venturini L, and Godoy H, "Mycotoxin T-2 and Aflatoxin B1 as Immunosuppressors in Mice

Chronically Infected with *Toxoplasma gondii*," *J Comp Pathol*, 115 (3), October 1996, pp. 229–237.

Verma RJ, Choudhary SB, "Hypercalcaemia During Aflatoxicosis," *Med Sci Res*, 1995.

Vijayaraghavan R, Husain K., Kumar P, Pandey KS, Das Gupta S, "Time Dependent Protection by Carbamates Against Inhaled Sarin Aerosols in Rats," *Asia Pac J Pharmacol*, 7 (4), 1992, pp. 257–262.

Vojvodic V, Milosavljevic Z, Boskovic B, Bojanic N. "The Protective Effect of Different Drugs in Rats Poisoned by Sulfur and Nitrogen Mustards," *Fund Appl Toxicol*, 5, 1985, pp. S160–S168.

Volpe LS, Biagioni TM, and Marquis JK, "*In Vitro* Modulation of Bovine Caudate Muscarinic Receptor Number by Organophosphates and Carbamates," *Toxicology and Applied Pharmacology*, 78, 1985, pp. 226–234.

Vranken MA, De Bisschop HC, Willems JL, "'In Vitro' Inhibition of Neurotoxic Esterase by Organophosphorus Nerve Agents," *Arch Int Pharmacodyn*, 260, 1982, pp. 316–318.

Wachtel C, ed., *Chemical Warfare*, Brooklyn, NY: Chemical Publishing Co., Inc., 1941.

Walday P, Aas P, and Fonnum F, "Inhibition of Serine Esterases in Different Rat Tissues Following Inhalation of Soman," *Biochem Pharmacol*, 41, 1991, pp. 151–153.

Wall HG, "Development of Brain Lesions in Rats Surviving After Experiencing Soman-Induced Convulsions: Light and Electron Microscopy," *Fifth Annual Chemical Defense Bioscience Review*, Columbia, Md.: Johns Hopkins University, Applied Physics Laboratory, 1985.

Walton M, MacGibbon G, Young D, Sirimanne E, Williams C, Gluckman P, and Dragunow M, "Do c-Jun, c-Fos, and Amyloid Precursor Protein Play a Role in Neuronal Death or Survival?" *Journal of Neuroscience Research*, 53, 1998, pp. 330–342.

Wang C, and Murphy SD, "Kinetic Analysis of Species Difference in Acetylcholinesterase Sensitivity to Organophosphate Insecticides," *Toxicol Appl Pharmacol*, 66, 1982, pp. 409–419.

Wang J, Wilson JR, and Fitzpatrick DW, "Central Effects of T-2 Toxin, a Trichothecene Mycotoxin," abstract, *Soc Neurosci*, 18, 1992, p. 1600.

Wang LY, Hatch M, Chen C, et al., "Aflatoxin Exposure and Risk of Hepatocellular Carcinoma in Taiwan," *Int J Cancer*, 67, 1996, pp. 620–625.

Wannemacher R, Bunner D, Pace J, Neufeld H, Brenecke L, and Dinterman R, "Dermal Toxicity of T-2 Toxin in Guinea Pigs, Rats, and Cynomolgus Monkeys," Fort Detrick, Md.: U.S. Army Medical Research Institute of Infectious Diseases, DTIC ADA133130, 1983.

Wannemacher RW Jr., and Wiener SL, "Trichothecene Mycotoxins," in Sidell, Takafuji, and Franz (1997), pp. 655–676.

Wasserman GM LTC, et al., "A Survey of Outpatient Visits in a United States Army Forward Unit During Operation Desert Shield," *Mil Med*, 162, 1997, pp. 374–379.

Watson AP, Ambrose KR, Friffin GD, Leffingwell SS, Munro NB, and Waters LC, "Health Effects of Warfare Agent Exposure: Implications for Stockpile Disposal," *Environ Prof*, 11, 1989, pp. 335–353.

Watson AP, and Griffin GD, "Toxicity of Vesicant Agents Scheduled for Destruction by the Chemical Stockpile Disposal Program," review, *Environ Health Perspect*, 98, 1992, pp. 259–280.

Watson BW, George B, Tsouras P, and Cyr BL, *Military Lessons of the Gulf War*, London: Greenhill Books, 1991.

Watson SA, Mirocha CJ, and Hayes AW, "Analysis for Trichothecenes in Samples from Southeast Asia Associated with 'Yellow Rain,'" *Fund Appl Toxicol*, 4, 1984, pp. 700–717.

Wecker L, Mrak RE, and Dettbarn WD, "Evidence of Necrosis in Human Intercostal Muscle Following Inhalation of an Organophosphate Insecticide," *Fund Appl Toxicol*, 6, 1986, pp. 172–174.

Wellner RB, Hewetson JF, and Poli MA, "Ricin Mechanism of Action, Detection, and Intoxication," *J Toxicol-Toxin Rev*, 14, 1995, pp. 483–522.

Wells WJEG, and MacFarlan CW, *Phosgene Oxime (Dichloroformoxime)*, Part II: *Toxicity: Median Lethal Concentration for Mice and Vesicant Action on Man*, Edgewood Arsenal, Md.: War Department, Chemical Warfare Service, 1938.

Wende O, *Skin Damage Caused by Chemical Warfare Agents*, DTIC ADB026006, 1977.

West SG, "Rheumatic Disorders during Operation Desert Storm," *Arthritis Rheum*, 36 1993, pp. 251–253.

White LE, and Price JL, "The Functional Anatomy of Limbic Status Epilepticus in the Rat, I. Patterns of 14C-2-deoxyglucose Uptake and fos Immunocytochemistry," *J Neurosci*, 13, 11, November 1993, pp. 4787–4809.

Whorton MD, and Obrinsky DL, "Persistence of Symptoms After Mild to Moderate Acute Organophosphate Poisoning Among 19 Farm Field Workers," *J Toxicol Environ Health*, 11, 1983, pp. 347–354.

Wickelgren I, "Rat Model for Gulf War Syndrome?" *Science*, 278, 1997, pp. 1404–1405.

Wilhelmsen CL, and Pitt ML, "Lesions of Acute Inhaled Lethal Ricin Intoxication in Rhesus Monkeys," *Vet Pathol*, 33, 1996, pp. 296–302.

Willems JL, Nicaise M, and De Bisschop HC, "Delayed Neuropathy by the Organophosphorus Nerve Agents Soman and Tabun," *Arch Toxicol*, 55, 1984, pp. 76–77.

Willems JL, Palate BM, Vranken MA, and De Bisschop HC, "Delayed Neuropathy by Organophosphorus Nerve Agents," *Proceedings of the International Symposium on Protection Against Chemical Warfare Agents*, Stockholm, Sweden, June 6–9, 1983, pp. 95–100.

Wilson A, "The Effects on Man of DFP and Other Anticholinesterases," *Chem Ind*, 1, 1954, pp. 2–8.

Wilson BW, Kawakami TG, Cone N, et al., "Genotoxicity of the Phosphoramidate Agent Tabun (GA)," *Toxicology*, 86, 1994, pp. 1–12.

Wintermeyer SF, Pina JS, Cremins JE, and Heier JS, "The Inpatient Experience of a U.S. Army Combat Support Hospital in the Persian Gulf During Non-Combat and Combat Periods," *Mil Med*, 159, 1994, pp. 746–751.

———, "Medical Care of Iraqis at a Forwardly Deployed U.S. Army Hospital During Operation Desert Storm," *Mil Med*, 161, 1996, pp. 294–297.

Wittich AC, "Gynecological Evaluation of the First Female Soldiers Enrolled in the Gulf War Comprehensive Clinical Evaluation Program at Tripler Medical Center," *Mil Med*, 161, 1996, pp. 635–637.

Wolthuis OL, Benschop HP, and Berends F, "Persistence of the Anti-Cholinesterase Soman in Rats: Antagonism with a Non-Toxic Simulator of This Organophosphate," *Eur J Pharmacol*, 69, 1981, pp. 379–383.

Wolthuis OL, Groen B, Busker RW, and van Helden HP, "Effects of Low-Doses of Cholinesterase Inhibitors on Behavioral Performance of Robot-Tested Marmosets," *Pharmacol Biochem Behav*, 51, 1995, pp. 443–456.

Wolthuis OL, Philippens IHCHM, and Vanwersch RAP, "On the Development of Behavioral Tolerance to Organophosphates IV: EEG and Visual Evoked Responses, Pharmacol," *Biochem Behav*, 39, 1991, pp. 851–858.

Woodard CL, Calamaio CA, Kaminskis A, Anderson DR, Harris LW, and Martin DG, "Erythrocyte and Plasma Cholinesterase Activity in Male and Female

Rhesus Monkeys Before and After Exposure to Sarin," *Fundam Appl Toxicol*, 23, 1994, pp. 342–347.

Worek F, Widmann R, Knopff D, and Szinica L, "Reactivating Potency of Obidoxime, Pralidoxime, H1-6 and HL07 in Human Erythocyte Acetyl-cholinesterase Compounds," *Archive Toxicology*, 72, 1998, pp. 237–243.

World Health Organization, *Health Aspects of Chemical and Biological Weapons, Report of a WHO Group of Consultants*, Geneva: World Health Organization, 1970.

Writer JV, DeFraites RF, and Brundage JF, "Comparative Mortality Among U.S. Military Personnel in the Persian Gulf Region and Worldwide During Operations Desert Shield and Desert Storm," *JAMA*, 275 (2), January 10, 1996, pp. 118–121.

Yamakido M, Ishioka S, Hiyama K, and Maeda A, "Former Poison Gas Workers and Cancer: Incidence and Inhibition of Tumor Formation by Treatment with Biological Response Modifier N-CWS," abstract, *Environ Health Perspect*, 104 (Suppl 3), 1996, pp. 485–488.

Yap HY, Murphy WK, DiStefano A, Blumenschein GR, and Bodey GP, "Phase II Study of Anguidine in Advanced Breast Cancer," *Cancer Treat Reps*, 63, 1979, pp. 789–791.

Yarom R, Sherman Y, More R, Ginsburg I, Borinski R, and Yagen B, "T-2 Toxin Effect in Bacterial Infection and Leukocyte Functions," *Toxic Appl Pharmacol*, 75, 1984, pp. 60–68.

Yasuda A, Yamaguchi T, Manabe Y, Ohkoshi K, Sakuma A, and Kusano Y, "Sarin Terrorism in Tokyo 3 Months Followup," abstract, *Invest Ophthalm Vis Sci*, 37, 1996, p. S943.

Yokoyama K, Araki S, Murata K, et al., "A Preliminary Study on Delayed Vestibulo-Cerebellar Effects of Tokyo Subway Sarin Poisoning in Relation to Gender Differences: Frequency Analysis of Postural Sway," *J Occup Environ Med*, 40, 1998a, pp. 17–21.

Yokoyama K, Araki S, Murata K, Nishikitani M, Okumura T, Ishimatsu S, Takasu N, and White RF, "Chronic Neurobehavioral Effects of Tokyo Subway Sarin Poisoning in Relation to Posttraumatic Stress Disorder," *Arch Environ Health*, 53 (4), July–August 1998b, pp. 249–256.

Yokoyama K, Ogura Y, Kishimoto M, et al., "Blood Purification for Severe Sarin Poisoning After the Tokyo Subway Attack," *JAMA*, 274, 1995, p. 379.

Yokoyama K, Yamada A, and Mimura N, "Clinical Profiles of Patients with Sarin Poisoning After the Tokyo Subway Attack," *Am J Med*, 100, 1996, p. 586.

Zarba A, Hmieleski R, Hemenway DR, Jakab GJ, and Groopman JD, "Aflatoxin B1-DNA Adduct Formation in Rat Liver Following Exposure by Aerosol Inhalation," *Carcinogenesis*, 13, 1992, pp. 1031–1033.

Zajtchuk R, Bellamy RF, eds., *Textbook of Military Medicine*, Washington, D.C.: Department of the Army, Office of the Surgeon General, Borden Institute, 1997.

Zilinskas RA, "Iraq's Biological Weapons, The Past as Future?" *JAMA*, 278, 1997, pp. 418–424.